NUTRITION AND RHEU

NUTRITION ◊ AND ◊ HEALTH
Adrianne Bendich, Series Editor

Recent Volumes

Handbook of Nutrition and Pregnancy, edited by **Carol J. Lammi-Keefe, Sarah Collins Couch, and Elliot H. Philipson,** 2008

Nutrition and Health in Developing Countries, Second Edition, edited by **Richard D. Semba and Martin W. Bloem,** 2008

Nutrition and Rheumatic Disease, edited by **Laura A. Coleman,** 2008

Nutrition in Kidney Disease, edited by **Laura D. Byham-Gray, Jerrilynn D. Burrowes, and Glenn M. Chertow,** 2008

Handbook of Nutrition and Ophthalmology, edited by **Richard D. Semba,** 2007

Adipose Tissue and Adipokines in Health and Disease, edited by **Giamila Fantuzzi and Theodore Mazzone,** 2007

Nutritional Health: Strategies for Disease Prevention, Second Edition, edited by **Norman J. Temple, Ted Wilson, and David R. Jacobs, Jr.,** 2006

Nutrients, Stress, and Medical Disorders, edited by **Shlomo Yehuda and David I. Mostofsky,** 2006

Calcium in Human Health, edited by **Connie M. Weaver and Robert P. Heaney,** 2006

Preventive Nutrition: The Comprehensive Guide for Health Professionals, Third Edition, edited by **Adrianne Bendich and Richard J. Deckelbaum,** 2005

The Management of Eating Disorders and Obesity, Second Edition, edited by **David J. Goldstein,** 2005

Nutrition and Oral Medicine, edited by **Riva Touger-Decker, David A. Sirois, and Connie C. Mobley,** 2005

IGF and Nutrition in Health and Disease, edited by **M. Sue Houston, Jeffrey M. P. Holly, and Eva L. Feldman,** 2005

Epilepsy and the Ketogenic Diet, edited by **Carl E. Stafstrom and Jong M. Rho,** 2004

Handbook of Drug–Nutrient Interactions, edited by **Joseph I. Boullata and Vincent T. Armenti,** 2004

Nutrition and Bone Health, edited by **Michael F. Holick and Bess Dawson-Hughes,** 2004

Diet and Human Immune Function, edited by **David A. Hughes, L. Gail Darlington, and Adrianne Bendich,** 2004

Beverages in Nutrition and Health, edited by **Ted Wilson and Norman J. Temple,** 2004

Handbook of Clinical Nutrition and Aging, edited by **Connie Watkins Bales and Christine Seel Ritchie,** 2004

NUTRITION AND RHEUMATIC DISEASE

Edited by
LAURA A. COLEMAN, PhD, RD

*Marshfield Clinic Research Foundation,
Marshfield, WI*

Foreword by
RONENN ROUBENOFF, MD, MHS

*Immunology Medical Research,
Biogen Idec, Inc.,
Cambridge, MA*

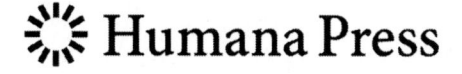

Humana Press

Editor
Laura A. Coleman
Marshfield Clinic Research Foundation
Marshfield, WI
coleman.laura@mcrf.mfldclin.edu

Series Editor
Adrianne Bendich
GlaxoSmithKline Consumer Healthcare
Parsippany, NJ

ISBN: 978-1-61737-862-1   e-ISBN: 978-1-59745-403-2

©2010 Humana Press, a part of Springer Science+Business Media, LLC
All rights reserved. This work may not be translated or copied in whole or in part without the written permission of the publisher (Humana Press, 999 Riverview Drive, Suite 208, Totowa, NJ 07512 USA), except for brief excerpts in connection with reviews or scholarly analysis. Use in connection with any form of information storage and retrieval, electronic adaptation, computer software, or by similar or dissimilar methodology now known or hereafter developed is forbidden.
The use in this publication of trade names, trademarks, service marks, and similar terms, even if they are not identified as such, is not to be taken as an expression of opinion as to whether or not they are subject to proprietary rights.
While the advice and information in this book are believed to be true and accurate at the date of going to press, neither the authors nor the editors nor the publisher can accept any legal responsibility for any errors or omissions that may be made. The publisher makes no warranty, express or implied, with respect to the material contained herein.

Printed on acid-free paper

9 8 7 6 5 4 3 2 1

springer.com

Dedication

This book is dedicated to Ben and Andrew, my dear boys,
and to Paul Coleman, my dear dad.

— Laura A. Coleman

Series Editor Introduction

The *Nutrition and Health*™ series of books, as an overriding mission, provide health professionals with texts that are considered essential because each includes (1) a synthesis of the state of the science; (2) timely, in-depth reviews by the leading researchers in their respective fields; (3) extensive, up-to-date, fully annotated reference lists; (4) a detailed index; (5) relevant tables and figures; (6) identification of paradigm shifts and the consequences; (7) virtually no overlap of information between chapters, but targeted, inter-chapter referrals; (8) suggestions of areas for future research; and (9) balanced, data-driven answers to patient/health professionals' questions that are based on the totality of evidence rather than the findings of any single study.

The series volumes are not the outcome of a symposium. Rather, each editor has the potential to examine a chosen area with a broad perspective, both in subject matter and in the choice of chapter authors. The international perspective, especially with regard to public health initiatives, is emphasized where appropriate. The editors, whose trainings are both research and practice oriented, have the opportunity to develop a primary objective for their book, define the scope and focus, and then invite the leading authorities from around the world to be part of their initiative. The authors are encouraged to provide an overview of the field, discuss their own research, and relate the research findings to potential human health consequences. Because each book is developed *de novo*, the chapters are coordinated so that the resulting volume imparts greater knowledge than the sum of the information contained in the individual chapters.

Nutrition and Rheumatic Disease, edited by Laura A. Coleman, is a very welcome addition to the *Nutrition and Health*™ series and fully exemplifies the series' goals. This volume is especially timely because the number of individuals suffering from rheumatic diseases continues to increase around the world. The last decade has seen an increased emphasis on the identification and characterization of bioactive, immunomodulatory molecules that can be used in the treatment of rheumatic diseases. At the same time, there has been an increasing awareness of the role of inflammation in the development of these diseases and the potential for nutrients with anti-inflammatory properties to help slow disease progression. This text is the first to synthesize the knowledge base concerning autoimmune rheumatoid diseases as well as osteoarthritis, inflammation, genetics, dietary components, and the most well-researched alternative and complementary therapies available to patients. As clearly indicated in the Foreword, written by the world-renowned physician scientist, Dr. Ronenn Roubenoff, this excellent volume will be of great value to the practicing health professional as well as those professionals and students who have an interest in the latest, up-to-date information on the science behind the prescription drug choices available to modulate the effects of rheumatic diseases.

The 15 chapters of *Nutrition and Rheumatic Disease* serve a dual purpose of providing an overview of the biology behind rheumatic disease, the epidemiology, the related nutritional issues, and an overall assessment of the nondrug substances that have been evaluated as adjuncts to treatment for those with rheumatic diseases. Substances reviewed include essential nutrients including vitamins A, B6, B12, folate, C, D, and E; minerals including calcium, zinc, iron, and selenium; and the essential fatty acids. Other substances that are included in the chapter reviews include, but are not limited to, antioxidants, creatine, anabolic steroids, herbal supplements, polyphenols, algae, gluten, glutamine, glucosamine and chondroitin, flax, and other sources of anti-inflammatory long-chain omega-3 fatty acids. The second purpose is to provide in-depth chapters that specifically target the most prevalent inflammatory diseases. There are individual chapters that look at osteoarthritis, systemic lupus erythematosus, gout, fibromyalgia, polymyositis and dermatomyositis, vasculitis, and Sjogren's syndrome, and a final chapter on chronic arthritides in children. Each chapter includes a review of current clinical findings associated with the consequences of inflammatory disease and puts these into historic perspective as well as pointing the way to future research opportunities.

Dr. Laura A. Coleman, who has edited the volume, is an internationally recognized leader in the field of nutrition and rheumatic disease as well as the clinical outcomes. She is an excellent communicator and has worked tirelessly to develop a book that is destined to be the benchmark in the field because of its extensive, in-depth chapters covering the most important aspects of the complex interactions between cellular functions, diet, and inflammation, and their impact on the diseases reviewed in this volume. The introductory chapters provide readers with the basics so that the more clinically related chapters can be easily understood. Dr. Coleman has chosen 29 of the most well recognized and respected authors from around the world to contribute the 15 informative chapters in the volume. Hallmarks of all of the chapters include complete definitions of terms with the abbreviations fully defined for the reader, and consistent use of terms between chapters. Key features of this comprehensive volume include the informative bulleted summary points and key words that are at the beginning of each chapter, appendices that include a detailed list of nutrition resources, and rheumatology resources including lists of relevant books, journals, and websites. The volume contains more than 40 detailed tables and informative figures, an extensive, detailed index, and more than 1100 up-to-date references that provide the reader with excellent sources of worthwhile information about rheumatic diseases, nutrition, and health.

Dr. Coleman has chosen chapter authors who are internationally distinguished researchers, clinicians, and epidemiologists who provide a comprehensive foundation for understanding the role of nutrients and other dietary factors in inflammatory diseases and related co-morbidities. Outstanding unique chapters include a comprehensive review of the effects of major histocompatability factors on the development of rheumatic disease; a full clinically relevant chapter on drug–nutrient interactions; another in-depth chapter on cachexia, which is of great relevance to the health professional treating patients with inflammatory disease; and another important chapter on exercise in rheumatic disease that includes clinically relevant pointers for practitioners as well as patients on exercise program initiation and maintenance. It is important to also point out that, unlike most volumes that review rheumatic diseases, this volume contains a chapter devoted to the development of rheumatic diseases in childhood and the unique nutritional needs of these growing children. Thus, the chapter authors have integrated the newest research findings so the reader can better understand the complex interactions that can result from the development of rheumatic disease.

In conclusion, *Nutrition and Rheumatic Disease*, edited by Laura A. Coleman, provides health professionals in many areas of research and practice with the most up-to-date, well-referenced volume on the importance of nutrition in determining the potential for rheumatic chronic diseases to affect overall health. This volume will serve the reader as the benchmark in this complex area of interrelationships between immune cells, lymphoid tissue, muscle, bone, cartilage, blood vessels, skin, and other relevant organ systems in the human body and the substances that we consume. Moreover, the interactions between inflammation, genetic factors, and the numerous co-morbidities are clearly delineated so that students as well as practitioners can better understand the complexities of these interactions. Dr. Coleman is applauded for her efforts to develop the most authoritative resource in the field to date, and this excellent text is a very welcome addition to the *Nutrition and Health*™ series.

Adrianne Bendich, PhD, FACN

Foreword

It has been known for centuries that disease and malnutrition go hand in hand. Illnesses such as cancer (cachexia), tuberculosis (consumption), typhoid fever, and cholera (dysentery) classically cause severe malnutrition. Conversely, famine has, throughout human history, led to epidemics as the population's immune function deteriorated.

However, only in the past century or so have chronic diseases emerged as the main medical problems of humans in developed nations. Not surprisingly, altered nutritional status is part and parcel of most of these diseases as well. Rheumatic diseases are among the most common chronic illnesses, yet only now has *Nutrition and Rheumatic Disease*—the first volume dedicated to the interplay of nutrition and the rheumatic diseases—been published.

Actually, it was Sir James Paget who first described "rheumatoid cachexia" in the 1870s in a paper describing the muscle wasting he observed around tuberculous joints, especially the hip and shoulder. Shortly thereafter—from the 1890s to the 1940s—came the "golden age" of nutrition, when the vitamins were discovered and nutrient requirements were worked out, with Nobel prizes awarded for many of these discoveries. During those years, nutrition was a major part of medical education. However, after World War II and the advent of the antibiotics and rapid advances in pharmacology, nutrition lost much of its place in medical education. Ironically, by the late 20th century, patients often were much more concerned about their nutritional status than were their physicians, and often more knowledgeable due to the Internet.

Today, there is clear evidence in both directions—chronic inflammation alters macro- and micro-nutrient status, and diet can have important effects on immune function. As Leon Gordis said, "nutrition is the ultimate environmental exposure. We all do it three times a day." Yet nutrition, like arthritis, is prone to exploitation by charlatans who make exorbitant claims for unproven remedies. This book is an important advance because it allows both patients and doctors to find in one place a detailed and thorough review of the state of the art in nutrition and the rheumatic diseases.

The relationship between patient and doctor in chronic diseases differs from that in acute illness. In acute illness, there is not much time to make decisions, and both knowledge and the need to act give nearly all the power to the physician. However, in chronic illness, both the effects of the disease and the pace of treatment are slower, allowing more time for reflection and joint decision-making between patient and doctor. In this more transactional setting, the patient's opinion, attitudes, and knowledge matter much more. Nutrition, being an area where patients claim both knowledge—whether correct or not—and interest, often becomes a battleground between doctor and patient.

It is the goal of this book to give patients and practitioners a sound scientific basis on which to base their approach to nutrition and the rheumatic diseases.

Finally, it is to the credit of Dr. Laura Coleman that this book has appeared, and those of us in both the nutrition and the rheumatology communities owe her a debt of gratitude for her efforts.

Ronenn Roubenoff, MD, MHS

Preface

Nutrition and Rheumatic Disease was born out of an article written nearly a decade ago on nutrition and connective tissue health *(1)*. Although historically, nutrition therapy for rheumatic diseases has been viewed with a fair amount of skepticism by the medical community, it has always been a topic of great interest to patients. Medical practitioners need information on how best to respond to patients' questions about what they should be eating in an attempt to control their disease symptoms. At the same time, however, it is difficult, if not impossible, for health care providers to remain at the forefront of knowledge for all aspects of nutrition and rheumatic diseases. The goal in editing this work, therefore, is to provide a comprehensive review of current knowledge regarding nutrition and dietary management for this complex set of conditions, from experts in each of the various rheumatic conditions.

Unike many other chronic diseases, there is no definitive diet to prescribe for patients with rheumatic disease. There is no "lupus diet," for example, the way there are diets for diabetes or cardiovascular disease, although there is more research for some conditions (e.g., rheumatoid arthritis, osteoarthritis, gout, or lupus) than for others (vasculitis or myositis). This is not only a challenge for medical providers, but also a frustration for patients who are vulnerable to influence from much of the misinformation that exists related to diet and disease. Arguably, nowhere is this more the case than in the field of complementary and alternative medicine, which is the focus of one of the general chapters in this volume. With Internet access and search engines nearly universal, and patients having the ability to obtain information but not necessarily having the skills or the knowledge to critically evaluate either the source of the information or the data itself, confusion results. Health care providers are in the position of having to clarify and simplify much of the seemingly conflicting information that patients obtain. *Nutrition and Rheumatic Disease* is intended to be this reliable source of sound advice that providers can pass along to their patients.

The field of rheumatic diseases includes a wide variety of pathological processes, although there are common features to a number of conditions. Inflammation is a central mechanism whereby much of the organ and tissue damage occurs, and pain is the most common manifestation of rheumatic disease. As a result, dietary interventions aimed at reducing inflammatory mediators in the body, such as the use of omega-3 fatty acids found in fish oils, are attractive to patients wanting to exert some control over their illness. Comprehensive reviews of the scientific literature by experts on each of the rheumatic diseases included in this work will help, we hope, to alleviate some of the inherent confusion surrounding the risks and benefits of various dietary therapies.

Also common to most of the rheumatic diseases is their episodic nature, making it difficult to attribute improvement in symptoms to any one intervention. The natural history of relapses and remissions in rheumatoid arthritis, for example, confounds studies attempting to examine the effect of diet alone on clinical symptoms.

This book is divided into two major parts (Part III consists of appendices): Part I includes general topics, such as an overview of immunology and rheumatic disease, nutrition assessment, epidemiology, drug–nutrient interactions, exercise, and complementary and alternative therapies. The goal in including these chapters is to provide a better understanding of a variety of topics that are applicable to the discussion of the specific rheumatic diseases that follow. One distinction that we have made is to include separate discussions on nutritional status versus dietary therapy for individuals with each rheumatic condition.

Part II focuses on specific rheumatic conditions, and includes chapters on rheumatoid arthritis, osteoarthritis, systemic lupus erythematosus, gout (the four most frequent serious rheumatic diseases), fibromyalgia, polymyositis, the vasculitides, Sjogren's syndrome, and juvenile arthritis. Within each of these disease-specific chapters, the authors provide an historical perspective, a discussion of the major clinical features, current management and treatment, a review of the literature related to nutritional status and diet, and dietary recommendations, based on current scientific evidence. Not only do these chapters include a critical evaluation of the literature, but they also are based on extensive clinical experience from each of the chapter authors; it is this combination that provides a unique perspective from which to address the role of nutrition in rheumatic diseases.

Part III consists of appendices that provide references for additional reading and Websites should readers need information that is beyond the scope of this book. Many of the chapters could be the focus of entire books themselves, and as a result, we have tried to limit discussion to the most practical and commonly misunderstood aspects of each topic. Although this book is oriented primarily toward practicing health professionals, others who may find it useful include research scientists, health policymakers, and individuals working in foundations supporting each of the rheumatic diseases, such as the Arthritis Association, Lupus Foundation, and others. These organizations are often the first place where patients turn when they are in need of information.

I thank Adrianne Bendich, Series Editor, and the staff at Humana Press for their guidance and patient assistance in helping to complete this work. I extend my deep gratitude to each of the authors for their hard work to complete these comprehensive chapters in the midst of maintaining busy clinical practices and research careers. I also offer my thanks to Dr. Ronenn Roubenoff for his, as always, insightful foreword.

Laura A. Coleman, PhD, RD

REFERENCE

1. Rall LC, Roubenoff R. Nutrition and connective tissue health. Nutrition Today 2000:35:142–150.

Contents

Dedication v
Series Editor Introduction.. vii
Foreword.. xi
Preface... xiii
Contributors.. xvii

PART I: INTRODUCTION TO RHEUMATIC DISEASES AND RELATED TOPICS

1 Overview of Immunology and the Rheumatic Diseases 3
   Elena M. Massarotti

2 Overview of Nutritional Assessment 15
   Shari Baird and Johanna Dwyer with the assistance of Emily Evans

3 An Overview of Rheumatic Disease Epidemiology 39
   Daniel J. McCarty and Erin K. Bundy

4 Drug–Nutrient Interactions in Rheumatic Diseases 57
   Sung Nim Han

5 Exercise in Rheumatic Diseases 69
   Lindsay M. Bearne and Mike V. Hurley

6 Complementary and Alternative Therapies 89
   Kevin Khaw and Sharon L. Kolasinski

PART II: RHEUMATIC DISEASES

7 Rheumatoid Cachexia 113
   Ronenn Roubenoff

8 Nutrition and Nutritional Supplements and Osteoarthritis 125
   Paola de Pablo, Grace Lo, and Timothy E. McAlindon

9 Nutritional Supplementation in Systemic Lupus Erythematosus 159
   Sangeeta D. Sule and Michelle Petri

10 Hyperuricemia, Gout, and Diet 169
Naomi Schlesinger

11 Fibromyalgia and Diet 183
Osmo Hänninen and Anna-Lissa Rauma

12 Nutrition and Polymyositis and Dermatomyositis 195
Ingela Loell and Ingrid Lundberg

13 Nutritional Issues in Vasculitis 215
Paul F. Dellaripa and Donough Howard

14 Sjögren's Syndrome and Its Implications for Diet and Nutrition 227
Carole A. Palmer and Medha Singh

15 Chronic Arthritides of Childhood 251
Basil M. Fathalla and Donald Goldsmith

PART III: NUTRITION AND RHEUMATIC DISEASE-RELATED RESOURCES

Appendix A: *Nutrition Resources* 279

Appendix B: *Rheumatology Resources* 281

Index 283

Contributors

Shari Baird, MS, RD • *Frances Stern Nutrition Center, Boston, MA*
Lindsay M. Bearne, PhD, MSC, MCSP • *Rehabilitation Research Unit, Dulwich Hospital, Dulwich, London, UK*
Erin K. Bundy, BS • *Marshfield Clinic Research Foundation, Marshfield, WI*
Laura A. Coleman, PhD, RD • *Marshfield Clinic Research Foundation, Marshfield, WI*
Paola de Pablo, MD, MPH • *Division of Rheumatology, Department of Medicine, Tufts-New England Medical Center, Tufts University School of Medicine, Boston, MA*
Paul F. Dellaripa, MD, FACP, FACR • *Division of Rheumatology, Immunology and Allergy, Brigham and Women's Hospital, Boston, MA*
Johanna Dwyer, DSC, RD • *Frances Stern Nutrition Center, Boston, MA*
Emily Evans, BS • *Frances Stern Nutrition Center, Boston, MA*
Basil M. Fathalla, MD • *Division of Rheumatology, St. Christopher's Hospital for Children, Philadelphia, PA*
Donald Goldsmith, MD • *Department of Pediatrics, St. Christopher's Hospital for Children, Philadelphia, PA*
Sung Nim Han, PhD, RD • *Department of Food and Nutrition, College of Human Ecology, Seoul National University, Seoul, Korea*
Osmo Hänninen, Prof Em., Dr Med Sci, PhD • *Department of Physiology, University of Kuopio, Kuopio, Finland*
Donough Howard, MD • *Division of Rheumatology, Lahey Clinic, Burlington, MA*
Mike V. Hurley, PhD, MCSP • *Rehabilitation Research Unit, Dulwich Hospital, Dulwich, London, UK*
Kevin Khaw, MD • *Department of Medicine/Rheumatology, University of Pennsylvania, Philadelphia, PA*
Sharon L. Kolasinski, MD • *Division of Rheumatology, Hospital of University of Pennsylvania, Philadelphia, PA*
Grace Lo, MD • *Rheumatologist, Tufts-New England Medical Center, Boston, MA*
Ingela Loell, BSC • *Rheumatology Unit, Karolinska University Hospital, Stockholm, Sweden*
Ingrid Lundberg, MD, PhD • *Rheumatology Unit, Karolinska University Hospital Stockholm, Sweden*
Elena M. Massarotti, MD • *Division of Rheumatology, Immunology and Allergy, Brigham and Women's Hospital, Boston, MA*
Timothy E. McAlindon, MD, MPH • *Division of Rheumatology, Department of Medicine, Tufts-New England Medical Center, Tufts University School of Medicine Boston, MA*

DANIEL J. MCCARTY, PhD • *College of Professional Studies, University of Wisconsin, Stevens Point, WI*
CAROLE A. PALMER, EdD, RD • *Division of Nutrition and Oral Health, Tufts University School of Dental Medicine, Boston, MA*
MICHELLE PETRI, MD, MPH • *Department of Medicine-Rheumatology, Johns Hopkins University School of Medicine, Baltimore, MD*
ANNA-LISSA RAUMA, PhD, RD • *Savonlinna Department of Teacher Education, University of Joensuu, Savonlinna, Finland*
RONENN ROUBENOFF, MD, MHS • *Immunology Medical Research, Biogen Idec, Inc., Cambridge, MA*
NAOMI SCHLESINGER, MD • *Department of Medicine, University of Medicine and Dentistry, New Brunswick, NJ*
MEDHA SINGH, DDS, MS • *Division of Nutrition and Oral Health, Tufts University School of Dental Medicine, Boston, MA*
SANGEETA D. SULE, MD • *Division of Rheumatology, Johns Hopkins University, Baltimore, MD*

I Introduction to Rheumatic Diseases and Related Topics

1 Overview of Immunology and the Rheumatic Diseases

Elena M. Massarotti

Summary

- The immune system is centrally involved in the pathogenesis of many rheumatic diseases, although the precise mechanisms by which the immune system becomes diseased remain undefined for most illnesses.
- A central theory governing autoimmunity is that disease results when a genetically susceptible individual is exposed to either a self-antigen or foreign antigen, resulting in an aberrant immune response.
- Autoantibody formation is characteristic of many rheumatic illnesses but many of these autoantibodies are not directly pathogenic.
- This chapter provides an overview of immunology and the rheumatic illnesses discussed in this volume, with a focus on autoimmunity.

Key Words: Autoimmunity; immunology; major histocompatibility complex; rheumatic illnesses

1. OVERVIEW OF IMMUNOLOGY AND THE RHEUMATIC DISEASES

Rheumatic diseases are comprised of a wide range of specific disease states and syndromes that directly or indirectly involve the joints, and are associated with "aches and pains." These diseases include but are not limited to regional pain syndromes like tendonitis or sprain, systemic inflammatory diseases like rheumatoid arthritis (RA) and systemic lupus erythematosus (SLE), infections directly involving joints and periarticular structures, and diseases in which the joints are "secondarily" involved as what may be seen in paraneoplastic syndromes. Multiple organ systems may also be involved in a single disease and different pathogenetic processes contribute to the clinical manifestations of each illness. For example, scleroderma, a systemic rheumatic disease, is associated with progressive thickening of the skin, arteriolar narrowing, joint pain, pulmonary hypertension, pulmonary fibrosis, glomerulosclerosis, and gastroesophageal reflux with abnormal peristalsis. Furthermore, although scleroderma may share some pathogenetic features with other rheumatic diseases, its pathogenesis is really quite unique from that seen in other systemic inflammatory rheumatic diseases as in RA and SLE. Osteoarthritis is also a rheumatic disease but does not have any systemic features, is primarily a degenerative disease of cartilage, and is not a disease characterized by defects in the immune system. Thus, grouping the rheumatic diseases into distinct pathogenetic modules can be challenging and no one organ system is uniformly involved in the manifestations of a particular disease.

The immune system plays a direct role in the pathogenesis of many rheumatic diseases. No unifying theory of immunopathogenesis governs the pathophysiology of immune-mediated rheumatic diseases. Although many of the specific cells and pathways involved in various rheumatic diseases have been defined, much remains unknown regarding the precise mechanism by which pathological events are triggered and developed within the human body. With this in mind, this chapter summarizes the rheumatic diseases in which the immune system is centrally involved and the role of the major histocompatibility complex (MHC) in diseases.

2. AUTOIMMUNITY

Autoimmunity can be defined as the immune response to self-antigens or foreign antigens, and autoimmune disease results from the pathological effects of this response on one or more organ systems *(1)*. Autoimmunity can result from several processes, including altered antigen presentation, increased T-cell help, and molecular mimicry. Autoimmunity has been shown to occur in normal individuals where antibodies or T cells react with self-antigen, resulting in self-reactivity without evidence of pathology. Loss of tolerance to self is at the crux of autoimmunity.

3. DISEASES WITH AUTOANTIBODIES

3.1. Autoantibody Formation

The formation of antibodies against self-antigens, or autoantibodies, is characteristic of many autoimmune diseases. Several theories have been put forth regarding how autoantibodies are generated, including polyclonal activation, molecular mimicry, apoptosis, altered self, and idiotype–anti-idiotype interactions *(1)*. Polyclonal activation of B cells is found in lupus and has been demonstrated with lipopolysaccharide, which can stimulate autoantibody formation against self-antigens *(2)*. Molecular mimicry refers to the generation of autoantibodies when an immune response to a foreign antigen cross-reacts with an epitope found on self-antigens *(3)*. Apoptosis, or programmed cell death, may contribute to autoantibody formation by the production of autoantigens in "apoptotic blebs" *(1)*. Altered self is said to occur with the binding of foreign and self-antigen, or with immunization of a foreign protein that then leads to autoimmunity to a homologous self-protein *(1)*. Idiotypes, which are antigenic determinants found on the variable region of antibodies, may mimic foreign antigens, and antibodies made against the foreign antigen could in turn react against idiotypes, generating anti-idiotype antibodies *(4)*.

Autoantibody formation occurs in some autoimmune diseases, and these diseases are not confined to rheumatology, per se. For example, nearly all patients with Hashimoto's thyroiditis, an endocrinological disorder associated with hypothyroidism, possess antibodies to two proteins found within human thyroid tissue: thyroid peroxidase and thyroglobulin. Celiac disease is a gastrointestinal illness manifest by malabosorption; affected patients contain antibodies to gliadin, a glycoprotein within gluten, and endomysium, which is a structure of the smooth muscle connective tissue. Destruction of pancreatic beta cells is seen in type 1 diabetes, with the production of autoantibody formation against islet cells, glutamic acid dehydrogenase, and insulin.

More than one autoimmune disease can also be present within an individual. It is not at all unusual, for example, for a patient with RA to have Hashimoto's thyroid disease, or for a patient with polymyositis to have manifestations of Grave's disease, another autoimmune thyroid disease leading to hyperthyroidism. Numerous other autoimmune diseases within other specialties other than rheumatology exist and can serve as models to better understand the pathophysiological events seen in rheumatic diseases.

Autoantibodies may be directly pathogenic, or may be epiphenomen, serving as disease markers, or have unclear implications in disease pathogenesis. For diseases like RA and SLE, their presence supports or reinforces the diagnosis at hand. For others, like Wegener's granulomatosis (WG), the antibody may be considered virtually diagnostic of the disease and may have a clearer role in the pathogenesis of the disease.

3.2. *Autoantibody Formation in SLE*

SLE is considered the prototypic autoimmune disease and is characterized by the marked production of autoantibodies; autoantibody formation is considered to be the hallmark of the disease, and is in part related to polyclonal stimulation of B cells. SLE is a multisystem disease that primarily affects women in the childbearing years, although men and both older and younger females are also affected. Antinuclear antibodies (ANAs) react against numerous nuclear antigens, and are identified in the serum of more than 95% of patients with SLE by the reaction with fluorescent anti-immunoglobulin antibodies *(5)*. Nuclear staining is ascertained with a fluorescence microscope, and different staining patterns are associated with different target antigens: diffuse or homogeneous (the nucleus is diffusely stained), speckled, nucleolar, or centromere. All patterns can be seen in patients with SLE, although the centromere pattern is highly characteristic of a form of scleroderma known as CREST or limited scleroderma. The detection of ANAs, however, is not "in and of itself" considered to be *diagnostic* for SLE because a positive ANA can be detected in about 2% of healthy individuals, especially young women *(6)*. Higher ANA titers tend to be more associated with SLE, but their presence must be interpreted clinically, with a careful history and physical examination.

ANAs in SLE are directed against self-antigens that are located in the nucleus, cell surface, and cytoplasm. Some antibodies are also directed against circulating antibodies and coagulation factors *(7)*. Antibodies directed against nuclear antigens are most characteristic of SLE, especially those directed against double-stranded DNA (dsDNA) and the nuclear antigen, Sm. Sm, a small nuclear ribonucleoprotein, is a component of the spliceosome, and is involved in RNA processing. Individual patients with SLE may express unique autoantibody profiles. For example, the presence of antibodies against dsDNA are highly correlated with the presence of glomerulonephritis, whereas antibodies directed against SSA/Ro, which are proteins complexed with RNA molecules, are associated with the neonatal lupus syndrome and Sjogren's syndrome (SS), a related autoimmune disease characterized by exocrine gland dysfunction resulting in manifestations such as excessive ocular and oral dryness. However, clinical situations also exist in which elevated dsDNA antibodies are not associated with nephritis, or any *clinical* disease activity. This is true of the other ANAs, too. Anti-Sm antibody titers tend to not correlate with disease activity, whereas antibodies to dsDNA in some patients may correlate with the intensity of the clinical manifestation with which it is associated for that individual patient. Anti-dsDNA antibodies can also fix complement, resulting in complement levels that correlate with disease activity—lower complement levels are associated with active disease, whereas rising or normal levels are seen with recovery or disease remission. Hypocomplementemia (low serum complement) is not uncommon with glomerulonephritis.

The pathogenecity of these autoantibodies also varies, and has been best studied with anti-dsDNA and the kidney in which anti-dsDNA antibodies and dsDNA form immune complexes that become deposited within the glomerulus and invoke renal injury by triggering inflammation. The contribution of other autoantibodies to the pathogenesis of disease manifestations in SLE is less well defined but clinical manifestations have been associated with the presence of certain antibodies (Table 1).

Immune complex formation is characteristic of SLE, but not all immune complex formation in SLE is associated with activation of complement and the measurement of serum immune complexes as a guide to assessing clinical activity is not clinically useful.

3.3. Autoantibody Formation in Sjogren's Syndrome

SS is a connective tissue disease with autoimmune features that primarily affects women in midlife and is characterized by lymphocytic infiltration of exocrine glands with resultant organ dysfunction. Disease, however, is not confined to the exocrine glands; patients with SS may develop a nonerosive arthritis, lymphadenopathy, vasculitic rash, leukopenia, thrombocytopenia, as well as other organ-specific dysfunction. Non-Hodgkin's lymphoma is also associated with SS. SS can occur alone, in the absence of a concomitant rheumatic disease (primary SS), or in association with a more well-defined connective tissue disease, most commonly SLE or RA (secondary SS). Autoantibody formation is highly characteristic of primary SS: approximately

Table 1
Autoantibodies and Disease Manifestations

Autoantibody	*Clinical Manifestations*
Anti-dsDNA	Renal disease; glomerulonephritis; specific for lupus
Anti-Ro; Anti-La	Sjogren's syndrome; neonatal lupus; congenital heart block; photosensitivity; subacute cutaneous lupus
Anti-RNP	Mixed connective tissue disease; Raynaud's phenomenon; myositis; interstitial lung disease
Anti-ribosomal P	Central nervous system disease; depression
Anti-Smith	Specific for lupus

80% of patients with primary SS have ANAs, with 50 to 90% of affected patients possessing antibodies against SSA/Ro and SSB/La (8). Autoantibodies in the sera of patients with SS react with a variety of nonorgan-specific antigens including extractable nuclear antigens and cytoplasmic antigens; antibodies directed against immunoglobulin can also be found. Hypergammaglobulinemia is common in SS, and rheumatoid factor (RF), which is an antibody directed against the Fc portion of immunoglobulin (Ig)G, is found in about 90% of patients with SS. SSA/Ro, a cytoplasmic antigen, consists of a 52-kDa and a 60-kDa polypeptide in association with cytoplasmic RNA. SSB/La is a 48-kDa protein bound to RNA III transcripts. Anti-SSA/Ro antibodies are associated with the development of neonatal heart block in about 3% of women affected with SS who possess these autoantibodies (9). Antibodies to SSB/La usually coexist with antibodies to SSA/Ro.

The histopathology of exocrine tissues reveals a focal mononuclear cell infiltrate that consist primarily of CD4+ T cells, macrophages, and mast cells (10) but the specific immunopathogenetic pathways leading to disease remain undefined.

3.4. Autoantibody Formation in Systemic Sclerosis (Scleroderma)

Like SLE and SS, systemic sclerosis, or scleroderma, is a connective tissue disease that primarily affects women and is also associated with the formation of ANAs in about 95% of affected individuals (11). The clinical hallmark of the disease is progressive skin thickening caused by excessive deposition of collagen with resultant fibrosis. The fibrotic process may involve multiple organs including the lungs, gastrointestinal tract, and heart. Immune and vascular-mediated mechanisms contribute to the clinical manifestations. Different forms of systemic sclerosis are associated with different autoantibody profiles; progressive systemic sclerosis, the more severe form, is associated with antibodies to DNA topoisomerase in about 40% of affected patients (11), whereas those patients affected with less severe skin involvement, as what is seen with limited scleroderma (previously known as the CREST syndrome) have titers of anticentromere antibodies approaching 90% (12). Other autoantibodies against RNA polymerase III and U3RNP have been shown to correlate with specific manifestations and ethnicities, reinforcing the genetic influence upon autoantibody formation. Patients with progressive systemic sclerosis who have antibodies to DNA topoisomerase, or anti-SCL-70, generally have a worse prognosis, but other autoantibodies identified in the sera of patients with scleroderma may not be associated with this degree of clinical significance. These include anti-endothelial antibodies and antimyenteric neuronal antibodies. Immune complex formation with activation of complement is generally not part of the immunopathogenesis of scleroderma, and it does not appear that anticentromere antibodies and antitopoisomerase antibodies are directly pathogenic as well.

3.5. Autoantibody Formation in Inflammatory Muscle Disease

The inflammatory muscle diseases comprise a group of heterogeneous diseases characterized by proximal muscle weakness and inflammation of skeletal muscle. Polymyositis and dermatomyositis, as well as the juvenile form of dermatomyositis, are immune-mediated diseases characterized by autoantibody formation. Antibodies to both nuclear and cytoplasmic antigens can be found in about 20% of patients with inflammatory muscle disease *(13)*. However, there are some myositis-specific antibodies (MSA) that are found exclusively in patients with inflammatory myositis, and can assist in the clinical definition of the myositis. Antisynthetase antibodies are directed against cytoplasmic ribonucleoprotein antigens that are involved in protein synthesis and are characteristic of polymyositis and dermatomyositis. Anti-Jo-1, which is directed against histidyl transfer RNA synthetase, is the most common MSA and is clinically associated with the presence of interstitial lung disease in patients with dermatomyositis. The antibodies are diagnostic markers, and their role in the immunopathogenesis of the diseases remains unclear. Like the other autonantibodies discussed, they do not appear to be directly pathogenic and do not appear to fix complement.

3.6. Autoantibody Formation in the Vasculitides

The term *vasculitis* signifies inflammation within blood vessels, and vasculitis can be seen with connective tissue diseases like SLE, SS, and RA. Additionally, distinct vasculitis syndromes have been defined and comprise a heterogeneous group of disorders with overlapping clinical features. These vasculitis syndromes have been historically grouped in a variety of ways: with respect to the predominant vessel size affected (small, medium, or large), by the histopathology of the affected vessel (e.g., necrotizing features, fibrinoid necrosis, leukocytoclastic), associated clinical manifestations, and serological markers. Biopsy of clinically affected tissue is usually required for the diagnosis of most types of vasculitis. The identification of antineutrophilic cytoplasmic antibodies (ANCAs) in 1985 has provided the clinician with a reliable serological diagnostic test for the necrotizing vasculitides, a group of disorders usually affecting medium-sized vessels that on histopathology show necrosis of blood vessel walls. These disorders include Wegener's granulomatosis WG, polyarteritis nodosa (PAN), microscopic PAN, and Churg Strauss disease.

Vasculitis may be caused by the deposition of immune complexes within vessel walls resulting in focal complement activation, recruitment of inflammatory cells, and narrowing of the vessel lumen. Immune complexes, however, are not always detected in the serum of affected patients but may be more common with certain types of vasculitis. The specific trigger for each of the vasculitic processes is not clear, and different models have been proposed for individual diseases.

The clinical presentation of the vasculitides in large part depends on the particular vessels involved. Diseases characterized by small vessel involvement may present with skin manifestations (purpura). For example, large vessel involvement is seen with giant cell arteritis (GCA) or Takayasu's arteritis, although the former is seen mostly in women over the age of 60, whereas the latter is seen in very young females. WG is predominantly a disease of middle-aged men, and is associated with upper respiratory tract manifestations in 80% of cases; the kidneys, lungs, and skin can also be involved. WG primarily affects medium-sized vessels, but small vessels can also be affected. Vasculitis is not uncommon in lupus, and may take a variety of forms. Purpura caused by inflammation within the small blood vessels of the skin, hemoptysis from vasculitis involving the vasculature in the pulmonary parenchyma, and cerebritis owing to small vessel involvement in the brain have all been described. Immune complex formation and deposition likely contributes to the pathogenesis of lupus vasculitis.

The association between autoantibodies and vasculitis is most clear with the necrotizing group of vasculitides with the discovery of ANCAs. Indirect immunofluorescence has identified two ANCA patterns: perinuclear (p-ANCA) and cytoplasmic or (c-ANCA). c-ANCA refers to cytoplasmic staining and is generally associated with antibodies against proteinase 3 (pR3), which is a serine protease found in the azurophil granules of neutrophils *(14)*. c-ANCA is fairly specific for WG, found in 50 to 70% of patients with WG; p-ANCA has also been seen in WG, but is less common. Enzyme-linked immunosorbent assay (ELISA) can be used to identify pR3. p-ANCA patterns result from an artifact of ethanol fixation, and target antigens associated with a p-ANCA pattern include myeloperoxidase (MPO), elastase, cathepsin G, and lactoferrin, among others *(14)*. MPO is the most common antigen associated with the p-ANCA pattern and is clinically associated with microscopic PAN and pauci-immunoglomerulonephritis; it too, can be identified with ELISA. There is good evidence that ANCAs have a direct pathogenic role in WG, with activation of neutrophils or monocytes by tumor necrosis factor (TNF)-α. This activation results in the movement of pR3 and MPO to the cell membrane; these molecules then interact with ANCA antibodies, and this interaction in turn causes degranulation of the white cells resulting in the production of reactive oxygen species that damage tissues *(15)*. However, ANCA titers may not predict disease relapse, and it remains unclear and controversial whether ANCA titers specifically correlate with disease activity.

Autoantibodies have also been seen with cryoglobulinemia, which can be seen with certain infections or other rheumatic diseases like lupus. Cryoglobulins are immunglobulins that precipitate in the cold, usually below 4° Celsius. They are categorized as type 1, 2, or 3, depending on the presence of a mononclonal component within the cryoglobulin itself. Type 1 cryoglobulins consist solely of a monoclonal component. Both type 2 and 3 cryoglobulins contain a polyclonal component, but type 2 cryoglobulins also contain a monoclonal component. Type 2 and 3 cryoglobulins can be detected in the sera of patients with systemic vasculitis caused by hepatitis C. In hepatitis C-associated cryoglobulinemia, an untoward immune response to hepatitis C infection results in the formation of immune complexes that deposit in the vessel wall. The immune complexes contain components of the hepatitis C virus, and monoclonal IgM RF *(16)*. The clinical manifestations of cryoglobulinemia caused by hepatitis C include skin disease with rash, and renal involvement owing to deposition of cryoglobulin complexes in the glomerulus, causing an abnormal urinalysis and renal function. Manifestations of cryoglobulinemia in lupus include skin and kidney disease, resulting from immune complex formation and activation of complement.

3.7. Autoantibody Formation Associated With Rheumatoid Arthritis

RA is the most common inflammatory arthritis and affects women greater than men, with a disease onset usually between the third and fifth decades. Untreated disease can lead to progressive joint destruction and disability. Extrarticular manifestations of RA occur and include secondary SS (manifest by dry eyes and mouth or the sicca complex), pericarditis, pleural effusions, and lymphadenopathy. RF, the immunoglobulin directed against the Fc portion of IgG, is found in about 80% of patients with RA. Higher titers are generally associated with more destructive disease but titers do not correlate with disease activity; patients with higher titers may have a worse prognosis. Seronegative patients (those who test negative for RF) may have a better prognosis. RF can be found in other chronic inflammatory diseases in which polyclonal B cell stimulation occurs. RF is found in normal elderly individuals. Although evidence of local immune complexes within synovial tissues containing RF exists, RA is not characterized by immune complex-mediated tissue injury with resultant hypocomplementemia.

In addition to RF, the sera of patients with RA also contain antibodies to cyclic citrullinated peptides (CCPs). Citrullinated extracellular fibrin found in RA synovium may act as an autoantigen that drives the local immune response, and elevated levels of anti-CCP have been seen with more progressive disease *(17)*. The relation between anti-CCP antibodies and disease activity has not been elucidated, and its formation in relation to disease onset and the formation of RF has not yet determined as well.

4. THE MHC AND RHEUMATIC DISEASES

Immune responses occur to antigens, and antigen-specific receptors, which share structural features with immunoglobulins, are located in the cell membranes of T and B cells. In order for T cells to process or "see" an antigen, the antigen must be "presented" by MHC molecules found on macrophages. MHC molecules are divided into two classes: class I and class II. MHC class I molecules present endogenous peptides, whereas class II molecules present exogenous peptides. The three-dimensional structure of the MHC molecules allows for the formation of a groove or cleft in which peptide is presented. The MHC molecules are genetically determined, and many autoimmune diseases are associated with different MHC alleles. One of the current prevailing theories regarding the development of autoimmune disease in general is that exposure to an unspecified antigen, in a genetically predisposed individual, results in disease. MHC alleles may confer susceptibility to diseases or specific subsets of diseases, or may define a specific autoantibody profile.

The class I MHC molecule is comprised of two subunits: the α chain, which is coded by genes in the HLA-A, B, and C loci, and $\beta 2$ microglobulin, which is not coded for by the MHC genes. Peptide processing within the cell leads to the formation of MHC and peptide fragment complexes that are then translocated to the cell surface for recognition by T cells. CD8, a T-cell coreceptor, binds to class I molecules on the cell surface. The formation of cytotoxic T cells results from the activation of CD8-positive T cells. Autoimmune disease is thought to follow aberrant antigen presentation by the CD8-positive T cell in the context of genetically determined Class I molecules. This interaction then leads to secretion of cytokines that help to promote the disease state.

The spondyloarthropathies are a group of inflammatory joint diseases manifest by spinal disease, peripheral joint arthritis, sacroiliitis, and extrarticular disease that are associated with the presence of the class I molecule, HLA B27. Ankylosing spondylitis is the prototypic spondyloarthropathy, and primarily affects men and is associated with the presence of HLA B27, a class I antigen, in more than 95% of affected patients. It remains one of the best examples of an association between a genetic marker and disease *(18)*. The specific mechanism by which HLA B27 invokes disease remains unclear. It has been proposed that HLA B27 participates in the presentation of an arthritogenic peptide, or does not clear specific intracellular organisms *(19)*.

The class II molecule is comprised of two MHC chains produced by different MHC genes (*HLA-DR, DQ,* and *DP*) and is found on B cells, dendritic cells, macrophages, activated T cells, and other cell types. Class II molecule-bearing cells process exogenous antigens and present these antigens to CD4-positive T cells, which in turn help to control both the cellular and immune response to antigen. Overall, MHC class II molecules have been shown to play a greater role in the immunopathogenesis of rheumatic diseases that possess autoimmune features.

4.1. MHC and SLE

Different sets of genes in different individuals contribute to the pathogenesis of lupus, and the MHC has been extensively investigated for its role in SLE. A relative risk of between 2 and 5 is found with the presence of HLA-DR2 and HLA-DR3, two class II molecules. Inherited complement deficiencies that are MHC-mediated also influence disease susceptibility. The relationship between specific disease manifestations and certain HLA alleles is less firm in lupus, probably because lupus is a disease characterized by an aberrant response to many self-antigens.

4.2. MHC and SS

White patients with primary SS express more HLA-DR3 and DLA-DQ2 alleles but different alleles are found in other ethnic groups *(7,20)*. Salivary and lacrimal gland epithelial cells of patients with SS present self-antigens to CD4-positive T cells because they express certain class II antigens. As a result, cytokines are induced, and stimulation of B cells occurs, leading to the immune abnormalities seen in SS.

4.3. MHC and Systemic Sclerosis

The role of MHC and scleroderma has also been extensively studied, showing some specific associations. A genetic susceptibility to scleroderma has been identified in Choctaw Native Americans, who have the highest prevalence of SS, and is associated with a specific haplotype on chromosome 15q *(21)*. Autoantibody profiles are associated with certain HLA alleles. In whites, HLA-DQB1 is associated with the presence of anticentromere antibodies, which are highly specific for limited scleroderma *(22)*.

4.4. MHC and Inflammatory Myositis

Certain MHC alleles are associated with specific muscle diseases or the expression of autoantibodies. HLA-DR3 appears to be associated with the development of polymyositis and juvenile dermatomyositis and the presence of HLA-DR52 is seen in patients who have antibodies to histidyl transfer RNA synthetase or Jo-1 *(23)*.

4.5. MHC and the Vasculitides

The association between genetic determinants of disease expression among the systemic vasculitides has been best studied in GCA, a large vessel vasculitis of unclear etiology affecting primarily women over the age of 60. High rates of GCA have been identified in Scandinavian populations, and the class II molecule HLA-DR4 has been correlated with increased risk of disease *(24)*. MHC associations are less well defined for other vasculitides.

4.6. MHC and RA

The role of the MHC in RA has been extensively studied; these studies have shown the clear association of HLA-DRβ1 alleles and the overexpression of RA. This association has been further honed, with the identification of the "shared epitope," a sequence of amino acids on the third hypervariable region of the HLA-DRβ1 allele in patients with RA *(25)*. Destructive disease is in particular associated with the presence of HLA-DRβ1, and different HLA-DRβ1 alleles have been associated with different manifestations of RA *(26)*. The utility of HLA-DR testing in assisting clinicians to identify patients at risk for more destructive disease who may need more aggressive treatment regimens remains unclear.

5. CYTOKINES AND RHEUMATIC DISEASES

Cytokines comprise a group of small proteins that mediate cell-to-cell communication and the immune response. They include growth factors, interleukin (IL) molecules, interferons (IFN), and other molecules. Cytokines react with specific cellular receptors and exert their effects on multiple cell types, including the cells from which they are released. Interactions between cytokines and their receptors result in the activation of intracellular pathways that in turn lead to other biological processes. Functional classes of cytokines include immunoregulatory cytokines, proinflammatory cytokines, and anti-inflammatory cytokines. Th (T helper)2 cells, which secrete the cytokines secrete IL-3, -4, -5, -6, -10, and -13, mediate the humoral immune response. The cell-mediated response is affected by cytokines produced by Th1 cells, which include IL-2, IFN-γ, IL-3, TNF-α, granulocyte macrophage colony-stimulating factor, and TNF-β. The identification of specific cytokines and their respective functions has helped scientists to piece together working models of the immunopathogenesis of some rheumatic diseases. To date, this has proved to be most fruitful for RA, in which the discovery of elevated levels of the pro-inflammatory cytokines TNF-α and IL-1 in the serum and synovial fluid of patients with RA has led to the development of targeted biological therapies in wide use today.

6. CONCLUSIONS

An aberrant immune response to self- and foreign antigens characterizes many of the autoimmune features of rheumatic diseases. Theories regarding the pathogenesis of this aberrant response include loss of tolerance, dysfunctional T-cell help, or molecular mimicry, in which shared features of the triggering antigen and self-antigen lead to an untoward immune response and resultant disease. The MHC plays a significant role in the development of many rheumatic diseases, governing the genetics of the immune response at the molecular level. Genetics influence the development of autoantibodies as well and many rheumatic diseases have multigenic processes at play. A single unifying theory of immunopathogenesis does not exist, but an abnormal immune response to antigen in a genetically predisposed individual is believed to lead to autoimmunity. The products of this interaction include various cytokines, which then trigger further immune and inflammatory mediated pathways inherent in each disease.

REFERENCES

1. Reeves WH, Richards HB, Satoh, M. Autoantibodies. In: Lahita R, ed. Textbook of Autoimmunity. Lippincott Williams and Wilkins, Philadelphia PA, 2000, pp. 81–100.
2. Dziarksi R. Preferential induction of autoantibody secretion in polyclonal activation by peptidoglycan and lipopolysaccharide: in vivo studies. J Immunol 1982;128:1018–1025.
3. Oldstone MBA. Molecular mimicry and autoimmune disease. Cell 1987;50:819–820.
4. Plotz PH. Autoantibodies are anti-idiotyope antibodies to antiviral antibodies. Lancet 1983;2:824–826.
5. Tan EM. Antinuclear antibodies: diagnostic markers for autoimmune diseases and probes for cell biology. Adv Immunol 1989;44:93–151.
6. Buyon JL. Systemic Lupus Erythematosus. Clinical and Laboratory Features. In: Klippel JH, ed. Primer on Rheumatic Diseases, 12th Ed. Arthritis Foundation, Atlanta Georgia 2001, pp. 335–346.
7. Pisetsky DS. Systemic Lupus Erythematosus. Epidemiology, Pathology, and Pathogenesis. In: Klippel JH, ed. Primer on Rheumatic Diseases, 12th Ed. Arthritis Foundation, Atlanta Georgia 2001, pp. 329–335.
8. Bell M, Askari A, Bokman A, et al. Sjogren's syndrome: a critical review of clinical management. J Rheumatol 1999;26:2051–2061.
9. Julkunen H, Siren MK, Kaaja F, Kurki P, Friman C, Koskimies S. Maternal HLA antigens and antibodies to SSA/Ro and SSB/La. Comparison with systemic lupus erythematosus and primary Sjogren's syndrome. Br J Rheumatol 1995;34:901–907.
10. Pillimer S. Sjogren's Syndrome. In: Klippel JH, ed. Primer on Rheumatic Diseases, 12th Ed. Arthritis Foundation, Atlanta Georgia 2001, pp. 377–384.
11. Gilliland, B. Systemic sclerosis and related disorders. In: Harrison' On line, chapter 303, McGraw Hill, New York, 2006, http://www.accessmedicine.com/content.aspx?alD=94691
12. Steen VD. Autoantibodies in systemic sclerosis. Semin Arthritis Rheum 2005;35(1): 35–42.
13. Tanimoto K, Nakano K, Kano S et al. Classification criteria for the idiopathic inflammatory myopathies. Curr Opin Rheumatol 1997;9:527–535.
14. Hoffman G, Specks U. Antineutrophil cytoplasmic antibodies. Arthritis Rheum 1998;41:1521–1537.
15. Keogan MY et al. Activation of normal neutrophils by anti-neutrophil cytoplasmic antibodies. Clin Exp Immunol 1992; 90:228.
16. Vassilopoulos D, Calabrese LH. Hepatitis C virus infection and vasculitis: Implications of antiviral and immunosuppressive therapies. Arthritis Rheum 2002;46:585.
17. Van Gaalen FA, van Aken J, Huizinga TW, et al. Association between HLA class II genes and autoantibodies to cyclic citrullinated peptides [CCPs] influences the severity of rheumatoid arthritis. Arthritis Rheum. 2004; 50:2113–2121.
18. Reveille JD. Seronegative Spondyloarthropathies. In: Klippel JH, ed. Primer on Rheumatic Diseases, 12th Ed. Arthritis Foundation, Atlanta Georgia 2001, pp. 239–245.
19. Mear JP, Schreiber KL, Munz C, et al. Misfolding of HLA-B27 as a result of itsB pocket suggests a novel mechanism for its role in susceptibility to spondyloarthropathies. J Immunol 1999;163: 6665–6670.
20. Fox RI, Tornwall J, Michelson P. Current issues in the diagnosis and treatment of Sjogren's syndrome. Curr Opin Rheumatol 1999; 11:364–371.
21. Tan FK, Stivers DN, Foster MW, et al. Association of microsatellite markersnear the fibrillin 1 gene on human chromosome 15q and scleroderma in a Native American population. Arthritis Rheum 1998;41:1729–1737.
22. Reveille JD, Owerbach D, Goldstein R, Moreda R, Isern RA, Arnett FC.Association of polar amino acids at position 26 of the HLA DQB1 first domainwith the anticentromere antibody response in systemic sclerosis. J Clin Invest1992;89:1290–1213.

23. Wortmann RL. Inflammatory and metabolic diseases of muscle. In: Klippel JH, ed. Primer on Rheumatic Diseases, 12th Ed. Arthritis Foundation, Atlanta Georgia 2001, pp. 369–376.
24. Weyand CM, Goronzy JJ. Vasculitides. In: Klippel JH, ed. Primer on Rheumatic Diseases, 12th Ed. Arthritis Foundation, Atlanta Georgia 2001, pp. 397–405.
25. Gregersen PK, Silver J, Winchester RJ. The shared epitope hypothesis. An approach to understanding the molecular genetics of susceptibility to rheumatoid arthritis. Arthritis Rheum 1987;30:1205–1213.
26. Weyand CM, McCarthy TG, Goronzy JJ. Correlation between disease phenotype and genetic heterogeneity in rheumatoid arthritis. Ann Intern Med 1992;117:801–806.

2 Overview of Nutritional Assessment

*Shari Baird and Johanna Dwyer
with the assistance of Emily Evans*

Summary

- Nutritional status consists of more than dietary intake.
- Six key aspects of nutritional status assessment are ABCDEFs: anthropometry, biochemical tests, clinical indices, dietary status, environmental influences, and functional indices.
- Nutritional status assessment includes the ABCDEFs, but may require special adoptions for some of the arthritis and rheumatic diseases.

Key Words: Anthropometric; biochemical; clinical; dietary; dietary status; environmental; functional assessment; nutritional assessment, nutritional status

1. INTRODUCTION

This chapter summarizes nutritional status assessment with particular attention to arthritis and rheumatoid diseases. It discusses the difference between dietary and nutritional status and provides some historical perspectives on nutritional status assessment. The six essential components of nutrition assessment are discussed, with specific attention to the arthritic and rheumatoid diseases.

1.1. Distinction Between Dietary Status and Nutritional Status

Dietary status refers to the assessment of intakes of nutrients from food, beverages, and supplements in relation to a reference standard, such as the dietary reference intakes. *Nutritional status* is a broader term, and includes dietary intake, as well as biochemical, anthropometric, clinical, dietary, environmental, and functional measures. Nutritional status assessment involves evaluating their impacts on physiological needs, digestion, absorption, excretion, and measures of the body's storage and utilization of nutrients. Malnutrition may result from inadequate intake, malabsorption, excess excretion of nutrients, and inborn errors of metabolism. The individuals at greatest risk for under- and malnutrition are infants, children, pregnant women, the elderly, and persons living in poverty because of their unique physiological needs and their dependency. Overnutrition contributes to obesity and increases the severity of other diseases such as hypertension, atherosclerosis, and diabetes, and occurs among individuals of all ages.

From: *Nutrition and Health: Nutrition and Rheumatic Disease*
Edited by: L. A. Coleman © Humana Press, Totowa, NJ

1.2. Historical Perspective

Nutritional status assessment includes not only dietary but also anthropometric, biochemical, clinical, environmental, and functional assessment. These are the ABCDEFs of assessment. The field has developed rapidly over the past century. Now it is possible to take standardized anthropometric measurements and to assess various compartments of body composition using techniques such as dual-energy X-ray absorptiometry (DEXA) and bioelectrical impedance analysis (BIA), which are economical and available enough to be used clinically. There are also a variety of research techniques, including total body potassium, doubly labeled water, ^{13}C-leucine kinetics, and others, that may be used.

Biochemical assessment has become increasingly standardized as reference materials have become available, and automated assays have become popular. Biochemical tests that are specific and sensitive for various markers, such as C-reactive protein (CRP) to detect inflammation, are now widely used. Standard reference materials are now being developed for plasma 25-hydroxyvitamin D (OHD), for example, which will help to standardize assessment procedures for that nutrient.

Dietary assessment began in ancient times, but only when knowledge of food composition expanded in the 20th century was it linked to nutrients and other bioactive ingredients in food that affect health. Technological advances now include standardized biochemical measures for estimating biomarkers of nutrient intakes to supplement or corroborate dietary intake data. Microcomputers or computerized dietary analysis software now permit direct data entry using structured dietary recall interviews with appropriate prompts. Semi-quantitative food-frequency questionnaires (FFQs) are now available in computerized formats. Computerized nutrient analysis programs and automated data processing ease the burden of calculating nutrient intakes and rapidly provide summaries of the analyses, databases, and tables. These advances have helped to expand and standardize dietary assessment tools and extended their uses from the bedside to large surveys. Statistical techniques for analyzing dietary data have also been refined.

Clinical and functional tests have been better standardized in the past few decades, and now include both generic- and disease-specific quality-of-life measures. Environmental assessment is now also recognized as key to planning for the patient's physical and social well-being. Easy-to-use and standardized tests of functional status are now available.

The pressing challenges of the future include development of better methods for rapidly screening and assessing dietary intakes and incorporating results routinely into computerized databases and other communications to optimize patient care.

This chapter provides tools for selecting appropriate dietary and nutritional assessment methods for the purpose of evaluating and planning the diets of individuals with the arthritic and other rheumatic diseases.

2. ESSENTIAL COMPONENTS OF NUTRITIONAL ASSESSMENT

2.1. The ABCDEFs of Nutritional Status

Nutritional status is determined by assessing an individual's nutrition and health-related ABCDEFs. These include *a*nthropometry, *b*iochemistry, *c*linical evaluation, *d*ietary history, *e*nvironmental assessment, and *f*unctional status. Disordered nutritional status is identified by assessing all of these components together.

Nutritional status declines in a progressive fashion. The first stage is decreased dietary intake and cellular dysfunction that gives rise to biochemical abnormalities in body fluids, and progresses through the tissue-depletion stage, physiological abnormalities, nutrient-specific clinical abnormalities, organ damage, and ultimately, death. At the initial stage, careful probing of dietary intake and other aspects of nutritional status are helpful in discovering inadequate intake. When combined with anthropometric, biochemical tests, and clinical signs and symptoms, poor nutritional status may be detected earlier and appropriate interventions initiated.

3. ANTHROPOMETRIC MEASUREMENTS

Anthropometry involves making physical measurements of individuals and comparing these to standards that are age, gender, and racially appropriate. Anthropometric data are the most valuable when they are monitored long term.

The most common anthropometric measurements used for nutritional assessment include height, weight, waist and arm circumferences, and skinfold thickness. Chumlea et al. and Lohman et al. published reference standards and techniques for making appropriate measurements *(1,2)*. Population-based reference standards are available for both healthy adults and children *(3,4)*.

3.1. Height/Stature

Measurement of stature is critical because reported heights from patients are usually grossly overestimated *(5)*. Height is best measured directly using a stadiometer mounted on a wall. Measuring bars on beam balance scales are not accurate.

The individual must be able to stand upright. Infants, toddlers, and adults must be able to lay flat to measure recumbent length. When they are unable to do so, special measures must be used that provide an indirect estimate of height. Height is measured indirectly when individuals are wheelchair bound, bedridden, have extensive contractures, paralysis, scoliosis, or other conditions causing inability to stand erect or straight *(5)*. Indirect methods include recumbent length, knee height *(6)*, and arm span *(7)*. Recumbent length is measured using a tape measure to estimate height for individuals who do not have any deformities or contractures *(5)*. Knee height is measured using knee-height calipers, and tables are available for estimating stature from knee height. Standard equations for age, gender, and race are available to estimate height using this measurement *(5,6)*.

Stature may also be roughly estimated using the arm-span method *(7,8)*. Tables are available to estimate height from this measurement.

3.2. Weight and Body Mass Index

Weight is another anthropometric measure that is essential in nutritional assessment. It is more sensitive to rapid changes in nutritional status than height. Weight must be measured directly because it is usually underestimated when it is self-reported *(8)*. Weight is assessed by use of weight-for-height charts or body mass index (BMI) and is used in conjunction with clinical measures such as the presence of edema, wasting, and so on. Changes in body weight are also helpful.

The BMI is the most widely accepted reference standard for relative weight. BMI is calculated as the individual's body weight divided by the square of their height (kg/m^2)*(3)*. BMI is categorized as underweight (<18.5), normal weight (18.5–24.9), overweight (25–29.9), obese class I (30–34.9), obese class II (35–39.9), and severe obesity class III (>40) *[3]*.

Although it is useful, there are limitations to BMI as an indicator of fatness. Some people may be misclassified, particularly those who are obese but not particularly large, or those who are heavy from bone and muscle but are not obese. For example, an athlete may have a high BMI but little body fat, and a sedentary individual may have a normal BMI but excessive fat. Also, as people age, muscle is lost, fat accumulates, and composition alters, but weight may be stable *(8)*. This may result in errors in assessing fatness status. In patients with arthritis, relative immobility and muscle wasting combined with edema may lead to failure to recognize excessive fatness or other changes in body composition that occur with the illness. Therefore, other methods may also be needed. A weight history and weight monitoring are helpful in reducing such errors. An obese individual with a recent weight loss may still be overweight but may be at risk for malnutrition and should be monitored. Other nutritional assessment techniques, such as biochemical, clinical, dietary, and functional assessments, may also help in determining the cause of the weight change and developing the plan of care.

It is also important to evaluate changes in weight over time. Loss of weight may be caused by wasting, with losses of both fat and lean tissue, and gains in weight are usually caused by changes in fat tissue. Loss of weight resulting from loss of bone is usually a slow process. However, rapid changes in weight also often occur with alterations in water balance *(8)*. When weight changes are used in conjunction with clinical measures such as presence of edema or ascites and wasting, some estimates of true changes in fat stores can be made. Weight gain of both fat and fluid is also promoted by some medications such as steroids (prednisone) and other drugs *(9–11)*. Weight loss reflects loss of adipose and lean tissue.

The weight history is another key component of anthropometric assessment in chronic disease. Changes from usual reported body weight should be assessed. When weight loss or gain is evident, monitoring should intensify, and causes should be determined and corrected. It is important to determine whether the weight loss or gain was intentional or unintentional because unintentional changes are often due to the result of disease or drug use. Significant weight loss is a loss of 5% of usual weight over a 1–month period or 10% over a 6–month period; severe weight loss is a loss of more than 5% over a 1– month period or more than 10% over a 6–month period *(5)*. Changes in functional status and health outcomes are often present among individuals with severe weight loss *(8)*. These should be documented, as they are important in determining quality of life and care plans.

Undernutrition is also sometimes assessed using percent of usual body weight. Individuals at a current weight of 85 to 90% of their usual reported body weight are considered to have mild malnutrition *(5)*. Moderate malnutrition is defined as an individual at 75 to 84% of their usual reported weight, and individuals are considered to be malnourished when they are at less than 75% of their usual weight. Although these are rough rules of thumb, they are useful clinically.

3.3. Fatness

The limitations in BMI exist because of the many individual variations in body composition. Additional measures may be needed for greater accuracy to measure fatness in research studies that require additional precision and accuracy. Other methods for determining body fat distribution and fat mass include circumferences, skinfold thickness, BIA, and DEXA.

Body weight includes skeletal mass, fat mass, and fat-free mass (e.g., muscle, organs). Both the absolute amount of fat and fat distribution may be relevant. Age, gender, and genetics all contribute to body fat accumulation. Changes in weight may reflect an accumulation or depletion of fat stores in the subcutaneous, visceral, and intramuscular body fat compartments, but especially in the subcutaneous fat deposits. Changes in fat tissue are also accompanied by changes in lean body mass *(8)*. Men, elderly individuals, and the obese tend to have a more central distribution of body fatness than women, young people, and lean individuals, respectively *(8)*. Obese, elderly, and physically inactive individuals tend to have a higher proportion of central fat.

3.3.1. WAIST CIRCUMFERENCES USED TO ASSESS BODY FAT DISTRIBUTION

Circumference measurements are often used because they are simple and detect changes in fat distribution that are associated with disease risk. Waist circumference is used to measure excess abdominal adiposity, which is associated with risk for diabetes and metabolic syndrome *(5)*. Waist circumference is measured with standardized techniques using a plastic, non-elastic tape at the umbilicus level and parallel to the floor *(3)*. Men with a waist greater than 102 cm (40 in) and women greater than 88 cm (35 in) are considered at increased risk for morbidity for diabetes, hypertension, and cardiovascular disease *(3)*. The advantage to waist circumference is that it includes a measure of both intra-abdominal and subcutaneous fat. However, it does give some estimate of body fat distribution. Nevertheless, like BMI, some individualization is required because both muscle and bone will influence values at some sites such as the calf and upper arm *(8)*. Other circumference measurements include hip, chest, thigh, iliac crest, calf, and upper arm, but these are rarely used.

3.3.2. SKINFOLDS

Skinfold thickness measurements, combined with the associated circumference measurements, are used to estimate subcutaneous fatness and sometimes within standardized equations to get a rough estimate of body fat. The most common measurements are at the mid-arm (triceps) and at the scapula (subscapular skinfold), although the calf and thigh may also be used. The skinfold thickness measures subcutaneous adiposity, whereas the mid-arm circumference measures the bone and muscle at the site. Skinfold measurement is taken on the right side of the body *(5)*. A plastic, non-elastic measuring tape should be used to locate and mark the midpoint to be measured. Using the left hand, the skin should be pinched with the thumb and index finger about .05-in above the mark. With the right hand, the skinfold thickness is measured at the site to the nearest millimeter, for about 4 sec after releasing the lever. At least one additional measurement should be taken about 15 sec later. If the skinfold remains depressed, edema may be present.

Standardized age- and gender-based equations are used for triceps skinfold and mid-arm measurements to estimate body composition *(5,8)*. The major problem with skinfold measurement is that it is inaccurate and difficult to reproduce. Also, this measurement is difficult to perform in clinical situations. Therefore, skinfold measurement is not routinely used in clinical practice.

3.4. Muscle and Bone

3.4.1. BIOELECTRICAL IMPEDANCE ANALYSIS

BIA is a reliable method for estimating body composition. Bioelectrical impedance equipment functions by sending an electrical current between the electrodes placed on the wrist and hand and the ankle and foot. The electrical current has a higher conductivity in muscle than fat. Estimates of both body fat and lean tissue can be made using BIA. The bioelectrical impedance method's benefits are that it is safe and noninvasive, the equipment is portable, and the results are available quickly with standardized calculations *(5)*. However, it is not without its problems. Abnormal water balance may influence the results *(5)*, and some patients with arthritis who are taking drugs such as prednisone may have altered water balance *(10,11)*. Additionally, the equations for estimating lean mass may not be appropriate when patients are wasted or water balance is abnormal.

3.4.2. DUAL-ENERGY X-RAY ABSORPTIOMETRY

DEXA uses low-dose radiation to measure both body fat and bone mineral density. The DEXA is easy to complete and involves little participation from the individual. The report is generated by the DEXA scanner and evaluated by a radiologist or skilled technician to provide the body composition data. As with BIA, water balance and abnormal hydration of the lean or fat tissue, and abdominal size, will influence results *(5,8)*. Accuracy decreases when scanning either very small infants or very large individuals such as obese adults *(8)*.

3.5. Edema

Edema is common in the diseases discussed in this volume. It may be caused by malnutrition (e.g., protein calorie malnutrition), drugs (e.g., glucocorticoids), or disease (cardiovascular and renal diseases). Patients who are edematous often complain of swelling of the hands and feet, making rings and shoes tight. Very rapid weight gain (e.g., in days), or rapid weight gain following the administration of certain drugs, such as corticosteroids, is also a sign of edema. Skin turgor and pitting are clinical evidence of edema. If the area is pressed and leaves a dent for 5 seconds or more, edema is likely to be present. However, such signs are only present when edema is pronounced.

4. BIOCHEMICAL INDICES

Biochemical and laboratory methods are also helpful in assessing nutritional status. Laboratory tests may be performed on various body fluids such as blood, urine, feces, and saliva, as well as on the skin, hair, and nails. The biochemical test may be for a specific nutrient or its metabolite. Care should be taken when evaluating a biochemical test to consider the disease, whether a fasting state is required, whether there are diurinal variations, and medication or supplement intakes that may influence the laboratory results. Also, each laboratory or functional test should be evaluated for its accuracy, precision, specificity, and sensitivity for the nutrient or metabolite in question. For example, a low ferritin value is not only an indication of potential iron deficiency, but may also be low because of protein calorie malnutrition. Although biochemical tests may reflect a more rapid change in nutritional status than other assessment techniques, it is important to consider the data collected from nutritional assessment components, anthropometric, dietary, clinical, and functional indices. For example, serum albumin is often decreased because of inflammation and wasting rather than low dietary intake of protein.

4.1. Key Indicators of Nutritional Status

4.1.1. SERUM PROTEINS

Visceral proteins are proteins synthesized in the liver that circulate in plasma *(12)*. They include albumin, transferrin, transthyretin (prealbumin), retinol-binding protein, and CRPs, among others. Visceral proteins are sometimes used as a measure of total body protein status. These visceral proteins are also acute- or negative-phase proteins and change according to stress and inflammation. Some somatic proteins may be used to estimate muscle. They include urinary creatinine, serum creatinine, and urinary 3-methylhistidine. These indices are sometimes used to assess protein and muscle status, but they are rather nonspecific *(12,13)*.

Many of the acute- and negative-phase reactants are used to assess the short-term visceral protein status in individuals. This section focuses on albumin and transthyretin because they are the most common biomarkers for protein used in clinical practice.

4.1.1.1. Serum Albumin. Serum albumin is commonly used in clinical settings to assess protein status in individuals, although it is of only limited utility because it is affected by many other factors, including the presence of inflammation. Although it is true that serum albumin decreases with protein restriction, it changes little with energy restriction *(12)*. Serum albumin is a negative acute-phase reactant and affected by inflammation. It has a relatively long half-life of about 20 days and it changes only slowly *(12)*. Low levels of serum albumin are associated with liver disease, pregnancy, increased capillary permeability, and overhydration. High values are associated with dehydration *(13)*. Therefore, it is a poor marker for protein and energy status.

4.1.1.2. Transthyretin (Prealbumin). Transthyretin is a transport protein that binds with thyroxin and retinol-binding protein *(12)*. It is another negative acute-phase reactant, and decreases in response to stress and infection, but it is also altered by zinc status *(12)*. Liver disease decreases levels, whereas pregnancy increases levels *(13)*. The advantages to using transthyretin are its short half-life, which is about 2 days *(12,13)*, making it more sensitive to changes. However, it also has all of the disadvantages that have been described for serum albumin, including lack of specificity and high cost *(12)*.

4.1.1.3. Serum Creatinine. Creatinine is found primarily in the muscles and is sometimes used as an indicator of muscle mass and adequate energy status. Low values are associated with muscle loss from a calorie deficiency *(14)*. Serum creatinine is affected by disease and diet. A high consumption of muscle meats that contain creatine in the diet may give rise to high serum creatinine. Dehydration, muscle wasting, renal failure, and congestive heart failure may also increase the serum creatinine level; therefore, the indicator is rather nonspecific *(13)*.

4.1.1.4. Urinary Creatinine. Creatinine levels may also be measured in the urine and compared to a standard. A complete 24-hour urine collection is best, but collecting 24-hour urine samples may be difficult for ambulatory patients. Incomplete collection may result in low values. Collecting for more than 24 hours may give high results *(13)*. The skeletal muscle mass (in kilograms) is sometimes very roughly estimated with this equation: the 24-hour urinary creatinine (grams per day) is multiplied by 18.9 and 4.1 is added *(12)*. Urinary creatinine levels are increased with exercise and with high meat intake *(13)*. Levels are decreased with renal and heart failure.

4.1.1.5. Urinary 3-Methylhistidine. Urinary 3-methylhistidine is found only in muscle and is associated with muscle mass. It cannot be recycled in the body, and therefore, is excreted in the urine *(12)*. A complete 24-hour urine 3-methylhistidine collection is required to obtain estimates of muscle mass. As with creatinine, consumption of muscle meats will also increase the level of urinary 3-methylhistidine excretion, so a meat-free diet must be followed during, and for several days prior, to collection.

4.1.2. CALCIUM

Serum calcium levels may be measured using total calcium or ionized calcium tests, but both are tightly controlled and change little in response to diet; hence, they are rarely used for nutritional status assessment. Calcium is primarily transported in the blood either freely or bound with albumin, and it is involved in muscle contraction and blood clotting *(13)*. The primary reserves for calcium are in the bones and teeth. The regulation of calcium and phosphorus levels in the blood is influenced by vitamin D, calcitonin, and parathyroid hormone *(15)*. If serum calcium falls, calcitonin, parathyroid hormone, and vitamin D levels immediately respond and increase to enhance calcium absorption and its release from bone, and decrease excretion, until serum levels are within normal limits. Serum calcium is elevated in individuals with hyperparathyroidism, vitamin D intoxication, some cancers *(12,13)*, and immobility *(13)*. Decreased serum calcium levels are associated with hypoparathyroidism, vitamin D deficiency, renal failure *(12, 13)*, and osteomalacia *(13)*.

4.1.3. VITAMIN D

The best measure of vitamin D is 25-hydroxyvitamin D in plasma. A standard reference material is now being developed.

4.1.4. IRON

There are many types of nutrition-related alterations to red blood cell and hemoglobin synthesis, including iron-deficiency anemia, folate-related anemia, and vitamin B_{12}-deficiency anemia. Both folate- and vitamin B_{12}-deficiency anemias are macrocytic anemias. Both serum folate and vitamin B_{12} levels must be measured. Iron-deficiency anemia is a microcytic, hypochromic anemia. Other non-nutritional conditions may contribute to microcytic or macrocytic anemias and should be considered when evaluating the biomarkers.

The early stages of iron-deficiency anemia are reflected by decreased serum iron, ferritin, and transferrin saturation, and an increase in total iron-binding capacity *(12,13)*. The late stages of iron-deficiency anemia reflect decreased hemoglobin, hematocrit, mean cell volume, mean cell hemoglobin, and mean cell hemoglobin concentration *(12,13)*, and increased red cell distribution width *(13)*.

4.2. Comorbidities

4.2.1. ANEMIA OF CHRONIC DISEASE

During chronic inflammatory states, serum ferritin levels are elevated or normal, and therefore, serum ferritin is not a specific marker for iron-deficiency anemia when inflammation is present, as it often is in those suffering from arthritis *(10,12,13)*. If anemia of chronic disease is present, increased ferritin levels are not representative of iron-deficient status. For example, individuals with arthritis who are truly iron-deficient may have elevated or normal serum ferritin levels. It is important to evaluate each biochemical test and disease state to determine if iron supplementation is warranted.

4.2.2. HYPERGLYCEMIA

Fasting blood glucose helps to identify abnormal glucose metabolism owing to diabetes or drugs. Hemoglobin A_{1c} provides a longer term indicator of blood glucose levels.

4.2.3. HYPERLIPIDEMIA

Total cholesterol, high-density lipoprotein, low-density lipoprotein, and triglycerides provide indicators of lipid abnormalities, if they are present. These tests are particularly important for those with obesity, a family history of heart disease, atherosclerosis, or diabetes. It is important to ensure that individuals fast for 12 hours before the blood draw.

4.2.4. MARKERS OF INFLAMMATION

Many of the acute-phase proteins are used to assess the presence of inflammation. The most common indicator is CRP (C-reactive protein) *(16)*.

4.3. Medications With Nutritional Implications

Medications and dietary supplements may influence the absorption, utilization, metabolism, and excretion of nutrients, and thus, nutritional status. Polypharmacy increases the risk of poor nutritional status in elderly, immunocompromised, and already malnourished, chronically ill, individuals. A common medication and nutritional interaction is between the anticoagulant, warfarin, and vitamin K, which compete with each other for the same binding site in the coagulation cascade *(17)*. Patients with rheumatoid arthritis (RA) may be prescribed corticosteroids (e.g., prednisone, hydrocortisone), which may cause deficiencies in folate, vitamin D, calcium, and potassium *(18,19)*, hyperglycemia, negative nitrogen balance *(19)*, and nausea *(18,19)*. Individuals taking nonsteroidal anti-inflammatory drugs (NSAIDs) are at increased risk for folate and iron deficiency *(18)*, as well for processes inhibiting intake such as nausea, vomiting, and constipation *(19)*. Immunosuppressive drugs are associated with anorexia, nausea, diarrhea, and altered taste, in addition to calcium deficiency *(17–19)*. Patients with RA taking methotrexate are also at an increased risk for folate deficiency.

5. CLINICAL INDICES

Clinical assessment usually includes a review of information obtained from both the physical examination and personal and family medical histories to see if they reveal factors that might predispose the patient to malnutrition. Clinical manifestations occur late and are nonspecific, and may also be related to other conditions or multiple nutrient deficiencies.

The physical examination usually includes evaluating patients to visually inspect hair, eyes, lips, mouth, nails, and skin, and to detect signs of muscle wasting in the temporal and clavicle area. Relevant medical history includes prior surgeries, medical problems, history of alcohol use and smoking habits, current prescribed medications, and use of dietary supplements and other over-the-counter medications. It is also important to identify symptoms that influence intake and increase risk of malnutrition such as anorexia, taste changes, problems chewing or swallowing, nausea, vomiting, diarrhea, and signs of poor wound healing. These signs and symptoms may be caused by a disease, medication, or nutritional deficiency.

5.1. Comorbidities

The presence of other diseases often increases risk for malnutrition. The presence of end-stage renal disease and hemodialysis promote fluid accumulation, hypoparathyroidism, bone demineralization, hyperphosphatemia, and hypocalemia. Crohn's disease results in malabsorption in the gastrointestinal (GI) tract and malnutrition for several nutrients. Some diseases have symptoms that may appear similar to those resulting from nutritional deficiencies. For example, patients with Sjögren's syndrome (SS) often have dry eyes; this is rarely caused by vitamin A or riboflavin deficiencies. Patients with SS also often have angular cheilosis but again, this is likely to be caused by the disease, and not a sign of deficiency for pyridoxine (vitamin B_6). Biotin and riboflavin deficiencies include scaly, red rashes on the face and around orifices, which should be not be confused with the facial rash often found on patients with systemic lupus erythematosus.

6. DIETARY INTAKE

6.1. Need for Assessment of Total Dietary Intake (Food, Supplements, and Nutrient-Containing Medications)

Diet is often an earlier sign of malnutrition or overnutrition than anthropometric, biochemical, clinical, or functional indices. But dietary assessment is difficult and must be done carefully to distinguish under- or malnutrition owing to diet alone (a primary deficiency) from that resulting from other causes (secondary deficiency) *(20)*. Primary deficiency results from inadequate intake, which may be influenced by socioeconomic status and conditions such as alcohol abuse or eating disorders. Secondary nutrient deficiencies result from increased physiological needs, increased nutrient losses in feces and urine, and other causes.

A complete dietary assessment includes obtaining information on other factors that may influence dietary intake, including changes in appetite, taste and smell changes, food allergies, food intolerances, dental problems, problems chewing and swallowing, oral sores and health, dietary restrictions (i.e., fad diets or medical nutrition therapy), the use of over-the-counter medications that may contain nutrients, and the use of dietary supplements, especially those containing nutrients. In planning interventions it may also be helpful to know about shopping and cooking habits and the frequency of meals consumed away from the home *(5)*.

Medications and dietary supplement intakes are important to consider when assessing dietary intake. Some medications provide nutrients, such as antacids containing relatively large amounts of calcium. There may be sources of amino acids, sugar, and vitamins and minerals in other medications as well. Dietary supplement intake of vitamins and minerals and other nutrients should also be included in assessing nutrient intakes. The use of other supplements, especially botanicals, may be helpful in assessing interactions with medications.

Different methods are used to collect dietary intake. They may be retrospective or prospective in nature. The common methods in the clinical setting include retrospective methods such as the 24-hour recall, usual intakes, and FFQ, and prospective methods such as food records.

6.2. Assessment Methods

6.2.1. 24-Hour Recalls

The 24-hour recall method is a retrospective dietary intake method. The individual (or if a child is the patient, the parent or caretaker) is asked about intake over the last 24 hours. Probing is usually done to help the individual remember foods or beverages he or she may have forgotten. Memory aids and tools are used to promote an accurate estimation of portion sizes, including measuring cups and spoons, photographs of food in a known portion size, and food models. The individual should not be "led" to an assumed or socially acceptable answer; instead, open-ended questions should be asked.

Computerized dietary assessment programs are now available for research purposes with a multiple-pass interview style that decreases underreporting *(21)*. In the first pass, the individual recalls food and beverage intake for the designated time period. During the second pass, the interviewer prompts the patient to describe cooking methods, snacks, condiments, additions to beverages, brands, and between-meal beverages. The third pass is when the amount of foods and beverages are determined. Finally, in the fourth and final pass, the interviewer questions the consumption of supplements and medications that contain nutrients.

The advantages to performing a 24-hour recall are (a) it is quickly administered, (b) it involves little respondent burden, (c) it is inexpensive for the interviewer, (d) it may be performed in individuals with low literacy, and (e) it does not influence changes in dietary intake because it involves a history of past intake *(5,21)*. The disadvantages include the reliance on memory, thus making it inappropriate for individuals with a poor memory, and the fact that some foods may be forgotten or purposefully omitted *(5,21)*. Because a computerized dietary assessment program is not used, it is also difficult to calculate nutrient intakes.

6.2.2. Food-Frequency Questionnaires

An FFQ is a retrospective method for assessing diet. There are many different FFQs, the most popular being the Harvard (Willett) semi-quantitative FFQ and the Block

FFQ, which are both proprietary. The National Cancer Institute has a semi-quantitative FFQ that is available for public use (Diet History Questionnaire).

FFQs are of two major types. Some simply present a list of common foods and ask the respondent to recall consumption of the food over the past year. Because portion sizes and frequency of consumption are not included, estimates of nutrient intakes are not possible, but this type of FFQ may be useful for obtaining a picture of food patterns. A second type of instrument is the semi-quantitative FFQ, which attempts to get some estimate of total nutrient intake by including on the food list not only the most commonly eaten foods in the United States, but also the portion sizes and frequency of consumption. This permits a rough estimate of nutrient intake, which may be useful in epidemiological studies in particular. Specialized FFQs or food records are also available to assess intakes of foods high in specific nutrients, such as calcium, vitamin D, or vitamin K.

FFQs are available as self-administered instruments or can be administered by an interviewer. Some computer-assisted methods are also available. The advantages to using an FFQ include (a) a low respondent burden, (b) it is more quickly administered than the 24hour recall, (c) it is self-administered, thus it does not require an interviewer, and (d) in many cases, it can be analyzed on a computer *(5,21)*. However, the questionnaire requires the individual to be literate, to understand portion sizes, and to be able to remember his or her usual eating habits and meal patterns *(5,21)*. Without adjustments for caloric intakes, intakes are usually grossly overestimated. There may also be biases with underreporting of socially unacceptable items or behaviors such as high-fat foods, alcohol, and so on.

6.2.3. Food Records

Food records are another method of collecting dietary intake for nutrient analysis. The individual, parent, or caretaker is asked to record the time of intake of all meals and snacks, beverages, supplements, and medications for 1 or more days. The individual records the brand names, cooking method, and ingredients of mixed dishes in household measurements *(21)*. Forgetting to record intake and inaccurate estimation of volume and weights of foods and beverages are disadvantages to this method *(5,21)*.) Also, many people change their food intake when they are recording because they want to appear to be eating appropriately or simply because they are more aware of their food intake; this may lead to inaccuracies. Additionally, respondent burden is high, there is a need for literacy, and, if nutrient intakes are desired, the process of analyzing the records can be very time consuming *(5,21)*. Advantages include (a) no need for reliance on memory, (b) more accurate estimated measurements of food, (c) insight into meal patterns, and (d) if multiple days are completed, a more accurate account of usual intake *(5,21)*.

7. ENVIRONMENTAL FACTORS

Environmental factors may influence intake and contribute to over- or malnutrition in individuals. Environmental assessment includes the identification of physical and social influences on intake.

7.1. Influences in the Physical Environment on Intake

Conditions within the household, access to food shopping and cooking facilities, and other factors may greatly influence intake. For those who have difficulties ambulating, the use of assistive devices should be queried because they can make the process of food preparation much easier. It may also be useful to identify the number of people in the home *(5)*, the person responsible for purchasing and cooking food, and whether there are facilities to store and cook foods properly during periods of illness when the person may be shut in the house *(5,22)*. Other factors to determine include whether a car is available and how far it is to the grocery or convenience store, availability of foods at nearby stores, and the patient's ability to commute to and transport food from the store to the home *(5)*. An environment that promotes physical activity also contributes to nutritional status. Exercise facilities in the nearby area should be identified.

7.2. Social Environment

Environmental conditions that may affect food intake include a person's culture, education level, and current employment *(5,18)*, as well as the presence of adequate finances to purchase food *(5)*. If necessary, efforts should be made to assist a patient with applications for food assistance programs (e.g., food stamps, Meals on Wheels *(5,18)*. Family support and frequency of communication and activity with family and friends also need to be assessed because they too can influence dietary intake *(18)*.

8. FUNCTIONAL STATUS

8.1. Activities of Daily Living

Activities of daily living (ADLs) include those activities that are regularly performed throughout the day and that are necessary to take care of oneself, including bathing, walking, getting up from or into a chair or bed, personal hygiene, toileting, and eating *(23)*.

Patients with arthritis may not be able to perform many of the ADLs. Individuals with RA *(24)* or scleroderma *(25)* may have hand joint deformities and may not be able to grip a kitchen utensil well enough to feed themselves. These patients may require assistive devices. In scleroderma, the mouth may become small, making it difficult for patients to feed themselves and consume adequate nutrients. In these cases, special measures may be needed *(25)*. Patients with osteoarthritis (OA) often mention buckling joints and thus may not feel comfortable walking distances or climbing stairs *(26)*.

8.2. Instrumental Activities of Daily Living

Instrumental activities of daily living (IADLs) include activities that are required to live independently. IADLs include shopping and preparing meals, performing household chores, managing finances, and personal medical care (i.e., reading and taking medications properly, obtaining proper medical care) *(23)*.

8.3. Range of Motion and Difficulties Performing Everyday Tasks

Arthritis is often associated with pain and swelling of joints, destruction of cartilage, loss in muscle function, and bone alterations or deformities that may limit the range of motion (ROM) in joints for patients. RA limits ROM from destruction of cartilage as the disease progresses *(24)*. OA of the knee often limits ROM caused by bone enlargement and cartilage destruction *(26)*. It is helpful to review information about ROM in assessing the individual patient's ability to carry out ADLs and IADLs.

8.4. Health-Related Quality of Life

8.4.1. GENERIC QUALITY-OF-LIFE INDICATORS

Evaluation of quality of life includes assessing physical ability and functional activity as well as the health-related emotional and social implications. Quality of life is often assessed using self-administered questionnaires. Generic quality-of-life assessment tools include the Short-Form (SF) 36, the shorter versions SF 12 and SF 8 *(27)*, and the Health Assessment Questionnaire *(28)*. The Health Assessment Questionnaire was originally designed for patients with RA, but has since been used in the National Health and Nutrition Examination Survey follow-up, and for individuals with HIV and disabled workers *(28)*.

Quality-of-life questionnaires are also available specifically for pediatric or adolescent patients. The most common measures include the Childhood Health Questionnaire, Pediatric Quality of Life Inventory Scales, and Quality of My Life Questionnaire *(29)*.

8.4.2. ARTHRITIS-SPECIFIC QUALITY OF LIFE

Disease-specific quality-of-life questionnaires have been designed for many rheumatoid diseases. Table 1 lists the disease-specific quality-of-life measures for arthritis and related diseases. They are particularly useful because they provide specific information that is directly related to the disease.

Table 1
Some Disease-Specific Health-Related Quality-of-Life Questionnaires

Disease	*Disease-Specific (Reference)*
Fibromyalgia	Fibromyalgia Impact Questionnaire *(48–50)*
	Arthritis Impact Measurement Scales 2 *(50)*
Gout	Gout Assessment Questionnaire *(51)*
Juvenile arthritis	Juvenile Arthritis Quality of Life Questionnaire *(29)*
	Childhood Arthritis Health Profile *(29)*
Osteoarthritis	Arthritis Impact Measurement Scales 2 *(52)*
Rheumatoid arthritis	Arthritis Impact Measurement Scales 2 *(52)*
	Rheumatoid Arthritis Quality of Life Instrument *(53)*

9. SPECIFIC ASPECTS OF NUTRITIONAL STATUS ASSESSMENT FOR VARIOUS ARTHRITIC AND RHEUMATOID DISEASES

Specific rheumatic diseases are discussed briefly here, with particular focus on nutritional assessment. These conditions are discussed in more detail in the chapters that follow.

9.1. Rheumatoid Arthritis

Many of the problems in performing anthropometric measurements are discussed in the section on juvenile rheumatoid arthritis (JRA). The major problem is obtaining appropriate measurements.

Patients with RA are often underweight and malnourished. Indicators of malnutrition also include rheumatoid cachexia, which involves muscle wasting that is often replaced with fat *(30)*. There may be no change in weight but a change in body composition. Mid-arm muscle circumference, triceps skinfold measurements, and DEXA may be helpful in detecting or monitoring this. Roubenoff et al. found that most patients with RA have rheumatoid cachexia *(31,32)*. Even with good disease control and adequate caloric intake, skeletal muscle catabolism persists *(31,32)*. Assessment of caloric and protein intake is important because inadequate intakes will further accelerate muscle loss. Muscle wasting also affects functional status and mobility, which may impair food shopping, meal preparation, and cleanup.

Inflammatory indices such as CRP are elevated in RA *(16)*. As a result of the chronic inflammation, anemia of chronic disease is often present *(10,11,34)*. Medication-related effects on biochemical indices of folic acid and iron status are also common. Some medications such as methotrexate also affect calcium and vitamin D status *(17–19)*. Dietary and functional assessments should include attention to energy intake and problems related to obtaining, preparing, and eating food. Particular attention should be paid to pain and its effects on food intake. Dietary supplement use should also be assessed.

Environmental assessment should include attention to use of assistive devices. Also, the patient's social network is critical. Patients with social support may have a better quality of life, potentially moderating the impact of pain, depression, and physical disability *(33)*.

Functional assessment should focus on factors that impact the ADLs and IADLs as well as other aspects of health-related quality of life. Pain is a common problem in RA, greatly affecting health-related quality of life *(33)*.

9.2. Juvenile Rheumatoid Arthritis

JRA is the most prevalent chronic arthritis in children, ranging from 3.8 to 19.6 cases per 100,000 children in the United States *(11)*. The disease is chronic and characterized by an age of onset before 16 years of joint swelling, heat, and pain and stiffness of unknown origin *(10, 11)* that occurs for 6 weeks or more *(11)*. These signs and symptoms may change throughout the day and from day to day *(10)*. The complications of JRA can range from mild to severe *(10)*. Disease characteristics often include inflammation, fever, damage/deformity of joints, and altered bone growth *(10)*.

Approximately 10 to 30% of children with JRA develop serious disabilities in adulthood *(34)*. Anthropometric measurements may pose problems in JRA. Contractures and abnormal bone growth may alter a child's stature *(10,34)*. In abnormal bone growth, one bone may be longer than another at times of accelerated growth and later become stunted. If the abnormal bone growth occurs in the leg, the child may compensate by bending the longer leg until the hips are level. Standing height may also be difficult to obtain in children with contractures and limited ROM in the legs or back *(10,34)*, and alternative methods of estimating height are necessary. Either arm-span or knee-height measurements are appropriate depending on the location of contractures and range in motion of joints.

Between 22 and 32% of individuals with JRA are below the fifth percentile of stature for age, indicating severe protein and calorie malnutrition *(11)*. Growth charts for stature for age, weight for age, and weight for stature are important tools for monitoring growth retardation and body composition changes.

Body fat and muscle distribution are also altered in patients with JRA. Children with JRA may have normal fat stores, but about one-third suffers from sarcopenia or muscle wasting, reflected in mid-arm muscle circumference below the fifth percentile *(12,44)*.

Biochemical indices may be affected by the disease. Anemia is common in patients with JRA, and may be caused by chronic inflammation, iron-deficient status, or as a side effect of medications *(10,11,34)*. Biochemical indices for iron-deficiency anemia should be monitored and assessed to determine the cause and intervention for the anemia. Medications prescribed to treat the disease may cause folic acid and iron deficiency, or GI distress. Patients with JRA are frequently prescribed NSAIDs such as ibuprofen or aspirin *(10,11,34)*. Chronic use of large doses of aspirin is sometimes associated with a deficiency in folic acid, iron, and vitamin C *(18)*, as well compromised intake from nausea, vomiting, stomach pain, and bleeding *(10,11)*.

Methotrexate, an immunosuppressive drug, may be taken if the patient is not responding appropriately to NSAIDs *(34)*. Folic acid and calcium deficiency may result from taking methotrexate. Intestinal complications that include anorexia, nausea, diarrhea, and altered taste may inhibit food intake *(18,19)*.

Glucocorticosteroids may be an alternative if the patient does not respond to NSAIDS. This drug is associated with vitamin D and calcium deficiencies and osteopenia *(10,11,18,19,34)* and may promote short stature in children. Other possible nutritional problems include low folic acid and potassium levels *(18,19)*, glucose intolerance *(10)*, hyperglycemia, and negative nitrogen balance *(19)*, which may contribute to muscle loss, sodium and water retention, edema, and hypertension *(10,11)*.

Gold compounds and D-penicillamine are therapies for children with JRA and extensive complications. Side effects that affect nutritional status include mouth sores, bone marrow damage and altered iron status *(10,34)*, and blood and protein loss in urine *(34)*. D-penicillamine may compromise dietary intake as a result of loss of taste and stomach disturbances and also may be associated with proteinuria *(10)*.

Dietary intake and status may be influenced by many manifestations of the disease, and therefore dietary intake is important to obtain. It may be helpful to get an estimate of intake on both "sick days" and "well days," and to plan recommendations keeping these realities in mind. Many children complain of poor appetite *(10)*. As previously discussed, some medications affect appetite, alter taste, and cause GI disturbances such as nausea and diarrhea. Energy and protein malnutrition may be found in 10 to 50% of children with this disease *(11)*.

Physical problems with dietary intake are also manifestations of the disease. Arthritis in the temporomandibular joint develops in approximately 18 to 30% of children with JRA *(10)*. This may make chewing difficult. Children may have a limited ROM in the jaw, may have a small mouth opening, and may experience pain when opening the mouth. Jaw function is compromised in the 20 to 30% of children who have abnormal jaw development *(10)*, and a small jaw or teeth misalignment can result in dysphagia (difficulty swallowing) *(10,11)*.

The disease may compromise functional status and ADLs. Painful, inflamed joints, contractures, and abnormal bone growth can make it difficult to complete ADLs including personal hygiene, using utensils for eating, toileting, and walking *(10,11)*. Patients may be depressed and embarrassed, negatively impacting their social life *(10,11)*.

9.3. Gout

Prevalence of reported gout is estimated at up to 3% of the population *(35)*. Gout is more prevalent in men than women *(18,19)* with an age of onset after 40 years *(18,35,36)*. Women are more likely to develop gout later in life (after menopause) than men, and the upper extremities are more often affected *(35,37)*. A purine metabolism disorder, high serum uric acid levels, and monosodium uric acid crystal deposition in and around the joints characterize gout *(18,35,36)*. The signs and symptoms of progression of crystal deposits, or tophi, in the joints include fever *(35,36)*, inflammation *(18,35,36)*, swelling and intense pain *(18,19,35,36)*. The most common joint affected is the big toe *(18,19,35)*, followed, in order of prevalence, by the insteps, ankles, heels, knees, wrists, fingers, and elbows *(36)*.

The disease may make it difficult to obtain accurate anthropometric measurements. As the crystals continue to deposit in the joints, deformities may occur *(35,36)*. Large tophi on the heels may make it difficult to accurately measure a standing height. Additionally, tophi deposits in the knees can reduce ROM in the knees making it difficult to stand erect *(38)*. The arm span may be difficult if large tophi are formed on the elbow and ROM is limited. Alternative methods of estimating height may be required depending on the manifestations of the disease.

Body weight and composition are associated with incidence of gout. Body weight and BMI are predictors of serum uric acid levels *(18,36)*. Fatness and obesity increase risk of developing gout and gout attacks. Central fat distribution may be measured using waist circumference and risk is increased with a waist circumference of more than 100 cm for men 88 cm for women *(39)*.

Nutrition-related biochemical indices might be affected by gout. CRP, the biomarker for inflammation, may be elevated when systemic inflammation and fever are present *(35)*. Medications may also affect nutritional status, particularly folic acid and compromised intake from GI disturbances. Patients with gout are often prescribed medications for inflammation and uric acid control. Drugs that influence uric acid synthesis or excretion include probenecid, sulfinpyrazone, and allopurinol *(19,35,36)*.

NSAIDs such as ibuprofen, aspirin, and naproxen are the first drugs of choice for inflammation *(19,35,36)*. The potential nutritional implications from NSAIDS include folic acid and iron deficiencies *(18)*, and compromised intake from nausea, vomiting, and constipation *(19)*. Other anti-inflammatory drugs prescribed for gout include colchicine and corticosteroids. About 80% of patients experience side effects of nausea, vomiting, and diarrhea when taking colchicine *(35)*. Nutritional deficiency of vitamin B_{12}, sodium, and potassium are also related to colchicine *(18)*. Corticosteroids increase the risk of folic acid, vitamin D, calcium, and potassium deficiencies *(18,19)*, hyperglycemia, and increase the risk of negative nitrogen balance *(19)* and compromised intake from nausea *(18,19)*.

Comorbid diseases also affect nutritional status. Central obesity and serum uric acid levels are associated with insulin resistance, hypertension, high serum lipids, and renal failure. The greatest complication in progression of gout is renal failure and calculi *(18,19,35,36,39)*. Additionally, patients often have high blood pressure, dyslipidemia, insulin resistance, and high blood sugar *(18,19,35,36)*.

Dietary assessment is important in patients with gout. When gathering dietary intake data, it is important to determine intake of alcohol, nonalcoholic beverages, and purine-rich foods. Alcohol intake is associated with high serum uric acid *(18,35,36,39)*. Adequate hydration is important if the patient is at risk for renal calculi *(18,19)*.

Purine metabolism produces uric acid as an end product. Dietary intake of purine-rich foods may contribute to as much as one-third of the serum uric acid *(18,19, 36,39)*. However, dietary intake of purine-rich foods and the impact on serum uric acid is controversial. Elevated serum uric acid is caused by inadequate renal excretion (~90% of the serum level) and excess synthesis (~10% *(18,19,36,39)*). Dietary intake contributes to excess synthesis; thus, dietary intake of purine-rich foods will have relatively little impact on serum uric acid levels. It may still be important to determine intake of purine-rich foods because individuals may be more sensitive to these foods and have a greater reaction, or they may be able to take lower drug doses.

Functional status may also compromise dietary intake and nutritional status. Joint swelling, tophi, and pain may limit ROM. These patients may not be able to prepare meals, grip utensils to eat, or even write. Tophi deposition in the knees *(38)*, feet, or ankles may impair walking. Deformities may also influence the individual's social life.

9.4. Systemic Sclerosis

Within the United States, the prevalence of systemic sclerosis is estimated at 240 cases per 1 million adults *(40)*. The disease occurs in females more than males. Disease onset is usually between the ages of 35 and 65 years. Systemic sclerosis includes limited and diffuse scleroderma. Both involve fibrosis of the skin but limited scleroderma only includes thickening of the skin in the face and neck and below the elbows and knees. In contrast, diffuse scleroderma also includes fibrosis of skin in the trunk and above the elbows and knees and dysfunction in the GI tract, kidney, heart, and lungs. Nutritional status may be affected in a number of ways in this disorder.

Disease manifestations make it difficult to obtain anthropometric measurements in some patients, particularly those with diffuse disease. Thickening of the skin in the lower extremities and trunk may limit ROM. It may be difficult to obtain accurate stature measurements if the patient is unable to stand upright. Alternative methods to estimate stature, including knee height and arm span, may be helpful; the choice depends on whether the patient has limited ROM below the knee, or if hand contractures are present.

The disease itself often affects biochemical indices. Biochemical indices are also affected by drugs that alter nutritional status of some nutrients, particularly folic acid, the fat-soluble vitamins, and calcium. GI dysfunction often leads to malabsorption and malnutrition in patients with scleroderma *(25,41)*, resulting in fat-soluble vitamin and calcium deficiencies *(42)*. Enteral or parenteral nutrition may be required if a patient is unable to maintain weight or if a patient has significant intestinal dysfunction *(41)*. Patients with systemic sclerosis may be prescribed NSAIDs or corticosteroids for bone and muscle pain *(42)*, thereby increasing risk of compromised folic acid status and iron deficiencies *(18)*, as well as nausea, vomiting, constipation *(19)* and gastroesophageal reflux *(42)*. These patients are also frequently given corticosteroids for muscle pain *(42)*, however, these drugs increase risk of compromised folate, vitamin D, calcium, and potassium nutritional status *(18,19)* as well as hyperglycemia, increased risk of negative nitrogen balance *(19)*, and nausea *(18,19)*.

Dietary intake is affected in a number of different ways by the disease. Skin fibrosis of the fingers may make it difficult to eat and write or to handle objects in shopping or cooking. Merkel et al. studied patients with systemic sclerosis who had Raynaud's phenomenon to assess hand function *(43)*. Raynaud's phenomenon involves vasoconstriction with resulting symptoms of cold hands and feet and changes in skin color on the fingers and toes *(25)*. The patients with moderate to severe Raynaud's phenomenon had greater difficulty in performing activities that involved hand use (i.e., gripping items, eating, and dressing themselves) compared with other ADLs (i.e., walking, arising, and hygiene) *(43)*. Reduced grip may increase difficulty in preparing food and fibrosis in the face may limit movement of the lips and mouth *(25)*. Hand disability may result from tight skin *(43)*, swelling, hand contractures *(25)* or ulcerations *(25,43)*; eating dysfunction seems to be the most closely associated hand disability *(43)*. From 10 to 90% of these patients have gastric dysfunction *(41,44)*, including dysphagia, gastroesophageal reflux, and delayed motility and transit time that may occur in any section of the GI tract *(25,41)*. Other signs and symptoms include early satiety, nausea, vomiting, diarrhea *(25,41)* and constipation *(41)*. Fecal incontinence *(25,41)* or urgency *(41)* may be a sign or symptom of dysfunction in the lower gut. This may have a negative impact on ADLs and the patient's social life.

9.5. Polymyositis

Polymyositis is an idiopathic inflammatory myopathy. Estimates of its prevalence are unknown *(45)*, but it is estimated to be up to 10 cases per 1 million people *(46)*. Polymyositis generally occurs in adults anytime over the age of 18 years *(45)*.

The disease manifests with proximal muscle weakness developing in a few weeks or months *(45–47)*. The muscle weakness is symmetrical and the pelvis and shoulder muscles are most commonly affected in these patients, but the neck muscles, primarily the flexor muscles, can also become weak and this is found in about 50% of the patients *(46)*. Patients with polymyositis often complain of stiffness, muscle and joint pain, tenderness, and fatigue, and they show signs of fever and weight loss *(45,46)*.

The weight loss in polymyositis may result in part from the muscles being in differing stages of synthesis and degradation. Degraded muscle fibers may be replaced with fibrous connective tissue, fat, or simply atrophy *(46)*. The muscle loss causes wasting. The stiffness and muscle weakness also make it difficult to take anthropometric measurements in some patients. The patient's neck flexor muscles may be so weak that raising the head to stand erect for a standing height is not possible. It may be difficult to obtain an accurate arm span with weak shoulder muscles. The knee-height measurement may be appropriate for these patients depending on muscle function and ROM.

Generally, these patients are initially prescribed corticosteroids such as prednisone *(45–47)*, increasing risk for folate, vitamin D, calcium, and potassium deficiencies as well as nausea *(18,19)*. Nausea may compromise an individual's desire to eat, further compromising nutritional status. Corticosteroids may also contribute to further muscle wasting, weakness and loss *(46)*.

Immunosuppressive drugs, particularly azathioprine and methotrexate, may be prescribed if the corticosteroids do not sufficiently improve muscle strength *(45–47)*. Side effects of these drugs often compromise nutritional status when the patient experiences anorexia, nausea, diarrhea, and altered taste. Calcium deficiency may also occur *(19)*. Methotrexate specifically increases risk of folate deficiency *(18,19)*.

As polymyositis progresses, cardiac and pulmonary muscle may become weak *(46)*. Patients may show signs and symptoms of hypoxemia and dyspnea *(46)*, which may decrease food intake owing to shortness of breath. Renal failure may develop with severe muscle degradation *(46)*.

Dysphagia is common in patients with weakened esophageal and pharyngeal muscles, and may increase risk of aspiration *(45–47)*. Food intake may become compromised because of limited food choices. It is important for dysphagia to be documented in the medical chart and for corrective actions to be taken.

Patients with polymyositis often report difficulty in performing some ADLs *(45–47)*. They may complain of cramping and fatigue when climbing stairs. Pelvic muscle loss may result in difficulties in toileting and rising from a sitting position. If the shoulder is affected, patients may find it difficult to groom themselves.

9.6. Sjögren's Syndrome

Dietary and nutritional assessment in SS focuses mainly on assessing the oral effects of the disorder, which include xerostomia (lack of saliva), making eating and chewing difficult and increasing the risk of dental caries. It is also important to assess dietary supplement use.

9.7. Other Rheumatic and Arthritic Diseases

OA is an extremely common rheumatic disease that has nutritional implications largely caused by mechanical and ROM problems related to the deterioration of joints and deformities of the bone at the joint. The major nutritional assessment challenges are anthropometric—obtaining sound estimates of fatness status and stature. Careful assessment of the ADLs and IADLs is also warranted because many activities related to obtaining and preparing foods may be affected.

Fibromyalgia is a disease that has few implications for nutritional assessment other than the need to assess the extent to which pain affects food intake and food-related activities. During flares the individual may be unable to eat at all or may only be able to eat very small amounts of food. Also important is an assessment of nutritional implications of the pain on health-related quality of life, ADLs, and IADLs.

Systemic lupus erythematosus is a disease that is much more common in women then men. Dietary and nutritional assessments are similar in most respects to other rheumatic disease. The unique feature of assessment in systemic lupus erythematosus is the need for very careful assessment of kidney function because the disease affects the kidneys and may eventually lead to kidney failure.

10. CONCLUSION

Patients with rheumatic disease are at risk of compromised nutritional status for a variety of reasons. Careful consideration of a patient's nutritional status using basic principles of assessment, and addressing problem areas, can contribute to a patient's overall well-being.

REFERENCES

1. Chumlea WC, Roche AF, Mukherjee D. Nutritional Assessment of the Elderly Through Anthropometry. Ross Laboratories, Columbus, OH, 1987.
2. Lohman TG, Roche AF, Martorell R. Anthropometric Standardization Reference Manual. Human Kinetics, Champaign, IL, 1988.
3. National Institutes of Health. The Practical Guide: Identification, Evaluation, and Treatment of Overweight and Obesity in Adults, 2000. NIH, Bethesda, MD,;2007, p. 88.
4. Centers for Disease Control. 2000 CDC Growth Charts. 2000;2007. http://www.cdc.gov/growthcharts/
5. Hammond KA. Dietary and Clinical Assessment. In: Mahan LK, Escott-Stump S, ed. Krause's Food, Nutrition, & Diet Therapy, 11th ed. Saunders, Philadelphia, PA, 2004, pp. 407–435.
6. Chumlea WC, Guo SS, Steinbaugh ML. Prediction of stature from knee height for black and white adults and children with application to mobility-impaired or handicapped persons. J Am Diet Assoc 1994;94:1385–1388,1391.
7. Jarzem PF, Gledhill RB. Predicting height from arm measurements. J Pediatr Orthop 1993;13: 761–765.
8. Heymsfield SB, Baumgartner RN. Body composition and anthropometry. In: Shils ME, Shike M, Ross AC, Caballero B, Cousins RJ, eds. Modern Nutrition in Health and Disease, 10th ed. Lippincott Williams & Wilkins, Philadelphia, PA, 2005, pp. 751–770.
9. Hill JO, Catenacci VA, Wyatt HR. Obesity: etiology. In: Shils ME, Shike M, Ross AC, Caballero B, Cousins RJ, eds. Modern Nutrition in Health and Disease, 10th ed. Lippincott Williams & Wilkins, Philadelphia, PA, 2005, pp. 1013–1028.
10. Garceau AO, Dwyer JT, Holland M. A practical approach to nutrition in the patient with juvenile rheumatoid arthritis. Clin Nutr 1989;8:55–63.
11. Purdy KS, Dwyer JT, Holland M, Goldberg DL, Dinardo J. You are what you eat: healthy food choices, nutrition, and the child with juvenile rheumatoid arthritis. Pediatr Nurs 1996;22:391–398.
12. Carlson TH. Laboratory data in nutrition assessment. In: Mahan LK, Escott-Stump S, eds. Krause's Food Nutrition, & Diet Therapy, 11th ed. Saunders, Philadelphia, PA,2004, pp. 436–454.
13. Pagana KD, Pagana TJ. Blood studies. In: Mosby's Manual of Diagnostic and Laboratory Tests, 2nd ed. Mosby, St. Louis, MO, 2002, pp. 9–485.
14. Heimburger DC. Adulthood. In: Shils ME, Shike M, Ross AC, Caballero B, Cousins RJ, eds. Modern Nutrition in Health and Disease, 10th ed. Lippincott Williams & Wilkins, Philadelphia, PA, 2005, pp. 830–842.

15. Gallagher ML. Vitamins. In: Mahan LK, Escott-Stump S, eds. Krause's Food, Nutrition, and Diet Therapy, 11th ed. Saunders, Philadelphia, PA, 2004, pp. 75–119.
16. Libby P, Ridker PM, Maseri A. Inflammation and atherosclerosis. Circulation 2002;105:1135–1143.
17. Chan LN. Drug–nutrient interactions. In: Shils ME, Shike M, Ross AC, Caballero B, Cousins RJ, eds. Modern Nutrition in Health and Disease, 10th ed. Lippincott Williams & Wilkins, Philadelphia, PA, 2005, pp. 1539–1553.
18. Morgan SL, Baggott JE. Nutrition and diet in rheumatic diseases. In: Shils ME, Shike M, Ross AC, Caballero B, Cousins RJ, eds. Modern Nutrition in Health and Disease, 10th ed. Lippincott Williams & Wilkins, Philadelphia, PA, 2005, pp. 1326–1338.
19. Dorfman L. Medical nutrition therapy for rheumatic disorders. In: Mahan LK, Escott-Stump S, eds. Krause's Food, Nutrition & Diet Therapy, 11th ed. Saunders, Philadelphia, PA, 2004, pp. 1121–1142.
20. Gibson RS. Introduction. In: Principles of Nutritional Assessment, 2nd ed. Oxford University Press, New York, 2005, pp. 1–26.
21. Gibson RS. Measuring food consumption of individuals. In: Principles of Nutritional Assessment, 2nd ed. Oxford University Press, New York, 2005, pp. 41–64.
22. Nelms M. Assessment of nutrition status and risk. In: Nelms M, Sucher K, Long S, eds. Nutrition Therapy and Pathophysiology. Thompson Brooks/Cole, Belmont, CA, 2007, pp. 101–135.
23. American Occupational Therapy Association. Occupational therapy practice framework: domain and process. Am J Occup Ther 2002;56:609–639.
24. Anderson RJ. Rheumatoid arthritis: clinical and laboratory features. In: Klippel JH, Weyand CM, Wortmann RL, ed. Primer on the Rheumatic Diseases, 11th ed. Arthritis Foundation, Atlanta, GA, 1997, pp. 161–167.
25. Wigley FM. Systemic sclerosis and related syndromes: clinical features. In: Klippel JH, Weyand CM, Wortmann RL, eds. Primer on the Rheumatic Diseases, 11th ed. Arthritis Foundation, Atlanta, GA, 1997, pp. 267–272.
26. Hochberg MC. Osteoarthritis: Clinical Features and Treatment. In: Klippel JH, Weyand CM, Wortmann RL, eds. Primer on the Rheumatic Diseases, 11th ed. Arthritis Foundation, Atlanta, GA, 1997, pp. 218–221.
27. Mayer EK, Purkayastha S, Athanasiou T, Darzi AW. Redefining quality of care. J R Soc Med 2007;100:122–124.
28. Bruce B, Fries JF. The Stanford Health Assessment Questionnaire: a review of its history, issues, progress, and documentation. J Rheumatol 2003;30:167–178.
29. Duffy CM. Measurement of health status, functional status, and quality of life in children with juvenile idiopathic arthritis: clinical science for the pediatrician. Pediatr Clin North Am 2005;52: 359–372.
30. Walsmith J, Roubenoff R. Cachexia in rheumatoid arthritis. Int J Cardiol 2002;85:89–99.
31. Roubenoff R, Roubenoff RA, Ward LM, Holland SM, Hellmann DB. Rheumatoid cachexia: depletion of lean body mass in rheumatoid arthritis. Possible association with tumor necrosis factor. J Rheumatol 1992;19:1505–1510.
32. Roubenoff R, Roubenoff RA, Cannon JG, et al. Rheumatoid cachexia: cytokine-driven hypermetabolism accompanying reduced body cell mass in chronic inflammation. J Clin Invest 1994;6: 2379–2386.
33. Jakobsson U, Hallberg IR. Pain and quality of life among older people with rheumatoid arthritis and/or osteoarthritis: a literature review. J Clin Nurs 2002;11:430–443.
34. Cassidy JT. Rheumatic diseases of childhood. In: Harris, Edward D., Jr., Budd RC, Genovese MC, Firestein GS, Sargent JS, Sledge CB, eds. Kelley's Textbook of Rheumatology, 7th ed. Saunders, Philadelphia, PA, 2005, pp. 1579–1592.
35. Kim KY, Schumacher HR, Hunsche E, Wertheimer AI, Kong SX. A literature review of the epidemiology and treatment of acute gout. Clin Ther 2003;25:1593–1617.
36. Wortmann RL, Kelley WN. Gout and hyperuricemia. In: Harris, Edward D., Jr., Budd RC, Genovese MC, Firestein GS, Sargent JS, Sledge CB, eds. Kelley's Textbook of Rheumatology, 7th ed. Saunders, Philadelphia, PA, 2005, pp. 1402–1426.
37. De Souza, Alexandre W. S., Fernandes V, Ferrari, Antonio J. L. Female gout: clinical and laboratory features. J Rheumatol 2005;32:2186–2188.

38. Yu KH, Lien LC, Ho HH. Limited knee joint range of motion due to invisible gouty tophi. Rheumatology 2004;43:191–194.
39. Fam AG. Gout, diet, and the insulin resistance syndrome. J Rheumatol 2002;29:1350–1355.
40. Mayes MD. Scleroderma epidemiology. Rheum Dis Clin North Am 2003;29:239–254.
41. Sallam H, McNearney TA, Chen, J. D. Z. Systemic review: pathophysiology and management of gastrointestinal dysmotility in systemic sclerosis (scleroderma). Aliment Pharmacol Ther 2006;23:691–712.
42. Steen VD. Systemic sclerosis and related syndromes: treatment. In: Klippel JH, Weyand CM, Wortmann RL, eds. Primer on the Rheumatic Diseases, 11th ed. Arthritis Foundation, Atlanta, GA, 1997, pp. 273–275.
43. Merkel PA, Herlyn K, Martin RW, et al. Measuring disease activity and functional status in patients with scleroderma and Raynaud's phenomenon. Arthritis Rheum 2002;46:2410–2420.
44. Marie I, Levesque H, Ducrotte P, et al. Gastric involvement in systemic sclerosis: a prospective study. Am J Gastroenterol 2001;96:77–83.
45. Dalakas MC, Hohlfield R. Polymyositis and dermatomyositis. Lancet 2003;362:971–982.
46. Wortmann RL. Inflammatory diseases of muscle and other myopathies. In: Harris, Edward D., Jr., Budd RC, Genovese MC, Firestein GS, Sargent JS, Sledge CB, eds. Kelley's Textbook of Rheumatology, 7th ed. Saunders, Philadelphia, PA, 2005, pp. 1310–1332.
47. Di Martino, Stephen J., Kagen LJ. Newer therapeutic approaches: inflammatory muscle disorders. Rheum Dis Clin North Am 2006;32:121–128.
48. Burckhardt CS, Clark SR, Bennett RM. The Fibromyalgia Impact Questionniare: development and validation. J Rheumatol 1991;18:728–733.
49. Bennett R. The Fibromyalgia Impact Questionnaire (FIQ): a review of its development, current version, operating characteristics and uses. Clin Exp Rheumatol 2005;23:S154–S162.
50. Mannerkorpi K, Ekdahl C. Assessment of functional limitation and disability in patients with fibromyalgia. Scand J Rheumatol 1997;26:4–13.
51. Colwell HH, Hunt BJ, Pasta DJ, Palo WA, Mathias SD, Joseph-Ridge N. Gout Assessment Questionnaire: initial results of reliability, validity and responsiveness. Int J Clin Pract 2006;60:1210–1217.
52. Meenan RF, Mason JH, Anderson JJ, Guccione AA, Kazis LE. AIMS2. The content and properties of a revised and expanded arthritis impact measurement scales health status questionnaire. Arthritis Rheum 1992;35:1–10.
53. De Jong Z, Van Der Heijde, D., McKenna SP, Whalley D. The reliability and construct validity of the RAQol: a rheumatoid arthritis-specific quality of life instrument. Br J Rheumatol 1997;36:878–883.

3 An Overview of Rheumatic Disease Epidemiology

Daniel J. McCarty and Erin K. Bundy

Summary

- Heterogeneity in clinical presentation and variability in disease course of rheumatic diseases pose a significant problem in describing the epidemiology of these conditions.
- Despite these limitations, our understanding of the epidemiology of rheumatic diseases has dramatically improved in the past several decades.
- Rapid advances in genomic technology and lowered cost of genotyping are leading to exciting new knowledge of the genetics underlying rheumatic disease.
- These exciting findings may help identify subphenotypes, predict drug response, as well as clarify the role of genetic and environmental disease risk factors.
- Hopefully, in the near future, these findings may result in promising new prevention strategies and treatments to reduce the suffering from rheumatic disease.

Key Words: Epidemiology; incidence; methods; osteoarthritis; prevalence; rheumatic diseases; SLE; rheumatoid arthritis

1. INTRODUCTION

Gouty arthritis was recognized as a specific disease by the ancient Egyptians, and many of the characteristics of gout suffers were described by Hippocrates in the fifth century BC *(1)*, but our knowledge of the epidemiology of most rheumatic diseases began only in the last half of the 20th century. Unlike cardiovascular disease, diabetes mellitus, and many cancers, the heterogeneity in clinical presentation and variability in disease course of rheumatic diseases pose a significant problem in describing the epidemiology of these conditions. This chapter presents an overview of some of the important issues in rheumatic disease epidemiology and it provides a summary of epidemiologic features of major rheumatic diseases.

2. OVERVIEW OF EPIDEMIOLOGICAL METHODS

Epidemiology is often referred to as the basic science of public health. It is broadly defined as the study of the distribution and determinants of health-related events or conditions in populations *(2)*. The goal of the epidemiologist is to identify risk factors

From: *Nutrition and Health: Nutrition and Rheumatic Disease*
Edited by: L. A. Coleman © Humana Press, Totowa, NJ

for a disease or health event so that these may be modified for prevention. Types of prevention are defined in Table 1 *(2,3)*.

Primordial prevention, a relatively new concept coined by Strasser *(4)*, includes efforts directed to the general population that prevent the emergence of disease risk factors. These can include changes in social or environmental conditions that favor the development of disease risk factors. An example of a primordial prevention to reduce the incidence of osteoarthritis (OA) could include a community-wide health lifestyles promotion program aimed at encouraging physical activity and healthy eating to prevent overweight and obesity. Because many diseases share the same risk factors, primordial prevention efforts can have a wide impact on multiple diseases.

Primary prevention protects health by eliminating or modifying risk factors in susceptible people. Using antibiotics to treat strep throat is an example of a primary prevention of rheumatic heart disease. Secondary prevention refers to early detection of a disease for prompt intervention and treatment to minimize disability. This type of prevention could include early detection of repetitive strain injuries to prevent further tissue damage. Finally, tertiary prevention is actions to prevent or minimize the impact of long-term complications and disability of a disease. Hip replacement to reduce pain and provide improved mobility from degenerative joint disease is an example of a tertiary prevention effort.

2.1. Primary Epidemiological Study Designs

In working toward the ultimate goal of preventing disease, epidemiologists use a variety of study methods to understand the frequency of disease, uncover risk factors, and design interventions to modify disease risk factors. These study designs, some of which are shown in Table 2, have various strengths and limitations. Epidemiologists

Table 1
Epidemiological Definitions of Prevention

Types of Prevention	*Definition*	*Example*
Primordial	Preventing the emergence and establishment of environmental, socioeconomic, behavioral conditions known to increase the risk of disease	Population-wide healthy lifestyles promotion program to encourage physical activity and prevent obesity
Primary	Protecting health by eliminating or modifying risk factors in susceptible people	Using antibiotics to treat strep throat to prevent rheumatic heart disease
Secondary	Detecting disease for early intervention and treatment to minimize disability	Early detection of repetitive strain injuries to prevent further tissue damage
Tertiary	Preventing or minimizing the impact of long-term complications and disability of a disease	Hip replacement to reduce pain and provide improved mobility from degenerative joint disease

Adapted from refs. *2* and *3*

Table 2
Primary Epidemiological Study Designs

Study Designs	Purpose	Cost	Strengths	Limitations
Descriptive	Disease surveillance / distribution of health conditions in a population	Moderate	Provides disease burden Important for public health planning Generate hypotheses	Generalizabiltiy of results to other populations Case finding may vary
Ecological	Identify potential factors associated with disease	Low	Hypothesis generation	Cannot infer causality Ecological bias
Case–control	Identify disease risk factors	Moderate	Good for studying rare diseases, Can help identify potential risk factors	Cannot predict the "risk" of developing the disease from these studies Can only estimate the size of the association between exposure and disease
Cohort	Identify disease risk factors	High	Temporal sequence between exposure and disease can be more clearly established. Allows the calculation of incidence rates and relative risks May allow for the examination of multiple effects of a single exposure Minimizes potential for selection bias of cases and controls	Time-consuming Expensive Loss to follow-up Generalizability of results
Randomized controlled trial	To test whether modifying a potential risk factor will alter disease outcome	High	Optimal design to determine causality	Loss to follow-up Generalizability of results

may progress from one study design to the next as they move from first describing the patterns of a disease in a population, then discovering disease risk factors, and finally to experimentally modifying the risk factors for disease prevention.

Epidemiological study designs are often grouped in the general categories of "observational studies" or "experimental studies." Observational studies include descriptive cross-sectional surveys, ecological studies, case–control and cohort studies. These studies describe the natural course of disease and they do not involve a planned intervention.

Descriptive studies are essential for estimating the distribution of disease and associated risk factors in populations. In general, they are moderately costly but yield important data for public health planning and evaluating disease trends that could help indicate disease etiology. Often they are conducted as cross-sectional studies at one period of time and provide estimates of disease *prevalence*, defined as the total number of individuals with the disease in a population at a given point of time. A second cross-sectional study conducted on the same population could allow the calculation of disease *incidence*, defined as the number of newly developing cases of a disease occurring in a defined population over a defined period.

Ecological studies, sometimes called correlational studies, use data from groups rather than individuals to identify correlations that could indicate potential risk factors *(2)*. These studies often use available data sources and are therefore very inexpensive to conduct. An example of an ecological study is an investigation of average ambient ultraviolet radiation at different latitudes in Australia with the prevalence of self-reported rheumatoid arthritis (RA) and other autoimmune diseases from the Australian National Health Survey *(5)*. Although ecological studies are an inexpensive means to identify potential risk factors, caution must be used in interpreting the correlation between aggregate-level data to avoid "ecological bias or fallacy" *(2)*. This bias occurs when an assumption is made that association observed at the aggregate level holds true at the case or individual level.

Case–control studies are designed to identify risk factors by comparing exposures or other characteristics of individuals with a disease or condition (cases) to those from a suitable comparison group without the disease or condition (controls). These studies are often called "retrospective studies" because the exposures or potential risk factors of interests are recalled or measured after the disease has occurred. In general, these studies are less expensive than cohort studies to conduct, but differential recall between cases and controls of past exposures can lead to bias. This kind of recall bias can lead to inaccurate associations of environment exposures with disease. Despite this potential bias, case–control studies are extremely helpful in identifying potential risk factors, especially for rare diseases.

Cohort studies involve measuring potential risk factors or exposures in disease-free individuals and then following these individuals over a period until some of them develop the disease of interest. These studies can be conducted prospectively in time or, if past exposure data are available, they can be conducted retrospectively. Because the study population is usually followed very closely over a long period, cohort studies can be quite expensive to conduct. However, cohort studies can provide estimates of the true relative risk of a factor with disease. A relative risk is the ratio of the incidence of disease for people with a risk factor divided by incidence of the disease in people without the risk factor *(2)*. A major advantage of cohort studies is that they can estimate the temporal sequence between exposure and disease. Randomized controlled trials (RCT) fall under the category of experimental epidemiological studies. These are experiments where subjects or groups of individuals with equal characteristics are randomly assigned to receive or not receive the therapy or intervention *(2)*. RCTs can be either clinical or community-based trials and they tend to be expensive to conduct. Because the study subjects are randomly assigned to a treatment or a control group and followed over time for health events, these studies are regarded as the most scientifically rigorous methods of hypothesis testing.

2.2. Epidemiology Subdisciplines

The study designs just reviewed form some of the basic tools in a field that is becoming increasingly specialized. Subdisciplines of epidemiology, like those shown in Table 3, each have developed very specific approaches to measuring and modifying disease risk factors, often incorporating newly developed technology and statistical methods.

For example, social epidemiology focuses on the complex social distribution and social determinants of health *(6)*. Social epidemiologists take a broad population and life-course perspective, building multilevel models incorporating community measures in addition to risk factors on the individual level. This discipline often focuses on health disparities and includes behavior and socioeconomic factors that are well known to associate with a wide range of diseases, including many rheumatic diseases such as RA and OA *(7)*.

Pharmacoepidemiology, a rapidly evolving branch of epidemiology, often utilizes genetic data along with traditional risk factors from groups of patients and controls to model variability in drug response with respect to efficacy, tolerability, and safety *(8)*. Given the wide pharmacotherapeutic options for treating rheumatic diseases and their variable effects on individuals, pharmacoepidemiology is an extremely important field for rheumatologists. For example, as reviewed by Solomon et al., pharmacoepidemiology is being applied to understand the potential cardiovascular risk associated with selective cyclooxygenase-2 inhibitors *(8)*. Understanding individual responses to medications is the first step to personalized medicine.

Environmental exposures have been implicated in the etiology of some chronic diseases, but quantifying these exposures is often extremely difficult. Environmental epidemiologists specialize in measuring the relationships between exogenous

Table 3
Examples of Epidemiology
Subdisciplines

Subdiscipline
Social/behavioral epidemiology
Pharmacoepidemiology
Environmental epidemiology
Genetic/molecular epidemiology

environmental agents and health *(9)*. For rheumatic diseases, tobacco smoke has been associated with an increased risk of developing RA and several other suspected environmental exposures have been investigated in systemic lupus erythematosus (SLE) including hair dyes and crystalline silica exposure *(9)*.

Genetic or molecular epidemiological studies seek to link a particular genotype or biological marker of a specific effect (i.e., gene expression) to a disease phenotype *(10)*. These types of studies combine principles of human and population genetics with classical epidemiological methods. They can be used to help determine disease etiology and also to improve our understanding of disease risk, classification, and progression. Genetic epidemiological studies determine the role of inherited causes of disease in families and in populations. Often, family or twin studies are used to first establish whether there is a genetic component to a disease. Next, segregation analyses are used to estimate the mode of genetic transmission and linkage and association studies are used to estimate the genetic locus and alleles associated with disease. Once the genes and alleles are identified, genetic epidemiologists also evaluate gene–gene and gene–environment interactions with disease risk. Genetic epidemiology is a particularly dynamic field that is being shaped by very rapid improvements in genotyping and bioinformatics technology, falling genotyping costs, and advances in statistical methods.

3. EPIDEMIOLOGICAL ISSUES IN STUDYING RHEUMATIC DISEASES

Although rheumatic diseases are often common and crippling, our knowledge of the epidemiology of these diseases is much less advanced than for other chronic diseases such as cardiovascular disease, diabetes, or many cancers. Rheumatic diseases are clinically complex and this presents many methodological challenges in studying these diseases. For example, unlike childhood-onset type 1 diabetes, which usually has a very clear clinical presentation (ketoacidosis) and standard treatment (insulin) allowing for relatively straightforward case identification, the majority of individuals with rheumatic diseases have extremely variable clinical presentations, multiple treatment options, and unpredictable disease courses. Some of the major methodological issues in rheumatic disease epidemiology are shown in Table 4.

Difficulties in classification of rheumatic diseases, including the slow and variable disease onset, variability in disease course, and multiple organ involvement, have limited the ability to conduct epidemiological studies. Fortunately, this problem is being addressed by the adoption of very specific criteria to classify cases. For example, the American Rheumatism Association's 1987 revised criteria for the classification of RA can be applied to classify a patient as having RA if that person has four of seven criteria (morning stiffness, arthritis of three or more joint areas, arthritis of hand joints, rheumatoid nodules, serum rheumatoid factor, radiographic changes *(11)*). The creation and continual refinement of these classification criteria to reflect new disease knowledge greatly improves the ability to conduct epidemiological studies and it allows study results to be more easily compared.

The difficulty in identifying individuals with rheumatic disease in populations is another limitation to better understanding the epidemiology of these disorders. Many

Table 4
Methodological Issues in Rheumatic Disease Epidemiology

Major Methodological Issues
Case identification
Often rare diseases
May not present for medical care
Disease classification
Slow and variable disease onset
Variability of disease course
Multiple organ involvement
Complex treatment/variable response to treatment
Complex disease etiology
Polygenic
May involve multiple environmental exposures

rheumatic diseases, such as SLE or scleroderma, are rare and affected individuals may delay seeking medical care in the early stages of disease resulting in an underestimate of true disease incidence and prevalence. The difficulty of diagnosis and variability in disease course and treatments can also affect the ability to identify and track cases for epidemiological investigations over time. For this reason, investigators often use multiple clinic and hospital sources for case ascertainment and employ disease registries to more easily track patients over time.

A final limitation is the very complex etiologies of rheumatic disease. Many of these conditions are thought to be polygenic and involve multiple environmental exposures, and this complicated etiology has resulted in the identification of few potentially modifiable risk factors for rheumatic diseases. The lack of previously identified risk factors can dissuade investigators from carrying out epidemiological studies.

4. BURDEN OF ARTHRITIC CONDITIONS

Classification criteria standardize case definitions and provide a more reliable phenotype for researching disease risk factors and clinical outcomes. However, rheumatic disease classification criteria are by definition restrictive (i.e., they often exclude more mild cases of disease) and applying these criteria may underestimate the overall burden of rheumatic disease in populations.

In the United States, the data from the National Health Interview Survey (NHIS) can be used to estimate the burden of arthritis and rheumatic disease *(12)*. The NHIS is an annual, household-based survey of a representative sample of the U.S. civilian, noninstitutionalized population. In 2005, information was collected on 31,326 adults. The NHIS recorded self-reported, doctor-diagnosed arthritis if respondents answered "yes" to the question, "Have you ever been told by a doctor or other health professional that you have some form of arthritis, rheumatoid arthritis, gout, lupus, or fibromyalgia?" Those who answered "yes" were then asked, "Are you limited in any way in any of your usual activities because of arthritis or joint symptoms?" Persons responding "yes" to both questions were defined as having an arthritis-attributable activity limitation.

Table 5 shows the self-reported burden of arthritic conditions in 2005. Prevalence estimates are presented overall and by gender, age group, race/ethnicity, education level, and body mass index (BMI) categories. Estimates are age-adjusted to the standard 2000 U.S. population to facilitate comparisons between demographic subgroups *(13)*. Approximately 21% of U.S. adults reported being told by a doctor or other health care professional that they had some form of arthritis, gout, lupus, or fibromyalgia. Furthermore, 27% reported pain or stiffness in or around a joint in the past 30 days that began more than 3 months ago. The age-adjusted prevalence was higher among females (24.4%) than males (17.9%) and the prevalence increased dramatically in the older age groups, peaking at 54% among those aged 75 years or older. Prevalence was lowest among Asian and Hispanics and highest among Native Americans and Alaska Natives. Arthritis diagnosis and chronic joint symptoms were also more common among individuals with the lowest education and income levels.

With an understanding of the overall burden of rheumatic disease in the population, the next section of this chapter presents a brief review of the epidemiology of three major rheumatic diseases: RA, SLE, and OA. For a more complete review of the epidemiology of these and other rheumatic diseases, refer to Silman and Hochberg *(14)*.

4.1. Rheumatoid Arthritis Epidemiology

RA is a chronic, idiopathic, inflammatory arthropathy with aspects manifested in autoimmunity *(15)*. Disease onset can occur at any age, but a majority of cases are diagnosed between ages 40 and 60. In 1987, the American College of Rheumatology (ACR) published the currently accepted diagnostic criteria for RA *(11)*. Unlike previous diagnostic guidelines, subgroups are not assigned according to severity.

RA prevalence is approx 2% in the United States *(15–17)* and prevalence among women is 2.5 times that of men *(3)*. In Europe, there is considerable variation in RA prevalence ranging from 0.3% in Italy to 1.1% in Northern Ireland *(15–17)*. This is similar to the variation documented for primarily white U.S. populations (0.5%–1.1%). Perhaps the broadest range occurs between populations of North American Natives, from 0.6% prevalence in the Yupick Eskimos to 6.8% in the Chippewa Indians. In contrast, Asia has less variation in RA prevalence, ranging from 0.2% in rural Indonesia to 0.6% in Japan *(15–17)*. Differences in study methodologies, such as variable case ascertainment and different population age structures, may account for some of the variation in reported RA rates. However, undetermined causal factors, such as infection, environmental exposures, genetics, predisposing standards of living, nutrition, or availability of health care could also be responsible.

Table 6 presents the incidence of RA from selected studies *(16)*. Overall RA incidence ranges from 24 to 50 cases per 100,000 persons and the incidence is generally twice a high in females as males.

Although RA remains idiopathic, certain patterns have been recognized and documented by epidemiologists. For instance, it has been shown that the serum titer of rheumatoid factor (RF) is proportional to the risk of developing RA *(24)*. Other trends, although not completely understood, include decreased risk with high serum antioxidants such as β-carotene and α-tocopherol, omega-3 fatty acids, or schizophrenia *(15,17)*.

Table 5
Frequency of Self-Reported Arthritis and Chronic Joint Symptoms in the United States in 2005[a]

Characteristic	Population (Age 18 Yr and Older)	Arthritis diagnosis[a] Crude Prevalence (%)	Arthritis diagnosis[a] Age-Adjusted Prevalence (%)	Chronic joint symptoms[b] Crude Prevalence (%)	Chronic joint symptoms[b] Age-Adjusted Prevalence (%)
Total	217,774	21.6	21.3	27.0	26.7
Male	104,919	17.4	17.9	24.7	25.0
Female	112,855	25.4	24.4	29.1	28.2
Age group (yr)					
18–44	110,431	7.8	7.8	15.5	15.6
45–64	72,296	28.7	28.8	35.2	35.2
65–74	18,446	46.7	46.8	45.1	45.1
75+	16,600	53.8	54.2	48.0	48.2
Race					
White	180,477	22.4	21.6	28.1	26.6
Black	24,817	19.0	21.2	22.5	27.5
Asian	8,155	10.6	12.6	14.0	15.1
American Indian/Alaska Native	1,469	21.1	26.8	28.6	32.0
Ethnicity					
Not Hispanic or Latino	190,004	23.0	22.0	28.5	27.6
Hispanic or Latino	27,770	11.5	16.9	17.0	21.3
Education Level					
Less than high school	29,595	30.0	25.9	33.1	30.3
High school diploma/GED	54,937	27.1	25.3	30.7	29.4
Some college	49,855	24.6	25.9	32.1	32.7
College diploma	52,705	17.9	19.9	23.9	25.4
Family Income ($)					
Less than 20,000	37,622	27.5	20.9	32.7	26.4
20,000–34,999	30,980	23.6	22.5	28.7	28.0
35,000–54,999	32,819	21.1	22.2	28.1	28.7
55,000–74,999	23,619	18.1	20.7	25.9	27.4
75,000 or more	50,211	17.6	19.8	24.7	26.0

Numbers are in thousands. Data source: 2005 National Health Interview Survey. Estimates are based on household interviews of a sample of the civilian noninstitutionalized population.

[a] Self-reported medically diagnosed arthritis, rheumatoid arthritis, gout, lupus, or fibromyalgia.

[b] Self-reported pain, aching, or stiffness in or around joints during the past 30 days (excluding back and neck pain) and joint symptoms that first began more than 3 months prior to interview.

From reference *12*.

Table 6
Incidence of Rheumatoid Arthritis in Selected Studies

Source	Location (Period)	Overall	Male	Female
Uhlig et al. *(18)*	Oslo, Norway (1988–1993)	26	14	37
Symmons et al. *(19)*	Manchester, UK (1990–1991)	–	14	36
Drosos et al. *(20)*	Northwest Greece (1987–1995)	24	12	36
Doran et al. *(21)*	Rochester, MN, USA (1955–2000)	50	30	60
Savolainen et al. *(22)*	Koupio, Finland (2000)	40	30	50
Soderlin et al. *(23)*	Kronoberg County, Sweden (1999–2000)	24	18	29

Incidence (per 100,000 population)

Adapted from reference *16*

Obesity, smoking, and certain infections are also examples of factors that may increase the risk of developing RA *(15,17,25,26)*.

Prior studies and clinical observations have documented spontaneous remission of RA during pregnancy, subsequent exacerbation of symptoms upon completion of gestation, and proinflammatory contributions from prolactin with breastfeeding *(15)*. A decline in symptom severity and delay of RA onset has been observed with the use of oral contraceptives *(15)*. Decreased fertility among women with RA both before and after disease onset has also been well established, and men with RA also have diminished circulating testosterone *(15)*. Therefore, regardless of gender, higher levels of reproductive hormones may provide an avenue by which primary prevention methods may be established *(27)*.

Twin studies have demonstrated a genetic component in RA risk *(15)*. A monozygotic twin has up to four times the risk of developing RA, given that his or her twin has the disease, when compared with dizygotic twins *(15)*. Additional studies of RA inheritance have been primarily based on the expression of the human leukocyte antigen (HLA) class II gene complex *(15)*. HLA class II molecules are heterodimeric peptides, with one α and one β chain, found on B lymphocytes and antigen-presenting cells of the immune system *(28)*. Located on chromosome 6, the HLA gene complex includes coding regions for three HLA class II subregions, named *DP*, *DQ*, and *DR*. The *DR* subregion, of particular interest in RA, encodes four β chains and one invariable α chain. There is a high degree of polymorphism in the genes encoding the β chains, leading to many subsets within the *DR* region.

Association of RA to alleles of the *HLA-DRB1* gene is now well established *(29,30)*. Furthermore, these markers correlate with disease severity *(31)* and early age of onset *(32)*. Padyukov et al. reported a very interesting gene–environment interaction between smoking and shared epitope genes in *HLA-DR4 (33)*. There are likely to be other associations within the HLA region, some of which appear to be protective for developing RA (i.e., *DQ* haplotypes) *(30)*.

In 2004, an association of a nonsynonymous single-nucleotide polymorphism (*R620W*) in the protein tyrosine phosphatase gene was reported for both type 1 diabetes and RA *(34)*. This exciting finding has subsequently been widely replicated in other populations and the same polymorphism has also been associated with juvenile idiopathic arthritis, SLE, Grave's and Addison's diseases *(30)*. It calls into question whether there are common genetic risk factors underlying many autoimmune diseases *(30)*. Other genetic associations with RA have also been reported including *CTLA4, PAD14, FCRL3* and *MHC2TA* (reviewed in *30*). Additionally, many pharmacogenetic studies are underway to determine the genetic influences on treatment response, particularly toward understanding the pharmacogenetics of methotrexate response *(30)*. With the advent of affordable genome-wide association studies, these investigations may soon yield further exciting results.

4.2. Systemic Lupus Erythematosus Epidemiology

SLE is an uncommon chronic inflammatory disease that usually affects the connective tissues but can involve multiple organ systems. The pathogenesis of SLE is believed to involve abnormalities of the immune system. SLE is often not easily characterized or diagnosed as its clinical course can vary substantially between or even within individuals. This variation in onset and disease activity has formed a significant obstacle in describing the epidemiology of SLE.

Siegel and Lee conducted the first long-term epidemiological study of SLE in the early 1960s in New York City *(35)*. In this classic study, Siegal and Lee established their own classification criteria and employed multiple sources to identify cases of SLE in a defined area of Manhattan. Results from this study confirmed that age and gender and environmental influences, such as sun exposure and certain drug use, were related to SLE. One of the most intriguing findings was a threefold increase in the incidence of SLE in African-American females compared with white females.

Since this early investigation, there have been other reports of increased SLE rates in African-American females in Jefferson County, Alabama *(36)*; San Francisco *(37)*; Baltimore *(38)*; Allegheny County, Pennsylvania *(39)*; and Nottingham *(40)* and Birmingham *(41)*, England. The published incidence rates of SLE from selected population-based studies are summarized in Table 7. The crude rates are indicated, and the age-standardized rates and 95% confidence intervals are noted when available. Although many of the studies were conducted 25 years apart, and applied different classification criteria for SLE, the differences between the gender- and race-specific rates are remarkably similar.

For instance, in the New York City study *(35)* white females experienced 8.3 times the rate of SLE compared with white males and African-American females were found to have 3.2 times the rate of SLE as white females. In Allegheny County in Pennsylvania *(39)*, white women had 8.9 times the rate of SLE than white men and African-American women had 2.6 times the rate of disease compared with white women.

The overall incidence rates in European studies are all similar ranging from 3.3 in Iceland to 4.0 in Nottingham, England. White females had a 4.7 to 5.8 excess

Table 7
Incidence of SLE (per 100,000 Population) by Race and Gender for Selected Studies

Source	Location (Period)	Cases (n)	Overall Incidence[a]	Male White Incidence[a]	Male Black Incidence[a]	Female White Incidence[a]	Female Black Incidence[a]
Siegel and Lee (35)	Jefferson County, AL (1956–1965)	63	1.0	0.4	0.3	1.1	2.9
Siegel et al. (36)	New York, NY (1956–965)	98	2.0	0.3	1.1	2.5	7.9
Michet et al. (42)	Rochester, MN (1950–1979)	25	1.9 (1.2–2.6)	1.2 (0.2–2.2)	–	2.5 (1.4–3.6)	–
Hochberg (38)	Baltimore, MD (1970–1977)	302	4.6	0.4	2.5	3.9	11.4
Gudmundsson et al. (43)	Iceland (1975–1984)	76	3.3	0.8	–	5.8	–
Jonsson et al. (44)	Southern Sweden (1981–1986)	39	4.0 (1.6–6.4)	1.0	–	5.4	–
Hopkinson et al. (40)	Nottingham, England (1989–1990)	23	4.0 (2.4–5.7)	1.5 (0.0–2.9)	–	6.5 (3.6–9.5)	–
Nossent et al. (45)	Curaçao (1980–1989)	68	4.6 (0.4–8.8)	–	1.1 (0.9–3.1)	–	7.9 (2.3–13.2) 25.9
Johnson et al. (41)	Birmingham, England (1991)	33	3.8 (2.5–5.1)	–	–	4.5 (2.7–7.2)	22.8 (3.1–40.5)
McCarty et al. (39)	Allegheny County, PA (1985–1990)	191	2.8 (2.6–3.2)	0.4 (0.2–0.7)	0.7 (0.0–2.0)	3.5 (2.9–4.2)	9.2 (6.8–12.5)
Naleway et al. (46)	Rural Central Wisconsin (1991–2001)	44	5.1 (3.6–6.6)	1.9 (0.6–3.3)	–	8.2 (5.5–10.9)	–

[a] per 100,000
Crude incidence (confidence intervals in parentheses)
Age-standardized incidence

incidence in comparison to white males. Unfortunately, with the exception of the study from Birmingham United Kingdom, the populations where these investigations were performed did not contain enough ethnic diversity to explore racial differences in SLE.

The overall age-standardized incidence rates in the Baltimore study were remarkably similar to rates in Allegheny County. Figure 1 shows the age-specific incidence of SLE between African-American and white men and women from Baltimore and Allegheny County. For the most part, although different criteria were applied to classify cases, the gender- and race-specific rates are strikingly similar between the studies. In Baltimore, the incidence per 100,000 was 0.5 for white males and 3.9 for white females, which is virtually identical to the rates observed in these groups (0.4 and 3.5, respectively) in Allegheny County.

White female rates were also quite similar between the studies (Fig. 1), with virtually identical rates reported in the youngest age groups (0–14 and 15–24) and in the oldest age groups (55–64 and 65 and older).

There are many suspected risk factors for SLE including hormonal level, environmental exposures, viral infections, and genetics *(15)*. Hormonal factors, especially low androgen or high estrogen levels maybe associated with SLE and estrogen replacement therapy may increase disease risk *(48)*. Environmental exposure to silica dust, aromatic amine, hydrazines, solvents and cigarette smoke have all been associated with SLE *(15)*. Of these environmental factors, silica particles and smoking appear to have the strongest associations. Infectious agents may also be risk factors but their role need clarification *(15)*.

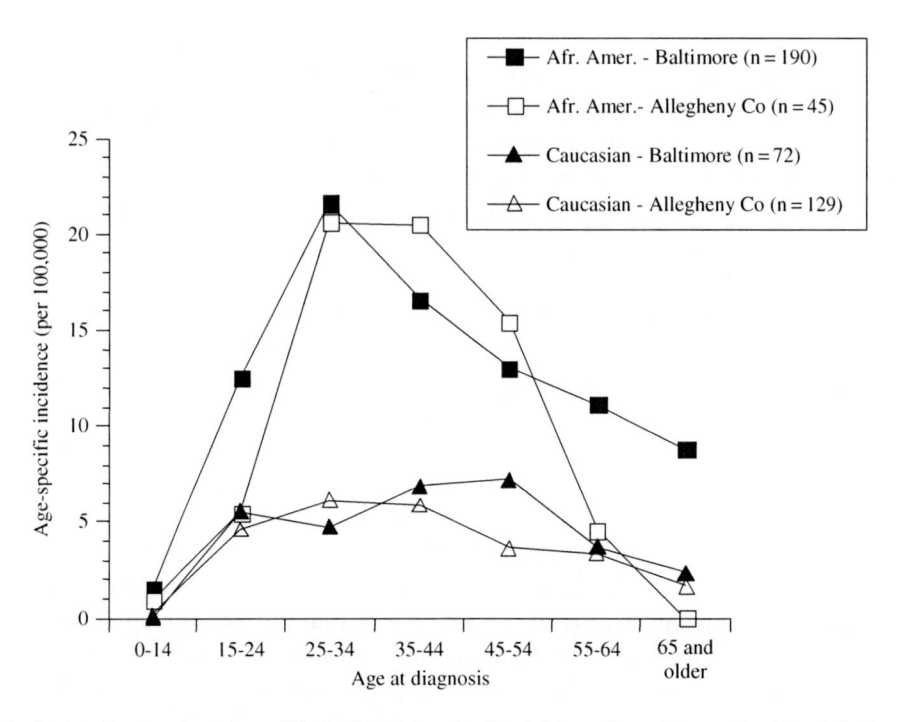

Fig. 1. Comparisons of age-specific incidence rates for African-American and white females with definite systemic lupus erythematosus.

Although most cases of SLE appear sporadic, SLE shows a strong familial aggregation, with higher frequencies among first-degree relatives *(15)*. These relatives may also have higher rates of autoimmune disease but this need confirmation in carefully conducted population-based studies.

Concordance rates are approximately 25 to 50% among monozygotic twins and 5% among dizygotic twins. Genome-wide linkage and association studies have successfully identified many genetic loci and genes associated with SLE, including several in the HLA region (*DR2* and *DR3* in particular). These findings are reviewed by Croker and Kimberly *(49)*. Whole genome-wide association studies will likely replicate many of these and identify new genetic associations. It is hoped that these studies may also identify SLE subphenotypes *(49)*.

4.3. Osteoarthritis Epidemiology

OA is the most common and one of the most expensive to treat forms of joint inflammation. Diagnostic criteria have been developed by the ACR, which distinguishes between the three main forms of OA—hip, knee, and hand—and primary or secondary etiology. Primary OA is an idiopathic designation, whereas secondary OA indicates joint trauma, additional arthropathies, congenital or developmental defects, or systemic disease *(50)*. And although all forms are classified as OA, distinct prevalence, incidence, and risk factors are documented for hip, knee, and hand OA.

Symptomatic hip OA prevalence within the United States has been found to be 3 – 6% for white populations, whereas the average is slightly lower in African-American, Asian, and East Indian populations *(51)*. Prevalence of symptomatic OA of the knee is approx 16% for United States adults, and has been shown to be higher for women, African-American populations, and the in general population with increasing age *(52)*. Symptomatic OA of the hand, as with OA of the hip, was shown to be less common in African-American populations. There are also no significant differences in the prevalence for men versus that of women. Overall, the prevalence of symptomatic OA of the hand among U.S. adults is approx 8% *(53)*.

The incidence, as well as prevalence, of OA of the hand, hip, and knee increases with age and women have higher rates than men, especially after age 50 *(15)*. Overall incidence rates within the United States, standardized for age and gender, have been found to be 0.88% per 1,000 people per year for hip OA, 2.4% per 1,000 people per year for OA of the knee, and 1% per 1,000 people per year for OA of the hand *(54)*.

As expected, each of the forms of OA has distinct risk factors in addition to various commonalities. The risk for developing OA of the hip is increased by chronic mechanical stresses such as climbing stairs, heavy lifting, operating heavy machinery as in farming, high exposure to sports or intense physical activity, and obesity *(55)*. Development of hip OA is invariable among people with congenital hip dislocation, Legg-Calvé-Perthes disease, or slipped femoral capital epiphysis *(56)*.

OA of the knee is most affected by obesity relative to hip and hand OA, with increased susceptibility if there is also weakness in muscles of the thigh. Obesity has also been shown to have a greater impact on the knee and the onset of OA in women, but exact causal evidence for this trend remains unclear *(57)*. Sports-related injuries, specifically cruciate ligament damage and meniscal tears, have also been strongly associated with OA development in the knee *(58)*.

OA of the hand has been shown to have a unique risk pattern. Given that OA is found in one joint within one digit, there is a significantly higher risk of developing OA in other digits at that joint, as well as developing OA in additional joints within the effected digit *(55)*. Also, long-term use of dexterity, especially with regard to the pincer grip, has been shown to correspond with increasing risk for OA of the hand *(15)*.

Several common risk factors encompassing hip, knee, and hand OA have also been established. Perhaps the most significant risk factor is aging, shown by a substantial increase in the development of OA after age 55 *(50)*. High levels of bone density, as well as low levels of serum vitamin D necessary for bone remodeling, also correspond with increased risk *(59,60)*. Multiple studies have been conducted to evaluate the effects of estrogen replacement therapy, oral contraceptives, and reproductive events with the risk for OA, with increasing evidence suggesting a protective effect of hormone replacement, but no definitive correlations have been established *(60–62)*.

A genetic component has also been identified in familial OA, characterized by early onset, consisting of an autosomal-dominant mutation in the gene-encoding type II collagen *(63)*. However, this connection was not observed in the general population, limiting its usefulness in a public health context. To date, researchers have not found highly indicative patterns of heritability. One study that examined families and twins to uncover any genetic patterns found that OA is actually heterogeneous and multigenetically inherited *(64)*.

In addition to minimizing any possible factors leading to an increased risk of OA, certain methods of prevention have been well documented. Increased intake of antioxidants, such as vitamins C and E, has been shown to decrease the risk of OA by combating common oxygen radicals that may cause significant tissue damage *(65)*.

Unfortunately, with the dramatic increase in the rates of overweight and obesity, the prevalence of OA will likely greatly increase. This underscores the urgency of clearly establishing OA risk factors early for disease prevention.

5. CONCLUSION

Our understanding of the epidemiology of, and risk factors associated with, rheumatic disease has dramatically improved in the past several decades. Rapid advances in genomic technology and lowered cost of genotyping are leading to exciting and explosive growth in the knowledge of the genetics underlying rheumatic diseases. These exciting findings may help identify subphenotypes, predict drug responses, as well as identify genetic risk factors for disease. Hopefully, in the near future, these findings will soon result in promising preventions strategies and treatments to reduce the suffering from rheumatic disease.

REFERENCES

1. Nuki G, Simkin PA. A concise history of gout and hyperuricemia and their treatment. Arthritis Res Ther 2006:8(suppl 1):s1
2. Last JM. A Dictionary of Epidemiology, 4th ed. Oxford University Press, New York, 2001.
3. Brownson RC, Remington PL, Davis JR, eds. Chronic Disease. Epidemiology and Control. American Public Health Association. United Book Press, Washington, DC, 1998.
4. Strasser T. Reflections on cardiovascular disease. Interdisc Sci Review. 1978;3:255–230.

5. Staples JA, Ponsonby AL, Lim LL, McMichael AJ. Ecologic analysis of some immune-related disorders, including type 1 diabetes, in Australia: latitude, regional ultraviolet radiation, and disease prevalence. Environ Health Perspect 2003;111(4):518–523.
6. Berkman LF, Kawachi I, eds. Social Epidemiology. Oxford University Press, New York, 2000.
7. Callahan LF. Social epidemiology and rheumatic disease. Curr Opin Rheumatol 2003;15:110–115.
8. Soloman DH, Avorn J. Pharmacoepidemiology and rheumatic disease:2001–2002. Curr Opin Rheumatol 2003;15:122–126.
9. Dooley MA, Hogan SL. Environmental epidemiology and risk factors for autoimmune disease. Curr Opin Rheumatol 2003;15:99–103.
10. Khoury MJ, Little J, Burke W: Human Genome Epidemiology: Scope and Strategies. In Khoury MJ, Little J, Burke W (eds): Human Genome Epidemiology. New York, Oxford University Press, 2004, pp 3–16.
11. Arnett FC, Edworthy SM, Bloch DA, et al. The American Rheumatism Association 1987 revised criteria for the classification of rheumatoid arthritis. Arthritis Rheum 1988;31:315–324.
12. Pleis JR, Lethbridge-Çejku M. Summary health statistics for U.S. adults; National health interview survey, 2005. National Center for Health Statistics. Vital Health Stat 2006;10(232).
13. Klein RJ, Schoenborn CA. Age adjustment using the 2000 projected U.S. population. Healthy People Statistical Notes, no 20. National Center for Health Statistics, Hyattsville, MD, 2001
14. AJ Silman, MC Hochberg, eds. Epidemiology of the Rheumatic Diseases, 2nd Ed. Oxford University Press, Oxford, 2001
15. Felson DT. Epidemiology of the rheumatic diseases. In: Koopman WJ, ed. Arthritis and Allied Conditions, 14th ed. Williams and Wilkins, Baltimore, MD, 2001.
16. Alamanos Y, Voulgari PV, Drosos AA. Incidence and prevalence of rheumatoid arthritis, based on the 1987 American College of Rheumatology Criteria: A systematic review. Semin Arthritis Rheum 2006;36:182–188.
17. Klippel JH, Stone JH, Crofford LJ, White P, eds. Primer on the Rheumatic Diseases, 12th ed. Atlanta, GA: Arthritis Foundation, 2001.
18. Uhlig T, Kvien TK, Glennas A, Glennas A, Smedstad LM, Forre O. The incidence and severity of rheumatoid arthritis, results from a county register in Oslo, Norway. J Rheumatol 1998;25:1078–1084.
19. Symmons DPM, Barrett EM, Bankhead CR, Scott DG, Silman AJ. The incidence of rheumatoid arthritis in the United Kingdom: Results from the Norfolk Arthritis Register. Br J Rheumatol 1994;33(8):735–739.
20. Drosos AA, Alamanos I, Voulgari PV, Psychos DN, Katsaraki A, Papadopoulos I, Dimou G, Siozos C. Epidemiology of adult rheumatoid arthritis in northwest Greece 1987–1995. J Rheumatol 1997;24(11):2129–2133.
21. Doran MF, Pond GR, Crowson CS, O'Falllon WM, Gabriel SE. Trends in incidence and mortality in rheumatoid arthritis in Rochester, Minnesota, over a forty-year period. Arthritis Rheum 2002;46:625–631.
22. Savolainen E, Kaipiainen-Seppanen O, Kroger L, Luosujarvi R. Total incidence and distribution of inflammatory joint diseases om a defined population: results from the Kuopio 2000 arthritis survey. J Rheumatol 2003;30:2460–2468.
23. Soderlin MK, Borjeson O, Kautiainen H, Skogh T, Leirisalo-Repo M. Annual incidence of inflammatory joint disease in a population based study in southern Sweden. Ann Rheum Dis 2002; 61911–61916.
24. Del Puente A, Knowler WC, Pettitt DJ, et al. The incidence of rheumatoid arthritis is predicted by rheumatoid factor titer in a longitudinal population study. Arthritis Rheum 1988;31:1239–1244.
25. Silman A, Bankhead C, Rowlingson B, et al. Do new cases of RA cluster in time or space? Int J Epidemiol 1997;26(3):628–634.
26. Hazes JMW, Dijkmans BAC, Vandenbroucke JP, et al. Cigarette Smoking and the onset of rheumatoid arthritis. Br J Rheumatol 1989;28(suppl 2):95.
27. Spector TD, Hochberg MC. The protective effect of the oral contraceptive pill on rheumatoid arthritis: an overview of the analytic epidemiological studies using meta-analysis. J of Clin Epidemiol 1990;43:1221–1230.
28. Wake CT. Molecular biology of the HLA Class I and Class II genes. Mol Biol Med 1986; 3(1):1–11.

29. Buckner JH, Nepom GT. Genetics of rheumatoid arthritis: is there a scientific explanation for the human leukocyte antigen assocation? Curr Opin Rheumatol 2002;14:254–259.
30. Oliver JE, Worthington J Silman AJ. Gentic epidemiology of rheumatoid arthritis. Curr Opin Rheumatol 2006;18:141–146.
31. Weyand CM, McCarthy TG, Goronzy JJ. Correlation between disease phenotype and genetic herogeneity in rheumatoid arthritis. J Clin Invest 1995;95:2120–2126.
32. Nepom BS, Nepom GT, Mickelson E, et al. Specific HLA-DR4-associated histocompatibility molecules characterize patients with seropositive juvenile rheumatoid arthrisits. J Clin Invest 1984;74:287–291.
33. Padyukov L, Silva C, Stolt P, et al. A gene–enviroment interaction between smoking and shared epitople genes in the HLA-DR provides a high risk of seropositive rheumatoid arthritis. Arthr Rheum 2004;50:3085–3092.
34. Begovich AB, Carlton VE, Honigberg LA, Schrodi SJ, Chokkalingam AP, et al. A missense single-nucleotide polymorphism in a gene encoding a protein tyrosine phosphatase (PTPN22) is associated with rheumatoid arthritis. Amer J Human Genet 2004;75(2):330–337.
35. Siegel M, Lee SL. The epidemiology of systemic lupus erythematosus. Semin Arthritis Rheum 1973;3:1–54.
36. Siegel M, Holley HL, Lee SL. Epidemiologic studies on systemic lupus erythmatosus. Comparative data for New York City and Jefferson County, Alabama, 1956–1965. Arthritis Rheum 1970;13: 802–811.
37. Fessel WJ. Systemic lupus erythmatosus in the community. Incidence, prevalence, outcome, and first symptoms; the high prevalence in black women. Arch Intern Med 1974;134:1027–1035.
38. Hochberg MC. The incidence of systemic lupus erythematosus in Baltimore, Maryland 1970–1977. Arthritis Rheum 1985;28:80–86.
39. McCarty DJ, Kwoh CK, Manzi S, Ramsey-Goldman R, Medsger TA, LaPorte RA. Incidence of SLE: Race and gender differences. Arthritis Rheum 1995;38(9):1260–1270.
40. Hopkinson ND, Doherty M, Powell RJ. The prevalence and incidence of systemic lupus erythematosus in Nottingham, UK, 1989–1990. Brit J Rheumatol 1993;32:110–115.
41. Johnson AE, Gordon C, Palmer RG, Bacon PA. The prevalnce and incidence of systemic lupus erythematosus (SLE) in Birmingham, England: relationship to ethnicity and country of birth. Arthritis Rheum 1995;38:551–557.
42. Michet CJ, McKenna CH, Elveback LR, Laslow RA, Kurkland LT. The epidemiology of systemic lupus erythematosus and other connective tissue diseases in Rochester, Minnesota, 1950 through 1979. Mayo Clin Proc 1985;60:105–113.
43. Gudmundsson S, Steinsson K. Systemic lupus erythematosus in Iceland 1975 through 1984. A nationwide epidemiological study in an unselected population. J Rheumatol 1990;17:1162–1167.
44. Jonsson H, Nived O, Sturfelt G, Solman A. Estimating the incidence of systemic lupus erythematosus in a defined population using multiple sources of retrieval. Br J Rheumatol 1990;29:185–188.
45. Nossent JC. Systemic lupus erythematosus on the Caribbean island of Curacao: an epidemiological investigation. Ann Rheum Dis 1992;51:1197–1201.
46. Naleway AL, Davis ME, Greenlee RT, Wilson DA, McCarty DJ. Epidemiology of Systemic Lupus Erythematosus in Rural Wisconsin. Lupus 2005;14(10):862–866.
47. Nivid O, Sturfelt G, Wolleim F. Systemic lupus erythematosus in an adult population in southern Sweden: incidence, prevalence and validity of ARA revised classification criteria. Brit J Rheumatol 1985;24:147–154.
48. Sanchez-Guerrero J, Liang MH, Karlson EW, et al. Post-menopausal estrogen therapy and the risk of developing systemic lupus erythematosus (SLE). Ann Intern Med 1995;122:430–433.
49. Croker JA, Kimberly RP. Genetics of susceptibility and severity in systemic lupus erythematosus. Curr Opinion in Rheumatol 2005;17:529–537.
50. Sharma L, Kapoor D, Issa S. Epidemiology of osteoarthritis: an update. Current Opinion in Rheumatology 2006;18:147–156.
51. Hoaglund FT, Steinbach LS. Primary osteoarthritis of the hip: etiology and epidemiology. J Am Acad Orthop Surg 2001;9(5):320–327.

52. Jordan JM, Helmick CG, Renner JB, et al. Prevalence of knee symptoms and radiographic and symptomatic knee osteoarthritis in African Americans and Caucasians: the Johnston County Osteoarthritis Project. J Rheumatol 2007;34(1):172–180.
53. Dillon CF, Hirsch R, Rasch EK, Gu Q. Symptomatic hand osteoarthritis in the United States: prevalence and functional impairment estimates from the third U.S. National Health and Nutrition Examination Survey, 1991–1994. Am J Phys Med Rehabil 2007; 86(1):12–21.
54. Oliveria SA, Felson DT, Reed JI, et al. Incidence of symptomatic hand, hip, and knee osteoarthritis among patients in a health maintenance organization. Arthritis Rheum 1995;38:1134.
55. Rooney BK, Silman AJ. Epidemiology of the rheumatic diseases. Curr Opin Rheumatol 1999;11: 91–97.
56. Gabriel SE. Epidemiology of the rheumatic diseases. In: Harris ED, Ruddy S, Sledge CB (eds). Kelley's textbook of rheumatology. Philadelphia: WB Saunders Company 2000;1:321–333.
57. Slemenda C, Heilman DK, Brandt KD, et al. Reduced quadriceps strength relative to body weight. A risk factor for knee osteoarthritis in women? Arthritis Rheum 1998;41(11):1951–1959.
58. Buckwalter JA, Lane NE. Athletics and osteoarthritis. Am J Sports Med 1997;25:873.
59. Dequeker J, Goris P, Utterhoeven R. Osteoporosis and osteoarthritis (osteoarthrosis). Anthropometric distinctions. JAMA 1983;249:1448.
60. McAlindon TE, Felson DT, Zhang Y, et al. Relation of dietary intake and serum levels of vitamin D to progression of osteoarthritis of the knee among participants of the Framingham Study. Ann Intern Med 1996;125(5):353–359.
61. Samanta A, Jones A, Regan M, et al. Is osteoarthritis in women affected by hormonal changes or smoking? Br J Rheumatol 1993;32:366.
62. Zhang Y, McAlindon TE, Hannan MT, et al. Estrogen replacement therapy and worsening of radiographic knee osteoarthritis: the Framingham Study. Arthritis Rheum 1998;41:1867–1873.
63. Palotie A, Ott J, Elim K, et al. Predisposition to familial osteoarthritis linked to Type II collagen gene. Lancet 1989;1:924–927.
64. Holderbaum D, Haqqi TM, Moskowitz RW. Genetics and osteoarthritis: exposing the iceberg. Arthritis Rheum 1999;42:397–405.
65. McAlindon TE, Jacques p, Zhang y, et al. Do antioxidant micronutrients protect against the development and progression of osteoarthritis? Arthritis Rheum 1996;39:648.

4 Drug–Nutrient Interactions in Rheumatic Diseases

Sung Nim Han

Summary

- Timing of medication in relation to mealtime influences absorption and bioavailability of drugs.
- Fish-oil supplementation can reduce prostaglandin production and proinflammatory cytokines. Nonsteroidal anti-inflammatory drug use can be modulated by fish-oil supplements.
- Folate status is important for prevention of methotrexate toxicity.
- Side effects of medication, pathological process of the disease, low appetite, and low mobility from active disease can contribute to poor nutritional status of patients with rheumatic disease.
- Optimal nutritional status should be maintained to achieve a positive treatment outcome and to reduce the risk for developing concurrent diseases.

Key Words: Antioxidant; fish oil; folate; methotrexate; nonsteroidal anti-inflammatory drugs; proinflammatory cytokines; prostaglandin E_2

1. INTRODUCTION

Rheumatic diseases include more than 100 diseases that are characterized by inflammation, pain, and degeneration of connective tissues and joints. Treatment plans for rheumatic diseases vary depending on the type of disease and the patient's condition. Medications for the treatment of rheumatic diseases are often used to relieve symptoms and prevent further worsening of the disease rather than to cure the disease. Lyme disease, infectious arthritis, and gout are some of the exceptions in which case symptoms of arthritis can be prevented or cured with early intervention and proper medications.

Drug–nutrient interactions can change both the therapeutic efficacy of medications and the nutritional requirements of patients. Therefore, understanding potential drug– and food– or nutrient interactions is crucial for maximizing biological effectiveness and minimizing the side effects of medications while ensuring optimal nutritional status of patients.

Medications most commonly used for the treatment of rheumatic diseases are nonsteroidal anti-inflammatory drugs (NSAIDs) to control pain and inflammation, corticosteroids to decrease inflammation and suppress the immune system, and disease-modifying anti-rheumatic drugs (DMARDs) to slow or prevent the damage to the joint. Anticytokine-based therapies have emerged recently and are often used in combination with conventional therapies. Potential drug–nutrient interactions are reviewed in relation to these different categories of therapies.

2. MECHANISMS OF DRUG–NUTRIENT INTERACTIONS

There are several mechanisms by which drug–nutrient interactions may result in altered therapeutic efficacy of drugs or altered nutrient requirements of patients.

2.1. Alteration of Pharmacokinetics by Food

Foods may interfere with or alter the absorption or metabolism of drugs and cause a change in pharmacokinetics *(1)*. Food can affect drug absorption and bioavailability by its effect on gastrointestinal (GI) physiology, including gastric emptying, acid secretion, intestinal motility, and bile secretion; and by physicochemical interactions between the drug and food components in the gut lumen and competitive inhibition between the drug and food components for absorption. Physicochemical interactions between nutrients and drug components include adsorption, complex formation, precipitation, and change in stability. Physicochemical interaction requires the simultaneous presence of the drug and the food component at the site of interaction. Therefore, timing of medication use in relation to food intake can influence the absorption of the drug. Additionally, the potential for a food–drug interaction is dependent on the region of the GI tract where the drug is absorbed. Drugs absorbed only in the upper intestine have a greater potential for reduced absorption when given with food *(2)*. Certain rheumatic disease medications such as methotrexate and penicillamine should be taken in a fasting state to prevent a decrease in absorption *(1)*.

2.2. Modulation of Biological Mediators of Rheumatic Diseases by Nutrients

Nutrients can modulate the course of therapy by their effects on biological mediators of rheumatic diseases such as cytokines and prostaglandins. Nutrients may have their own effect on the symptoms associated with rheumatic diseases, and as such, may influence the dose requirements of drugs. Nutrients may also affect side effects of the drugs to make the medication more or less tolerable. Omega-3 (n-3) fatty acids have been shown to have a significant impact on the production of eicosanoids and proinflammatory cytokines, which play a crucial role in the pathology of rheumatic diseases *(3)*.

2.3. Change in Nutritional Status by Drugs

Drugs can often change the nutrient status of the patient. Certain drugs have a direct antagonistic effect on a specific nutrient. Methotrexate is a well-known folate antagonist *(4)*. Drugs can also cause low levels of certain nutrients by interfering with nutrient absorption. Corticosteroids for the treatment of rheumatoid arthritis (RA) may impair intestinal calcium absorption *(5)*. Therefore, dietary intake and the nutritional status of patients should be monitored during the course of therapy to ensure adequate intake of nutrients and to prevent nutritional imbalance associated with drug therapy.

3. NONSTEROIDAL ANTI-INFLAMMATORY DRUGS

NSAIDs are often used for patients with a variety of rheumatic diseases to reduce the pain and inflammation. Naproxen (Aleve, Naprelan), ibuprofen (Advil, Motrin, Excedrin), and nabumetone (Relafen) are some of the NSAIDs commonly used. NSAIDs have not been shown to slow the progression of the disease; therefore, they should be used together with a DMARD for long-term care. Long-term administration of NSAIDs may cause GI ulcers, perforation, or hemorrhage *(6)*. Side effects of traditional NSAIDs have been attributed to the nonspecific inhibition of both forms of cyclooxygenase (COX): the constitutive form (COX-1) and the inducible form (COX-2). COX-1 is responsible for the production of prostaglandins (PG) necessary for normal physiological function of the GI tract and platelet function. COX-2 is inducible and is predominantly expressed in association with inflammation. COX-2-specific inhibitors, such as celecoxib, have been developed and introduced to provide anti-inflammatory activity with fewer GI side effects compared with traditional NSAID *(7)*.

3.1. Effects of Concomitant Food Intake on Bioavailability of NSAIDs

Effects of concomitant consumption of food on the bioavailability or absorption of NSAIDs seem to vary by the particular type of NSAID. Klueglich et al. *(8)* investigated the effect of food on ibuprofen pharmacokinetics in 38 adults. A lower peak plasma concentration and a delayed absorption of ibuprofen were observed when the drug was administered in a fed state (30 minutes after continental breakfast consumption) compared with a fasting state. On the other hand, Pargal et al. *(9)* reported a significant increase in the mean maximal plasma concentration and a delayed time to peak concentration of flurbiprofen (Ansaid) administered in a fed state. When administered with food, the maximum plasma concentration and the area under the plasma level curve of the metabolite of nabumetone increased *(10)*. The absorption of celecoxib, a specific COX-2 inhibitor, is minimally affected when administered with food. Although the time to reach maximal plasma concentration was delayed by 1 hour when administered with a high-fat food, the observed peak plasma concentration was increased by concomitant food intake. A longer intestinal transit time in the fed state may promote the opportunity for absorption of poorly soluble, highly permeable celecoxib, which can be absorbed throughout the GI tract. Therefore, in patients with arthritis, celecoxib can be given either with or without food. For acute therapy, it may be preferable that celecoxib is given in the fasting state to avoid the food-induced lag time in its absorption *(7)*.

3.2. Arachidonic Acid Metabolism and Prostaglandin Production

NSAIDs block inflammation by their action on COX, inhibiting PG synthesis. Therefore, any nutrients that can influence the production of PGs may interact with NSAIDs in patients with rheumatic disease. PGs are produced from arachidonic acid (AA) released from the plasma membrane by the action of phospholipase A_2. AA is transformed into PGG_2 by COX activity, and PGG_2 is converted to PGH_2 by the peroxidase activity of COX. PGE_2 is synthesized from PGH_2 by PGE synthase (PGES) (*see* Fig. 1). PGE_2 is one of the major mediators of inflammation, playing a role in the regulation of proinflammatory cytokine production and joint physiology *(11)*.

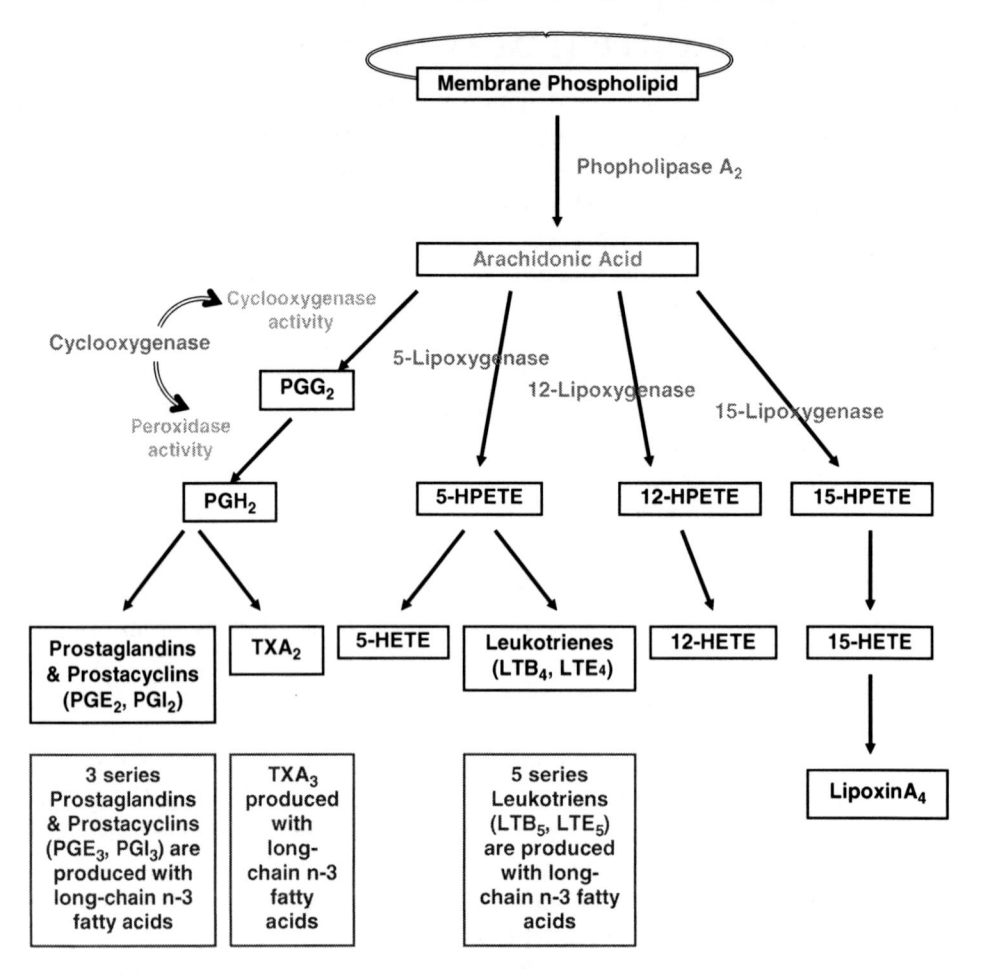

Fig. 1. Arachidonic acid (AA) metabolism. Prostaglandins (PG) are produced from AA released from the plasma membrane by the action of phospholipase A_2. AA is transformed into PGG_2 by cyclooxygenase (COX) activity, and PGG_2 is converted to PGH_2 by the peroxidase activity of COX. PGH_2 is converted to PGs, prostacyclins, and thromboxanes. PGE_2 is synthesized from PGH_2 by PGE synthase. Supplementation of n-3 fatty acids results in increased production of prostaglandins and thromboxanes in three series and leukotrienes in five series. HPETE, hydroperoxyeicosatetraenoic acid; HETE, hydroxyeicosatetraenoic acid; TXA, thromboxane A; LT, leukotriene.

High concentrations of PGE_2 in the synovial fluid of patients with RA have been reported *(12)*. The amount of AA in the membrane of inflammatory cells and the enzymatic activity of COX, a rate-limiting step in the production of PGE_2, are among the most important factors affecting the production of PGE_2. Dietary intake of fat can also influence the membrane phospholipid composition of inflammatory cells and result in changes in the synthesis of PGE_2. Decreased production of PGE_2 may occur with increased consumption of fish oil owing to decreased availability of substrate for synthesis of eicosanoids. In particular, eicosapentanoic acid (EPA) and docosohexanoic acid (DHA) are incorporated into the membrane at the expense of AA *(3)*. COX activity is determined by the level of the enzyme and requires the presence of oxidant hydroperoxide as an activator. Vitamin E has been shown to decrease COX activity by reducing the formation of peroxynitrite, a hydroperoxide involved in the activation of COX-2 *(13)*.

3.3. Clinical Benefits of n-3 Fatty Acids in Rheumatoid Arthritis

Dietary n-3 fatty acids are one of the most extensively studied dietary therapies in relation to rheumatic diseases. Significant clinical benefits of fish oil use for RA have been reported in many studies *(3,14–17)*. Fortin et al. *(15)* conducted a meta-analysis on 368 subjects from 10 trials and reported a modest but significant improvement in tender joint count and morning stiffness in patients with RA treated with dietary fish-oil supplementation for 3 months compared with placebo controls. In a more recent meta-analysis, MacLean et al. *(16)* evaluated results from 21 randomized controlled trials. They reported that there was no effect of n-3 fatty acids on patient reports of pain, swollen joint count, damage, and patient's global assessment. However, in a qualitative analysis of seven studies that assessed the effect of n-3 fatty acids on anti-inflammatory drug or corticosteroid requirements, six demonstrated a reduced requirement for these drugs. Cleland et al. *(17)* examined the effects of a long-term treatment (3 year) with fish oil in patients with RA. At 3 years, 18 patients who consumed either bottled fish-oil juice or fish-oil capsules (7 × 1 g capsules twice daily) to provide 4 to 4.5 g EPA and DHA daily and who maintained elevated plasma EPA levels (>5% of total plasma phospholipid fatty acids) were compared with 13 patients who did not take fish oil. Patients who took fish-oil supplements had 41% lower lipopolysaccharide (LPS)-stimulated whole blood production of PGE_2 and more frequent remission compared with patients who did not take fish oil. NSAID use was reduced by 75% from baseline in the fish-oil group while there was a 37% reduction in NSAID use in the group not consuming fish oil.

Although clinical benefits of fish-oil use in RA were shown to be robust, with improved control of symptoms and reduced need for NSAIDs, fish-oil supplementation can also adversely affect the immune function of patients, putting them at higher risk of infection. Consumption of a diet high in fish-derived n-3 fatty acid (1.23 g EPA and DHA per day [121–188 g fish per day]) for 6 months resulted in a lower cell-mediated immune response, as evidenced by lower proliferative response of peripheral blood mononuclear cells (PBMC) and lower delayed type hypersensitivity response, compared with adults who consumed diets low in fish (0.27 g EPA and DHA per day [33g fish per day]). In animal models, feeding fish oil was shown to impair host resistance against *Listeria* monocytogenes *(18)* and to delay virus clearance in mice infected with influenza virus *(19)*. Greater weight loss and suppression of appetite were observed following influenza infection in mice fed the fish oil diet for 14 days.

3.4. Impact of Vitamin E in Rheumatoid Arthritis

Supplementation of vitamin E in the diet has been shown to reduce PGE_2 production by spleen cells and macrophages in old mice by decreasing COX activity *(20,21)*. Using a macrophage cell line, Abate et al. *(22)* showed that vitamin E can enhance the inhibitory action of aspirin on PGE_2 production and COX-2 protein and mRNA expressions. However, the high level of vitamin E used (300 μM) in combination with aspirin in this study makes it hard to extend these findings to clinical practice. In a double-blind, placebo-controlled, randomized study, Edmonds et al. *(23)* investigated the effect of 3 months of vitamin E consumption (1,200 mg per day of *d*-α-tocopheryl acetate) on anti-inflammatory and analgesic parameters in patients with RA. Vitamin E did not have any effect on joint inflammation assessed by the Ritchie articular index, the duration of morning stiffness, or the number of swollen joints. Vitamin E significantly decreased pain parameters, suggesting some analgesic effects. However, it was not reported whether vitamin E treatment had any effect on NSAID use in this study.

4. CYTOKINE ANTAGONISTS

4.1. Role of Proinflammatory Cytokines in the Pathogenesis of Rheumatic Diseases

Cytokines, especially proinflammatory cytokines, play an important role in the pathogenesis of rheumatic diseases, including RA *(24)*. Patients with RA who have active disease have elevated interleukin (IL)-1β levels in plasma *(25)*, and elevated levels of tumor necrosis factor (TNF)-α in the synovial fluid. TNF-α and IL-1β in the synovial space increase collagenase production from chondrocytes in cartilage and activate osteoclasts in the bone. They also increase the expression of adhesion molecules on the endothelium contributing to the emigration of inflammatory cells and lymphocytes from the systemic circulation *(26)*. These factors contribute to the destruction of cartilage and bone, and the worsening of inflammation.

4.2. Anti-TNF-α-Based Therapies

Among the proinflammatory cytokines, TNF-α has emerged as a promising target for RA therapy because of (a) the dependence of other proinflammatory cytokines in rheumatoid synovial cultures on TNF-α, (b) upregulated expression of TNF-α and TNF-α receptor in synovial tissue, and (c) the effects of anti-TNF-α on reducing IL-1 production in synovial cultures and on ameliorating inflammation and joint destruction in animal models of arthritis *(27)*. There are two types of anti-TNF antibodies developed for use in RA, infliximab and adalimumab. Infliximab is a chimeric monoclonal antibody with mouse Fv1 and human immunoglobulin (Ig)G1, whereas adalimumab is a recombinant human IgG$_1$ monoclonal antibody. Both of these specifically, and with high affinity, bind to TNF-α with quite a long half-life of 10 to 12 days *(28,29)*. Another anti-TNF-based therapy is etanercept, a fusion protein constructed of the extracellular domain of human TNF receptor and the Fc fragment of human IgG, which has a fairly short half-life of 3 days *(29)*.

4.3. Modulation of Proinflammatory Cytokines by n-3 Fatty Acid Supplementation

Fish-oil supplementation can modulate inflammation by decreasing the production of proinflammatory cytokines. When nine young healthy subjects consumed 18 g of fish-oil concentrate per day (to provide ~2.75g EPA and 1.85 g DHA per day) for 6 weeks, IL-1β and TNF-α production by PBMC decreased by 43% (statistically significant) and 22% (statistically not significant), respectively *(30)*. Production of IL-1β and TNF-α decreased even further, by 61 and 40%, (both statistically significant compared with the baseline) 10 weeks after fish-oil supplementation was ended. Twenty weeks after the end of supplementation, the production of both cytokines returned to baseline levels. Even a more modest level of n-3 fatty acid consumption from dietary sources, rather than from a supplement, had a significant impact on the production of proinflammatory cytokines. Consumption of 1.23 g EPA and DHA per day from a diet high in fish for 6 mo resulted in a significant decrease in the production of IL-1β and IL-6 by PBMC in adults compared with those who consumed diets low in fish (0.27 g EPA and DHA per day *(31)*). In patients with RA, consumption of 130 mg/kg per day of n-3 fatty acids, for 26 weeks, decreased serum levels of IL-1β at 18 and 22 weeks after supplementation compared with those at baseline *(32)*. An inhibitory effect of fish oil on serum TNF-α concentrations was not demonstrated in this study as serum TNF-α levels increased from baseline in both fish-oil supplemented and placebo (corn oil) groups. However, changes in levels of proinflammatory cytokines at the site of inflammation, such as synovial tissue, may have provided more valuable information regarding regulation of proinflammatory cytokines by n-3 fatty acids in RA. These findings suggest that increased consumption of n-3 fatty acid from either dietary sources or supplements can influence the efficacy of anti-TNF antibody therapy. There is no study available yet in which the interaction between n-3 fatty acids and the efficacy of treatment with infliximab or adalimumab has been investigated. This is most likely owing to the short history of anti-TNF-α therapies.

5. DISEASE-MODIFYING ANTI-RHEUMATIC DRUGS

The bioavailability of methotrexate is greatly influenced by the concurrent consumption of food. Dupuis et al. *(33)* examined the bioavailability of oral methotrexate in 14 patients with juvenile RA in the fasting and fed states. The maximum serum methotrexate concentration was significantly lower after oral administration in the fed state (0.65 vs 0.39 µmol/L in fasting vs fed states, respectively), and it took longer to reach the maximum serum concentration (0.94 vs 1.32 hours in fasting vs fed states, respectively). The bioavailability of methotrexate decreased approx 20% when it was administered in the fed state.

5.1. Folate Status and Supplementation in Methtotrexate Treatment

Methotrexante is a known folate antagonist that inhibits dihydrofolate reducatase. It may also influence several other steps in folate metabolism and cause cellular depletion of folate and increased homocysteine levels. In fact, folate deficiency frequently occurs in patients with RA, which is further worsened by methotrexate therapy. A persistent increase in plasma homocysteine concentrations was also observed in patients treated with methotrexate *(4,34,35)*. Toxic effects associated with methotrexate therapy have been reported in 30 to 90% of patients; adverse effects are the main reason for discontinuing therapy. Toxic effects include GI intolerance, hematological abnormalities, alopecia, hepatotoxicity, and pulmonary toxicity *(35)*. A low dose of folate supplementation has been reported to reduce the side effects of methotrexate therapy. In a randomized, double-blind, placebo-controlled study, Morgan et al. *(35)* investigated the effect of weekly supplementation of 5 mg or 27.5 mg of folic acid on the toxicity and efficacy of low-dose methotrexate therapy in 79 patients with RA. Folic acid at either dose did not affect the efficacy as judged by joint indices and patient and physician assessment of disease. Folic acid-supplemented groups had significantly lower toxicity scores (duration of toxic events × intensity × clinical severity factor per 4 weeks in the protocol). Among 28 patients in the placebo group, dietary folate was negatively correlated with toxicity score. Negligible toxic effects were observed when dietary folate intake exceeded 400 μg per day. Hoekstra et al. *(36)* reported that the addition of folate to methotrexate treatment was strongly related to the lack of hepatotoxicity. In a 48-week randomized, placebo-controlled, multicenter trial, 411 patients with RA receiving methotrexate therapy were given 1 mg per day of folic acid, 2.5 mg per week folinic acid, or a placebo. An increase in transaminase activity was reduced significantly by folates. Concomitant use of NSAIDs was associated with increased efficacy. Ortiz et al. *(37)* compared the results from seven double-blind, randomized, placebo-controlled, clinical trials, in which patients with RA were treated with a low dose of methotrexate (< 20 mg per week) concurrently with folate supplementation. A 79% reduction in GI side effects was observed with folic acid supplementation. These studies suggest a protective effect of folate supplementation in reducing toxic effects (hepatotoxicity and GI abnormalities) associated with methotrexate therapy.

5.2. Interaction of Glutamine With Methotrexate

Glutamine is another nutrient that has been reported to have a significant interaction with methotrexate *(38–40)*. Charland et al. *(38)* reported that glutamine increases systemic methotrexate concentrations and decreases renal clearance of the drug. Animals on a 3% glutamine-supplemented diet for 35 days had a 25% lower mean methotrexate total serum clearance and 65% lower renal methotrexate elimination compared with animals on a control diet (3% glycine diet). An increased methotrexate concentration with glutamine supplementation may increase the risk for methotrexate toxicity if the methotrexate dose is not adjusted. On the other hand, Fox et al. *(39)* showed that a glutamine-supplemented elemental diet decreased intestinal injury and bacterial translocation in animals suffering from enterocolitis after methotrexate treatment. Lin et al. *(40)* reported that a glutamine supplemented diet (4 or 8%) improved the immune function of animals receiving a single methotrexate treatment.

6. NUTRITIONAL STATUS AND DIETARY MANAGEMENT

Maintaining an adequate nutritional status is important in order to achieve the best possible prognosis for patients with rheumatic diseases *(41,42)*. Rheumatic diseases are chronic inflammatory conditions that put patients at higher risk of oxidative stress; therefore, antioxidant nutrient requirements may increase. Medications can deplete or cause lower levels of certain nutrients. Methotrexate treatment decreases folate levels and corticosteroid treatment can cause low calcium and zinc status. Side effects of NSAIDs, such as ulceration and GI bleeding, can cause iron deficiency in patients. Symptoms of rheumatic diseases such as pain and joint problems may lower appetites or limit patients from getting access to a variety of fresh ingredients.

Table 1
Commonly Used Drugs in Rheumatoid Arthritis and Their Interactions With Nutrients

Drugs (Brand Names)	Interaction With Nutrients	Recommendations
NSAIDs Naproxen (Aleve, Naprelan), Ibuprofen (Advil, Motrin, Excedrin), Nabumetone (Relafen)	• Long-term administration may cause GI ulceration. • Absorption is delayed in fed state. • Long-term fish oil supplement can reduce the use of NSAIDs.	• Take with food to reduce GI irritation.
Celecoxib (Celebrex)	• Minimally affected by the concomitant food intake.	
DMARDs Methotrexate (Methotrexate, Rheumatrex)	• Bioavailability is greatly decreased with concomitant food intake. • Folate antagonist. Cause cellular depletion of folate and increased homocysteine levels. • Glutamine increases systemic methotrexate concentrations and decreases renal clearance of the drug.	• Folate supplementation can reduce side effects. • Ensure adequate vitamin B_{12} status to prevent the masking of vitamin B_{12} deficiency by folate supplementation.
Corticosteroid Dexamethasone (Decadron, Hexadron), prednisone (Deltasone)	• Increase appetite and weight. • Impair calcium absorption. • Cause increased risk for osteoporosis.	• Adequate intake of calcium and vitamin D should be encouraged.
Anticytokine Infliximab Adalimumab etanercept	• Fish oil supplement could affect the efficacy of anticytokine therapy owing to its effect on the production of proinflammatory cytokine production. However, there is no evidence available yet.	

DMARDs, disease-modifying anti-rheumatic drugs; GI, gastrointestinal; NSAIDs, nonsteroidal anti-inflammatory drugs

7. RECOMMENDATIONS

In order to assess all potential drug–drug and drug–nutrient interactions, health care providers should obtain a complete list of medications and dietary supplements. Concomitant consumption of food with medication can greatly influence absorption and efficacy of drugs. Specific instruction for the timing of medication is important for timely action and maximal absorption of drugs.

Folate deficiency is frequently observed in patients with rheumatic disease, especially those treated with methotrexate. Lower folate status can adversely impact toxic effects of methotrexate therapy, resulting in discontinuation of the therapy. Patients should be encouraged to consume a balanced diet to at least meet the recommended dietary allowance for folate (400 μg per day for adults) to minimize side effects of methotrexate. When it is hard to achieve proper levels of folate from the diet, folate supplementation, at an individually adjusted level, should be considered to provide some protection from toxicity of methotrexate therapy.

Evidence suggests that fish-oil supplementation can provide clinical benefit in improving symptoms associated with RA and in reducing the use of NSAIDs in patients with RA. However, levels or ranges of n-3 fatty acids that provide consistent clinical effects are not well defined. Dietary fish intake should be taken into account and changes in symptoms as well as use of NSAIDs should be closely monitored when fish-oil supplementation is considered.

Several factors can put rheumatic patients at higher risk for infections. Dietary fish-oil supplementation can suppress the immune functions. Anti-TNF therapy can increase the susceptibility to bacterial infections. Increased oxidative stress can result in lower immune functions. Strategies to maintain proper immune functions should be ensured. Drug–nutrient interactions of commonly used drugs in rheumatic diseases are listed in Table 1.

REFERENCES

1. Utermohlen V. Diet, nutrition, and drug interactions. In: Shils ME, Olson JA, Shike M, Ross AC (eds). Modern Nutrition in Health and Disease, 9th ed. Williams and Wilkins, Baltimore, MD 1999, PP. 1621–1641.
2. Fleisher D, Li C, Zhou Y, Pao LH, Karim A. Drug, meal and formulation interactions influencing drug absorption after oral administration. Clinical implications. Clin Pharmacokinet 1999;36:233–254.
3. Calder PC. n-3 polyunsaturated fatty acids, inflammation, and inflammatory diseases. Am J Clin Nutr 2006;83:1505S–1519S.
4. Haagsma CJ, Blom HJ, van Riel PL, et al. Influence of sulphasalazine, methotrexate, and the combination of both on plasma homocysteine concentrations in patients with rheumatoid arthritis. Ann Rheum Dis 1999;58:79–84.
5. Reid IR, Veale AG, France JT. Glucocorticoid osteoporosis. J Asthma 1994;31:7–18.
6. O'Dell JR. Therapeutic strategies for rheumatoid arthritis. N Engl J Med 2004;350:2591–2602.
7. Paulson SK, Vaughn MB, Jessen SM, et al. Pharmacokinetics of celecoxib after oral administration in dogs and humans: effect of food and site of absorption. J Pharmacol Exp Ther 2001;297:638–645.
8. Klueglich M, Ring A, Scheuerer S, et al. Ibuprofen extrudate, a novel, rapidly dissolving ibuprofen formulation: relative bioavailability compared to ibuprofen lysinate and regular ibuprofen, and food effect on all formulations. J Clin Pharmacol 2005;45:1055–1061.
9. Pargal A, Kelkar MG, Nayak PJ. The effect of food on the bioavailability of ibuprofen and flurbiprofen from sustained release formulations. Biopharm Drug Dispos 1996;17:511–519.

10. von Schrader HW, Buscher G, Dierdorf D, Mugge H, Wolf D. Nabumetone—a novel anti-inflammatory drug: the influence of food, milk, antacids, and analgesics on bioavailability of single oral doses. Int J Clin Pharmacol Ther Toxicol 1983;21:311–321.
11. Kojima F, Kato S, Kawai S. Prostaglandin E synthase in the pathophysiology of arthritis. Fundam Clin Pharmacol 2005;19:255–261.
12. Egg D, Gunther R, Herold M, Kerschbaumer F. [Prostaglandins E2 and F2 alpha concentrations in the synovial fluid in rheumatoid and traumatic knee joint diseases]. Z Rheumatol 1980;39:170–175.
13. Beharka A, Wu D, Serafini M, Meydani S. Mechanism of vitamin E inhibition of cyclooxygenase activity in macrophages from old mice: role of peroxynitrite. Free Rad Biol Med 2002;32:503–511.
14. Geusens P, Wouters C, Nijs J, Jiang Y, Dequeker J. Long-term effect of omega-3 fatty acid supplementation in active rheumatoid arthritis. A 12-month, double-blind, controlled study. Arthritis Rheum 1994;37:824–829.
15. Fortin PR, Lew RA, Liang MH, et al. Validation of a meta-analysis: the effects of fish oil in rheumatoid arthritis. J Clin Epidemiol 1995;48:1379–1390.
16. MacLean C, Mojica W, SC M, et al. Effects of Omega-3 Fatty Acids on Lipids and Glycemin Control in Type II Diabetes and the Metabolic Syndrome and on Inflammatory Bowel Disease, Rheumatoid Arthritis, Renal Disease, Systemic Lupus Erythematosus, and Osteoporosis. Agency for Healthcare Research and Quality,Rockville, MD, 2004.
17. Cleland LG, Caughey GE, James MJ, Proudman SM. Reduction of cardiovascular risk factors with longterm fish oil treatment in early rheumatoid arthritis. J Rheumatol 2006;33:1973–1979.
18. Irons R, Anderson MJ, Zhang M, Fritsche KL. Dietary fish oil impairs primary host resistance against Listeria monocytogenes more than the immunological memory response. J Nutr 2003;133:1163–1169.
19. Byleveld PM, Pang GT, Clancy RL, Roberts DC. Fish oil feeding delays influenza virus clearance and impairs production of interferon-gamma and virus-specific immunoglobulin A in the lungs of mice. J Nutr 1999;129:328–335.
20. Meydani SN, Meydani M, Verdon CP, Shapiro AA, Blumberg JB, Hayes KC. Vitamin E supplementation suppresses prostaglandine E_2 synthesis and enhances the immune response of aged mice. Mech Ageing Dev 1986;34:191–201.
21. Wu D, Mura C, Beharka AA, et al. Age-associated increase in PGE_2 synthesis and COX activity in murine macrophages is reversed by vitamin E. Am J Physiol 1998;275:C661–C668.
22. Abate A, Yang G, Dennery PA, Oberle S, Schroder H. Synergistic inhibition of cyclooxygenase-2 expression by vitamin E and aspirin. Free Radic Biol Med 2000;29:1135–1142.
23. Edmonds SE, Winyard PG, Guo R, et al. Putative analgesic activity of repeated oral doses of vitamin E in the treatment of rheumatoid arthritis. Results of a prospective placebo controlled double blind trial. Ann Rheum Dis 1997;56:649–655.
24. Brennan FM, Maini RN, Feldmann M. Role of pro-inflammatory cytokines in rheumatoid arthritis. Springer Semin Immunopathol 1998;20:133–147.
25. Eastgate JA, Symons JA, Wood NC, Grinlinton FM, di Giovine FS, Duff GW. Correlation of plasma interleukin 1 levels with disease activity in rheumatoid arthritis. Lancet 1988;2:706–709.
26. Dinarelllo CA, Moldawer LL. Proinflammatory and Anti-inflammatory Cytokines in Rheumatoid Arthritis: A Primer for Clinicians, 2nd ed. Amgen, Thousand Oaks, CA, 2000.
27. Feldmann M, Maini RN. Anti-TNF alpha therapy of rheumatoid arthritis: what have we learned– Annu Rev Immunol 2001;19:163–196.
28. Maini RN, Feldmann M. How does infliximab work in rheumatoid arthritis– Arthritis Res 2002;4(suppl 2):S22–S28.
29. Winthrop KL. Risk and prevention of tuberculosis and other serious opportunistic infections associated with the inhibition of tumor necrosis factor. Nat Clin Pract Rheumatol 2006;2:602–610.
30. Endres S, Ghorbani R, Kelley VE, et al. The effect of dietary supplementation with n-3 polyunsaturated fatty acids on the synthesis of interleukin-1 and tumor necrosis factor by mononuclear cells. N Engl J Med 1989;320:265–271.
31. Meydani SN, Lichtenstein AH, Cornwall S, et al. Immunologic effects of national cholesterol education panel Step-2 diets with and without fish-derived n-3 fatty acid enrichment. J Clin Invest 1993;92:105–113.

32. Kremer JM, Lawrence DA, Petrillo GF, et al. Effects of high-dose fish oil on rheumatoid arthritis after stopping nonsteroidal antiinflammatory drugs. Clinical and immune correlates. Arthritis Rheum 1995;38:1107–1114.
33. Dupuis LL, Koren G, Silverman ED, Laxer RM. Influence of food on the bioavailability of oral methotrexate in children. J Rheumatol 1995;22:1570–1573.
34. Berkun Y, Levartovsky D, Rubinow A, et al. Methotrexate related adverse effects in patients with rheumatoid arthritis are associated with the A1298C polymorphism of the MTHFR gene. Ann Rheum Dis 2004;63:1227–1231.
35. Morgan SL, Baggott JE, Vaughn WH, et al. Supplementation with folic acid during methotrexate therapy for rheumatoid arthritis. A double-blind, placebo-controlled trial. Ann Intern Med 1994;121:833–841.
36. Hoekstra M, van Ede AE, Haagsma CJ, et al. Factors associated with toxicity, final dose, and efficacy of methotrexate in patients with rheumatoid arthritis. Ann Rheum Dis 2003;62:423–426.
37. Ortiz Z, Shea B, Suarez Almazor M, Moher D, Wells G, Tugwell P. Folic acid and folinic acid for reducing side effects in patients receiving methotrexate for rheumatoid arthritis. Cochrane Database Syst Rev 2000:CD000951.
38. Charland SL, Bartlett DL, Torosian MH. A significant methotrexate-glutamine pharmacokinetic interaction. Nutrition 1995;11:154–158.
39. Fox AD, Kripke SA, De Paula J, Berman JM, Settle RG, Rombeau JL. Effect of a glutamine-supplemented enteral diet on methotrexate-induced enterocolitis. JPEN J Parenter Enteral Nutr 1988;12:325–331.
40. Lin CM, Abcouwer SF, Souba WW. Effect of dietary glutamate on chemotherapy-induced immunosuppression. Nutrition 1999;15:687–696.
41. Rennie KL, Hughes J, Lang R, Jebb SA. Nutritional management of rheumatoid arthritis: a review of the evidence. J Hum Nutr Diet 2003;16:97–109.
42. Kamanli A, Naziroglu M, Aydilek N, Hacievliyagil C. Plasma lipid peroxidation and antioxidant levels in patients with rheumatoid arthritis. Cell Biochem Funct 2004;22:53–57.

5 Exercise in Rheumatic Diseases

Lindsay M. Bearne and Mike V. Hurley

Summary

- Physical activity and exercise are safe and beneficial for the vast majority of people, including those with rheumatic disease.
- Exercise aids in the prevention and management of chronic ill health, including rheumatic conditions, coronary heart disease, diabetes, strokes, certain cancers, and improves psychological well-being.
- People should aim to do 30 minutes of moderate activity at least five times per week to gain health benefits.
- Prior to beginning an exercise regimen, patients should establish current physical abilities and activity levels, and then set realistic, appropriate goals that "nudge the boundaries" and can be monitored regularly.
- Within reason, the more exercise a person can do, the better, but only within the boundaries of maintaining safety and comfort.

Key Words: Arthritis; exercise; health benefits; physical activity

1. INTRODUCTION

The human body is designed to promote movement and function. All of the structures that comprise the joints—muscles, articular cartilage, ligaments, tendons, nerves, and bones—respond positively to movement. Additionally, physical activity has wider health benefits: improvement in general physical health; heart, respiratory, and vascular functions; prevention of certain cancers; weight control; improvement in sexual and mental health, self-confidence, self-esteem, independence, and social interactions.

Decreased mobility, on the other hand, contributes to muscle weakness, fatigue, joint stiffness, cartilage atrophy, loss of bone density, and a reduction in movement control, all of which can lead to pain, dysfunction, and disability. Moreover, reduced function and immobility are major risk factors for many acute and chronic conditions—diabetes, heart disease, high blood pressure, depression, and obesity. Therefore, an adequate level of habitual physical activity is vital for everyone, including people with arthritis.

Physical activity is defined as any bodily movement produced by skeletal muscles and resulting in energy expenditure *(1)*. Exercise is a subcategory of physical activity. It is planned, structured, and repetitive, and produces an improvement or maintenance of one or more facets of physical fitness (e.g., cardiovascular fitness, muscle strength

From: *Nutrition and Health: Nutrition and Rheumatic Disease*
Edited by: L. A. Coleman © Humana Press, Totowa, NJ

and endurance, flexibility and body composition) and psychological well-being *(2)*. Historically, exercise science investigated healthy, active, young males or athletes. Consequently, much of the information about fitness testing and the recommendations for exercise prescription to improve physical fitness indicated intensive exercise regimens were needed. However, studies are beginning to show that less fit, healthy people or people with musculoskeletal impairment and rheumatic disease do not need to participate in intense exercise programs to obtain health benefits *(2,3)*.

For people with rheumatic conditions, physical activity is as important as it is for the healthy population. Maintaining activity retains and restores physiological and pyschosocial function and health, so exercise forms an essential element for the management of rheumatic conditions.

This chapter provides a brief overview of the importance of exercise in the management of common rheumatic conditions. Our aim is to present general advice regarding exercise, and to show how exercise should be adapted to address an individual's specific problems and goals. It is important to remember that all patients with rheumatic disease are different, starting from a different baseline and with different needs.

2. EXERCISE SAFETY

For the vast majority of people with rheumatic disease, exercise can be performed safely. Nonetheless, safety is always a concern that should be discussed with patients, without raising (usually unnecessary) fears and anxiety. General advice is for patients to try exercising, start gently, and build slowly. People with joint problems or not used to exercising should always seek professional advice prior to starting an exercise regimen. Most people will find benefits, without adverse side effects, that will far outweigh the risks of inactivity.

Many individuals associate activity with pain and believe that this indicates that the activity is damaging their joints; consequently, they begin to avoid physical activity, which leads to muscle and general fitness de-conditioning. However, there is a growing body of research suggesting that exercise is safe for people with rheumatic conditions.

Early fears that exercise would exacerbate the symptoms of rheumatic disease, particularly in people with inflammatory arthritis, have been challenged by research demonstrating improvements in aerobic fitness, muscle strength, functional status, and disability following dynamic exercise programs *(4,5)*. Furthermore, these improvements were achieved with no exacerbation in joint symptoms or increase in biochemical markers of disease activity *(6,7)*. Additionally, no detrimental effects on joint structure in those with mild to moderate rheumatic disease have been identified *(8,9)*. Therefore, with a few exceptions (e.g., those people with severe joint damage secondary to inflammatory disease), exercise is safe for people with rheumatic conditions *(10,11)*.

It is important that patients are advised that initially, they may experience some discomfort during or following exercise. Advice for managing the increased symptoms and the resumption of exercise (*see* Patient Point 1) is needed. Teaching the principles of pacing and joint protection may be useful in preventing unnecessary pain that sometimes results from physical activity, which can discourage an individual from persevering with an exercise program. "Rest–activity cycling" encourages people to plan the time spent performing physical activities (pacing) or maintaining one joint position for a long time (joint protection) and intersperse the activity with periods of rest, stretching, or less strenuous activities, so that the risk of joint pain is reduced but the level of activity or exercise is maintained.

Patient Point 1: General Exercise Advice

There are a few basic principles that need to be remembered when completing any form of exercise.

- **Establish your current abilities**: Assess your usual activity level by recording your physical activity during a defined period (e.g., 2 days)
- **Goal setting**: Set realistic, achievable goals, deciding exactly what activity you will do, when and where you will do it and then focus on fulfilling these goals. Once these goals have been achieved, set more challenging targets
- **Safety**: Always ensure you are stable and safe when doing any exercise. Wear clothing that is appropriate to the climate and type of exercise you are doing (usually loose clothing is preferable). Complete a few warm-up exercises to get your body ready to exercise—this may include some stretching or flexibility exercises, too.
- **Progression**: Start a new exercise slowly and cautiously. Progress slowly, gradually increasing the time, frequency, and intensity of exercising, *do a little more each time*.
- **Work hard**: Work within your capabilities but near to your maximum without causing prolonged pain. Try to *nudge the boundaries* of your capabilities.
- **Pace yourself**: The exercises do not have to be done in one session, a few shorter exercises sessions are just good as one strenuous session. It is the cumulative total of exercise each day that is important.
- **Monitor yourself**: Post-exercise soreness is not uncommon when you start exercising or are returning to an exercise program— this generally starts after exercise and can last for a couple of days. This is not harmful. It is just your body getting used to working! However, if an activity causes pain, discomfort, or swelling for more than a couple of days, rest for a few days. As the pain or swelling settles, resume exercising gently, gradually building up the exercises as before and taking care to monitor the quality of the exercises. Leave out any specific activities that caused pain initially then add them back into the exercise program cautiously.

---

3. INITIATING AN EXERCISE REGIMEN

For the vast majority of people, exercise and physical activity carries little, if any, risk of harm if it progresses gradually. People with joint problems or those not used to participating in regular exercise should discuss what, when, and how they should exercise with a health care professional (physical or exercise therapist, nurse, physician). A person's current activity level, fitness, and general health should be considered when setting realistic and achievable goals. The level of exercising and these goals should be low at first and then gradually increased, for comfort, safety, and to prevent the patient from becoming disillusioned if he or she does not quickly reach unrealistic targets.

3.1. Assessment

Existing levels of physical activity can be assessed using measurement tools such as the Minnesota Leisure Time Physical Activity Questionnaire *(12)* or the Rapid Assessment of Physical Activity *(13)*. Alternatively, a simple way to estimate current activity levels is to keep a record of daily activities in an "activity diary." For more information see American College of Sports Medicine guidelines *(2,14)*.

An assessment of an individual's rheumatic disease (e.g., pain, inflammation, fatigue) and the extent of specific musculoskeletal dysfunction (weakness, loss of range of movement, proprioception, and balance impairment) can also be determined, using disease-specific, validated measures, before beginning exercise (e.g., 28 joint count for the assessment of tenderness and inflammation in patients with rheumatoid arthritis [RA; *(15)*]). However, the need to assess cardiorespiratory fitness depends on an individual's cardiovascular risk (*see* Practitioner Point 1). In general, men under age 50 and women under age 40 who have more than one risk factor should have a formal assessment of cardiorespiratory function before beginning a program involving moderate intensity exercise or physical activity.

Practitioner Point 1: Assessing Cardiovascular Risk

Men over age 50 and women over age 40 who have two or more of the following risk factors for cardiovascular disease should have their cardiorespiratory function assessed before undertaking a moderate exercise program:

- Hypertension (blood pressure > 160/90 mmHg)
- Serum cholesterol > 240 mg/dL (6.2 mmol/L)
- Cigarette smoking
- Diabetes mellitus
- Family history

For people who require cardiorespiratory testing:

- Maximal oxygen uptake ($\dot{V}O2_{max}$) testing (e.g., field, treadmill, cycle ergonomers, or step tests) offers high sensitivity in the diagnosis of coronary disease.
- In a clinical setting, submaximal testing may be easier to perform. These determine the heart rate response to a submaximal work rate from which a prediction of aerobic fitness (i.e., maximal oxygen uptake ($\dot{V}O2_{max}$) can be made.
- Several submaximal cardiorespiratory tests have been validated in people with rheumatic disease:
  - 5-minute walk test *(61)*
  - one-stage treadmill test *(62)*
  - 10-m shuttle walk test *(63)*

3.2. Self-Monitoring

People need to appreciate the difference between moderate and vigorous exercise so that they can exercise at an intensity that is suitable for their level of fitness. There are simple measures that can be used to gauge whether they are exercising appropriately.

The Rating of Perceived Exercise requires individuals to rate their perception of intensity of exercise on a 15-point scale. This scale relates well to the physiological and psychological responses to exercise *(16,17)*. In the initial stages of an exercise program, adhering to the "talk test" (a person should be able to carry on a conversation with someone else while exercising) indicates an appropriate intensity of exercise *(18)*.

Once baseline information has been collected and the goals of the exercise program identified between the health practitioner and the patient, a series of exercises may be prescribed and agreed on to achieve these aims. The frequency and intensity of exercise required must also be considered.

4. BENEFITS OF EXERCISE

Exercise has many benefits for patients with rheumatic disease, including improvements in movement, strength, endurance, proprioception, cardiovascular fitness, and function.

4.1. Exercise for Improving Joint Movement (see Patient Point 2, Practitioner Point 2)

An adequate range of motion in all joints is needed to maintain function, balance, and agility. Loss of joint movement is often associated with pain, muscle weakness, functional limitations, and increased risk of falls. In arthritic joints, restriction of movement may result from the following:

- capsular distension from increased amounts of synovial fluid or synovial tissue;
- contraction of the capsule, periarticular ligaments, or tendons; or
- loss of articular cartilage with varying amounts of fibrosis or osseous ankylosis.

Exercise and physical activity can help to reverse or minimize these effects, and intuitively, people realize that movement is beneficial for joints. However, concern and confusion may result if physical activity causes joint pain; even more so if rest eases it. In the absence of adequate education and advice, patients may interpret this as movement damaging the joint and surmise that reducing activity will prolong the life of the joint and modify (minimize) the disease process.

In fact, movement helps reduce joint effusion *(19)* and protects the smooth joint cartilage covering the bones involved in articulation. Regular motion, compression, and decompression are required to stimulate remodeling and repair *(20)*. Each day, weight-bearing and non-weight-bearing exercises and activities that move a joint through its full range of movement are necessary to maintain cartilage health *(21)*. Movement maintains and restores adequate compliance and flexibility of the periarticular structures (joint capsule, ligaments, tendons, muscles) which are important for protecting joints from damaging stresses.

Stretching and flexibility exercises are an important component of disease management in people with arthritis *(4,22)*. People with rheumatic conditions should perform stretching exercises at least two to three times per week. However, some rheumatic conditions, such as ankylosing spondylitis (AS), would benefit from patients performing stretching or flexibility exercises more regularly to prevent loss of spinal and thorax mobility, and hence breathing problems, which is a complication associated with AS *(11,23)*.

Stretches should be performed in a slow, controlled manner (without "bouncing") and be specific to a joint or muscle group *(24)*. Stretches should be performed after "warm-up" exercises, which are low-intensity exercises that prepare the body for more vigorous activity by increasing circulation, body temperature, and tissue extensibility. By doing so, warm-up exercises help to minimize the risk of musculoskeletal injury (e.g., muscle tears or joint sprains). Each stretch should be held for 10 to 30 seconds at the end of the range of movement and gradually progressed to greater joint range. Stretches may produce mild discomfort but should not cause pain. Joints that are hypermobile, deformed or subluxed, or vulnerable to injury as a result of effusion are easily overstretched and should be protected and exercised with care.

Patient Point 2: Stretching Exercises

Stretching or flexibility exercises improve joint mobility. There are several guidelines that should be followed when stretching:

- Stretching exercises should be completed after some **gentle warm-up exercises**. These are low-intensity exercises that prepare the body for exercise by increasing body temperature and increasing the extensibility of the tissues, thus preventing injury.
- All stretches should be performed in a **slow, controlled manner**.
- **Hold each stretch for 10 to 30 seconds** (don't "bounce") at the end of the joint range of movement.
- Complete stretching exercises **several times per week**, unless otherwise directed.
- Stretching exercises **may produce mild discomfort** but not pain.

4.2. Exercise for Improving Strength and Endurance (see Practitioner Point 3)

Inactivity leads to muscle weakness and wasting owing to a reduction in muscle fiber size, capillary density, and deposition of fat and connective tissue in muscles that are often not used enough *(25–27)*. Considerable weakness has been shown in people with early arthritic disease *(28)* as well as in those with long-standing disease *(5,6,29)*. Therefore, it is important for those with rheumatic disease to try to preserve or enhance their muscle strength by remaining as active as possible and/or completing strengthening exercises.

Practitioner Point 2: Stretching

There are several types of stretching exercises that can be prescribed.

- **Passive stretching exercises** are performed by a therapists/helper/carer to the end of range. The terminal position is held for an extended period of time (10–30 seconds).
- **Active assisted stretching** is performed by the individual with therapist/helper assisting with terminal stretch. The terminal position is held for an extended period of time (10–30 seconds).
- **Active stretching** is performed by the individual through full range of movement. The static stretch is held at or beyond initial limit to stretch periarticular structures and muscles to the point of mild discomfort (for 10–30 seconds).
- **Proprioceptive neuromuscular facilitation/muscle energy techniques** involve a combination of alternating contraction and relaxation of the agonist/antagonist muscle through the available range of motion to gradually increase range of movement.
- **Ballistic stretches** use repetitive bouncing movements to producing momentum that creates a muscle stretch. This can produce muscle soreness if the forces produced by the bouncing movement are too great. These are NOT suitable for patients with rheumatic conditions.

Practitioner Point 3: Muscle Strengthening

There are several types of muscle actions that can be used when prescribing strengthening exercises.

- **Isometric exercise** is when a muscle contraction occurs without joint movement. Therefore there is no change in the length of the muscle but tension increases.
- **Isotonic exercise** is when there is constant loading of the muscle with a variable velocity.
- **Isokinetic exercise** occurs when a muscle contraction is maintained with a constant joint angular velocity by accommodating resistance.
- **Isotonic exercise** and **isokinetic exercise** could occur with concentric muscle action (when the muscle shortens) or eccentric muscle action (when the muscle lengthens).

Any changes in muscle force production in the initial stages of training (6–10 weeks) are attributed to neural changes that result in a higher numbers of motor units being recruited and/or a higher rate of motor unit firing *(64)*. As the activation of the agonists is increased, a reduction of the antagonists occurs and coactivation of the synergists is improved.

As training continues further strength gains are achieved through hypertrophy of the muscle fibers, although an extended period of exercise is needed for training induced alterations in tendon, ligament, cartilage, and bone to occur.

Fortunately, the neuromuscular system has a considerable ability to adapt, and with careful planning and execution, rehabilitation of muscle wasting and weakness *and* the associated loss of function and disability can be achieved by applying different movements and resistance exercises (loading) to muscle groups *(6,29,30)*.

Different types of muscle actions (isometric, isotonic, and isokinetic) can be used to improve muscle functioning. The principle of "overload"—when the training load exceeds the daily load levels—should also be employed to achieve the changes in the structure and function of the muscles needed. Additionally, the frequency and a progressive increase in the overall amount (volume) of each training session are important variables to optimize training stimuli (specificity of training).

Strength-training specificity is important to consider, as different types of strengthening exercises produce different results. Strength training can be divided into three main components:

1. To increase the overall maximum strength of the muscle (i.e., increase the highest possible force a muscle or muscle group can produce during one maximal voluntary contraction) high loads (resistance) must be used. Typically, the maximum load an individual can lift once through range before fatiguing is determined (i.e,. 1 repetition maximum [RM]). The individual then exercises using a load of 60 to 85% of 1 RM, repeated three to eight times per set. This hypertrophic strength training increases muscle fiber size and is aimed at preventing muscle wasting and increasing muscle mass.
2. To increase power or explosive strength (the ability to produce a force as rapidly as possible or to move a load at a high velocity) lower loads (between 30 and 60% 1 RM) and 5–10 repetitions per set are needed but the contraction/movement velocities should be much higher than for typical strength training. This type of training can be used to improve functional activities such as standing up from a chair.
3. To improve endurance (the ability to sustain a medium or low submaximal contraction or complete repeated submaximal contractions for a long duration) use light loads (0-30% or 20-60% of 1 RM) but a high number of repetitions (10–15 repetitions per set). This type of exercise improves repetitive activities such as stair climbing, or enhances the ability to hold static postures for a long time.

Prescription of resistance exercises for patients with rheumatic disease should be based on careful assessment of an individual's current motor function (i.e., strength/endurance, etc.), rheumatic condition (i.e., level of disease activity) and consideration of the aims of the exercise program so that the appropriate activity, load, frequency, and intensity of exercise can be determined. Often, a mixture of exercise types may be needed to tackle weakness in many muscle groups that frequently occurs in systemic rheumatic conditions. Functional exercises such as sit to stand and step ups can be completed easily at home and the overload principle can be applied by progressively increasing the number of repetitions. Further progression can be achieved by lowering the height of a chair (sit to stand) or increasing the height of the step (step ups).

Exercise programs that incorporate strengthening are effective in people with rheumatic disease and in people with osteoarthritis (OA); progressive resistance exercise produces modest strength increases, which are important to people as they result in better function and performance of everyday activities *(31)*. This is mirrored in patients with RA and improvements in muscle strength following dynamic exercise programs at a variety of intensity levels have been shown in patients with long standing RA *(4,6)*, those with newly diagnosed RA *(28)*, and those with poorly controlled disease (i.e., those with a flare up of their disease *(32)*). These improvements, in turn, may allow easier performance of activities of daily living (e.g., sit to stand, walking) and maintenance of functional independence.

4.3. Exercise to Improve Proprioception

Proprioception, the awareness of ones body in space, is impaired by rheumatic disease as a result of altered joint biomechanics, muscle dysfunction, and articular destruction *(6,33)*. There are functional consequences of proprioceptive loss, such as altered gait in lower limb arthritis, causing increased ground reaction forces and exacerbating the arthritic process and symptoms *(33,34)*, and poor limb positioning during positioning tasks and an increased risk of falls.

Improvements in proprioceptive acuity have been demonstrated in some patients with arthritis following short exercise programs that include specific balance training (e.g., walking on a narrow line, balance board training, single-leg stand exercises with eyes open and closed *(33,34)*).

Some have suggested that a general functional and strengthening exercise program in patients with arthritis may be as effective as specific balance and proprioceptive exercises at improving proprioceptive awareness *(24)*, although it seems sensible to include specific balance training in those individuals who are particularly at risk of falling or sustaining serious injuries from falls, such as people with osteoporosis *(35)*.

4.4. Exercise for Modifying Risk Factors for Progression

Exercise has important effects on body composition that may alter the development and progression of some rheumatic diseases.

Obesity is a major risk factor in the development of lower limb OA. For every 1lb in body weight, the overall force across the knee in a single-leg stance increases 2 to 3lb *(36)*. Epidemiological studies indicate that low levels of physical activity are associated with greater body weight when compared to more active individuals *(37)*. These studies indicate that the percentage of body fat stored is greater in less active individuals and they are at increased risk of gaining weight, and therefore, developing OA. Consequently, dynamic exercise, through its effect on weight regulation and composition, in combination with appropriate caloric restriction, has a major role to play in modifying the risk of OA development and disease progression *(38)*. It is important to encourage individuals to appreciate the impact weight gain has on arthritis and obtain appropriate nutritional advice to assist weight control in those at risk.

In people with RA, the normal, age-related loss of muscle protein (*sarcopenia*) is accelerated by the inflammatory process, which results in the loss of lean body mass and increased body fat (cachexia). Even successfully treated patients with RA have a body cell mass (muscle and viscera) of 15% less than matched control subjects *(39)* and disease-modifying drug management alone does not improve body composition

(33,34). Exercise acts as an anabolic stimulus that reverses these changes *(30,41)*, thus, combining strengthening and aerobic training helps reverse the catabolic effects of inflammatory disease on muscle.

4.5. Exercise for Health Benefits (see Patient Points 3 and 4 and Practitioner Point 4)

Even when an individual's rheumatic disease is quiescent, exercise will improve their general health. Earlier, we described exercise as a subcategory of physical activity, however, within reason, any physical activity is good, so typical daily physical activities—manual work, walking, gardening, shopping, housework, and so on—can be seen as "informal" exercises that have health benefits.

Practitioner Point 4: NICE Guidelines *(58)*

Recent guidelines from the National Institute of Clinical Excellence (NICE) suggest practitioners should do the following:

- Identify inactive adults and advise them to aim for 30 min of moderate activity at least five times per week.
- Combine activity advice with written information on the benefits of exercise and local opportunities for people with rheumatic disease to be active.
- Provide healthy lifestyle advice and disease self-management techniques to maintain long-term motivation.
- Suggest activities that are accessible, convenient, and enjoyable to the participant—all factors directly related to exercise adherence.
- Recommend exercising in a group to provide important social reinforcement that helps adherence to exercise programs.

The intensity and duration of an activity determines the energy expenditure. The greater the intensity of the exercise, the less duration and frequency is required. Workloads of physical activities can be expressed as an estimation of oxygen uptake using metabolic equivalents. The energy requirements of everyday activities have been calculated so appropriate activities can be selected to take into account the individual's needs, preferences, and circumstances (*see* Table 1 *(42)*).

To attain health benefits, people need to accumulate 30 minutes of physical activity on most days of the week. This could be achieved by one 30-minute brisk walk, or two 15-minute walks, or three 10-minute walks. For those achieving this level of activity, additional benefits may be gained with a longer duration or higher intensity of exercise. However, people should begin exercising cautiously after having identified their current activity level, and gradually (over days and weeks) increase the duration and intensity of the activity. The aim is to "nudge the boundaries" of an individual's capabilities, challenging the individual to gently but gradually move a little further or work a little harder.

Table 1
Examples of Light and Moderate Physical Activities and the Metabolic Equivalents (METs)

Light Activity (~4 kcal/min)		*Moderate Activity (4–7 kcal/min)*	
	MET		MET
Baking	2.4	Cycling: 5.5 mph	4.4
Cooking	3.3	9 mph	6.8
Food shopping	4.2		
Mopping floors	4.2	Walking: 3mph	5.0
Swimming (slow)	4.2	3.5mph	6.1
Vacuuming	4.4	Uneven/hilly ground	5.5
Walking	2 mph = 3.6	Aerobic (low intensity)	6.7
	2.5 mph = 4.4		
		Resistance training (free weights)	5.8
Car washing	4.8		

The metabolic equivalents of activities of daily living.
1 MET is the unit equal to resting metabolic rate and is approx 3.5 mL of oxygen per kilogram body weight *(42)*.[4]
Data from McArdle WD et al Exercise physiology: Energy, Nutrition and Human performance. Baltimore, Williams & Wilkins, 1996, Appendix D

Patient Point 3: Exercise for Physical Health

When your rheumatic disease is quiescent, exercise can still provide health benefits.

- **Agree on goals** with your health care practitioner and integrate activities into everyday life.
- **Aim for 30 minutes** of moderate activity, at least 5 days a week.
- **Walking** is an excellent mode of exercise and it can be easily integrated into everyday life, for example, going for a brisk walk, walking rather than driving, getting off the bus earlier and walking.
- **Aquatic or stationary cycle exercise** may be useful for people with reduced ability to weight bear on the lower limbs.

Walking is the simplest way people can be more active. Walking is a safe, effective, and accessible form of exercise for people with arthritis, which can lead to improved aerobic capacity, strength, and physical performance *(43)*. Walking can be easily integrated into everyday life, and concerns that walking may be harmful for people with arthritis are being revised as impact forces generated by free speed walking are lower than those generated by other forms of exercise *(44)*. Impact forces can be reduced further by wearing training shoes (sneakers) or by placing viscoelastic materials or insoles in shoes *(45)*. However, biomechanical abnormalities, joint instability, or diminished proprioception must be addressed to ensure that faster walking speeds, achieved as pain reduces and function improves, do not increase inappropriate loading on the lower limb joints.

Patient Point 4: Pain Self-Management

Two things that may be helpful if you have pain:

- **Massaging or rubbing** a painful body part is a natural reaction to pain. Gently massaging painful joints or muscles for 5 to 10 minutes is a very effective and safe way to relieve pain.
- **Heat and cold** are often used to reduce pain, relax muscles, improve blood supply, and reduce swelling after activity.

Some people find that heat is most effective at relieving pain. Heat can be produced by commercially available hot packs, or a hot water bottle wrapped in a towel. Heat can also be used to warm up the muscles and joints prior to exercise.

Others find cooling a painful joint most effective for the reduction of inflammation and pain. This can be applied with commercially available cool packs and coolant sprays, or a homemade cool pack (a bag of frozen peas wrapped in a small wet towel).

When applying either heat or cool, position yourself comfortably so the joint to be treated is supported. Place a hot/cold pack on the painful joint for 10 to 15 minutes. The pain relief and muscle relaxation caused by the warmth/cooling will allow you to move easier.

More "formal" exercise (e.g., cycling, swimming) is excellent, but requires extra effort, equipment, facilities, and sometimes supervision. Recreational swimming or aerobic exercises in water are a possible alternative to walking for those with biomechanical abnormalities. Water exercises increase aerobic capacity and exercise tolerance, and keeps stiff, painful joints moving *(4)*. Many local pools run "aquatherapy" classes that provide controlled, water-based, exercise sessions. An additional benefit is that these classes provide peer support and social reinforcement, encouraging a long-term commitment to exercise.

Of primary importance is the need to find something that is enjoyable and easily achievable. Often, exercise is regarded as a chore requiring considerable effort, expert supervision, and the use of expensive, intimidating equipment and facilities. These are misperceptions and it is important that individuals are reassured that exercise does require effort, will power and determination, but does not require long bouts of exhausting, strenuous exercise, does not require joining a gym, and does not require expensive equipment.

5. PSYCHOSOCIAL EFFECTS OF PHYSICAL ACTIVITY AND EXERCISE

The biopsychosocial model of ill health accepts that there may be a biological cause of pain, but places great importance on the influence of people's health beliefs, understandings, experiences, emotions, and social environment on their reaction to pain and subsequent behavior *(46)*. This framework attempts to conceptualize a holistic

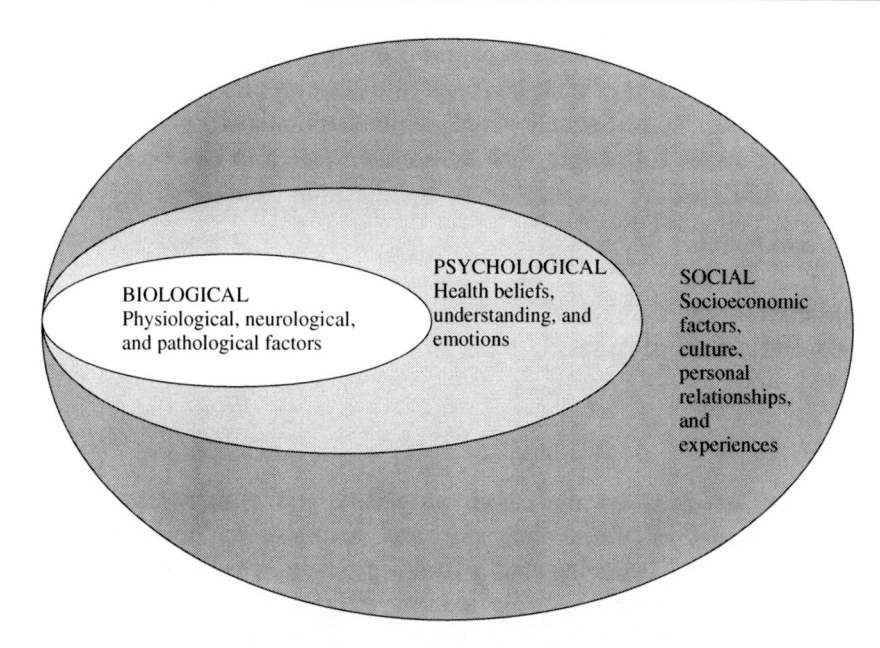

Fig. 1. A biopsychosocial model of rheumatic disease.

perspective for the assessment and treatment of musculoskeletal problems (Fig. 1). Instead of concentrating on "curing" the underlying pathology (grounded in the medical model), the biopsychosocial model emphasizes people's ability to cope and adjust to living with the consequences of ill health (*see* Practitioner Point 5). Thus, the effects and outcomes of rheumatic conditions are regarded as a complex interaction of the effects of physiological, psychological, and socioeconomic sequelae resulting from joint pain, damage, and disability (Fig. 2).

In order to identify and quantify the risk of psychosocial factors contributing to long-term disability in people with musculoskeletal conditions, a systematic assessment approach has been developed. The "yellow flag project" highlights factors that predict

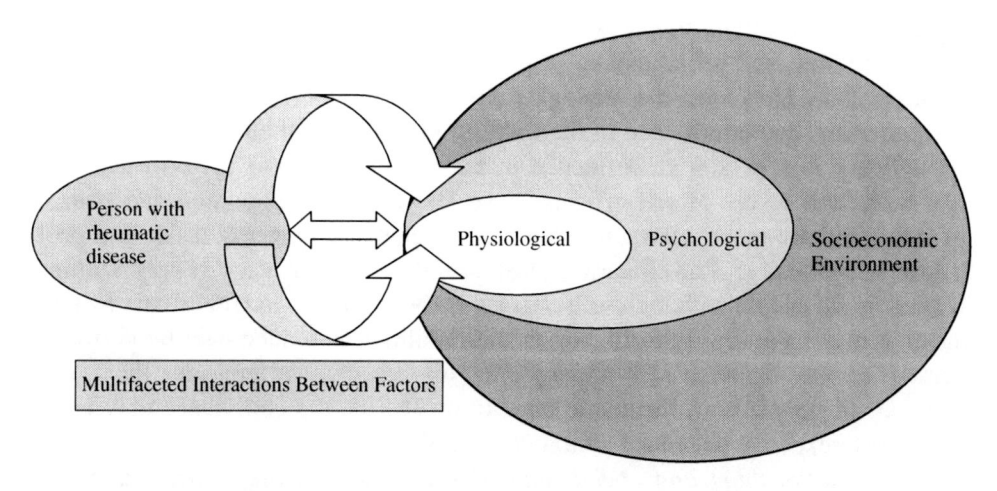

Fig. 2. Diagrammatic representation of the multifaceted, dynamic interactions between a person with rheumatic disease and environment.

poor outcomes in patients with low back pain and also provides suggestions for improved early behavioral management of acute low back pain that may prevent long-term problems *(47)*. These issues are also pertinent to people with other rheumatic diseases.

The important issues for people with musculoskeletal pain can be encapsulated in the mnemonic ABCDEFW:

Attitudes and beliefs
Behaviors
Compensation issues
Diagnosis and treatment issues
Emotions
Family
Work *(47)*

Attitudes and beliefs about the cause, prognosis, and effectiveness of treatment are key determinants of illness behavior and response to treatment. "Catastrophizing" health beliefs—believing that a health problem is inevitable, incurable and untreatable—are demoralizing, causing anxiety, helplessness and undermining self-confidence. These may be based on or propagated by people's previous experiences within the health care system or on cultural responses to disease. Beliefs about the extent to which pain can be controlled appear to be a powerful determinant of the development of incapacity and compliance with an activity-based treatment program. Pain locus-of-control scales *(48,49)* help to identify the extent people feel they are able to influence and control their pain and whether they are willing to take responsibility in the management of their condition. People's fear of pain and causing further damage makes them avoid what they perceive to be potentially "harmful" activities. These perceptions are usually erroneous, but if they are not challenged *"fear-avoidance"* behavior results in reduced mobility and functional activities leading to muscle weakness, fatigue, joint instability and stiffness, pain, disability, and social isolation.

Coping strategies are the efforts people make to minimize the effects of ill health. *Confronters*, or people who use active coping strategies (such as increasing physical activity, diverting attention) avoid catastrophizing (Fig. 3), have better control of pain, and better outcomes than people who use passive coping strategies (such as resting, avoiding activities, and relinquishing responsibility for pain control to others) known as *avoiders (50)*. However, the strategies employed vary based on people's beliefs, past experiences, and confidence in their ability to influence their problems.

Self-efficacy is a person's confidence in his or her ability to perform tasks *(51)*. People with high levels of self-efficacy have less anxiety, depression and pain, are more active and are more willing to attempt and persevere longer at tasks than people with low self-efficacy. Self-efficacy is task-specific and can vary greatly within an individual hence people with high self-efficacy in their abilities to reduce pain by taking medication may have low self-efficacy in their abilities to reduce pain by performing exercise (i.e., low exercise self-efficacy). In this context, we consider the *exercise self-efficacy* of people with rheumatic conditions, that is, the confidence they have in their ability to exercise to reduce pain and improve function.

People's *relationships and social networks* also have a major bearing on their physical, psychological, emotional, and social well-being. Peer support may have a

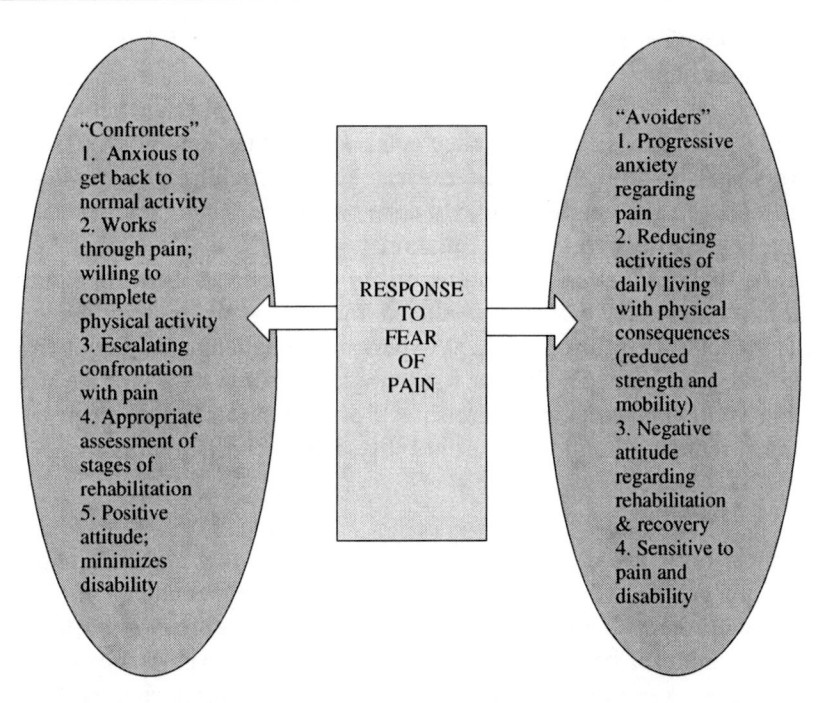

Fig. 3. Possible response to fear of pain in people with rheumatic conditions.

positive effect on an individual, encouraging and motivating the individual to be optimistic and proactive, although not all social interactions and relationships will have a desirable effect on people's illness beliefs and attitudes.

5.1. Interactions of Psychosocial Traits and Symptoms in People With Rheumatic Conditions

It is difficult to tease out the relative importance of psychosocial traits, as they are very labile and vary with the trait, situation, between people and within an individual over time. This variability is determined by an individual's psychological traits, external influences, and experiences. Positive experiences increase the chances of people doing something; poor experiences reduce the possibility.

Having a medical condition increases this complexity. People's psychosocial traits determine their perception and reporting of clinical symptoms and their reaction to these symptoms. For example, increasing pain and disability can adversely alter a person's health beliefs and ability to cope, leading to catastrophizing and adoption of fear-avoidance behaviors that is, inactivity, which exacerbates muscle weakness and joint instability and leads to further joint pain and damage. There is a complex "reciprocally deterministic" relationship between psychological traits and clinical symptoms.

The "plastic," dynamic nature of psychosocial traits on the perception and reporting of rheumatic symptoms presents opportunities to manage rheumatic conditions.

5.2. Education

Challenging erroneous ill-health beliefs by explaining that rheumatic conditions may be incurable but are not untreatable, that pain-related activity does not signal joint damage, and that movement is good for joints but prolonged inactivity bad, helps people re-evaluate their problems and reduce anxiety, catastrophizing, and fear-avoidance behaviors. Identification of specific fears around physical activity and work, for example by using the Fear Avoidance and Beliefs Questionnaire *(52)*, may enable health professionals to address specific exercise fears. Teaching pain-coping skills can enhance self-efficacy and enable people to cope better, increasing their sense of control and reducing helplessness and social isolation.

In particular, pain reduction and improvement in function following exercise-based rehabilitation programs is partially mediated by addressing unhelpful psychosocial traits and developing helpful ones. Such experiences challenge the belief that activity causes pain and joint damage, disrupt fear-avoidance behaviors, provide people with active coping strategies, enhance exercise self-efficacy, and enable them to do more for themselves, reducing helplessness, disability, and social isolation.

5.3. Positive Mastery

Psychological traits are often entrenched, and altering them usually requires more than just telling people what to do. Before they can be persuaded that something that conflicts with their beliefs is effective, useful, and safe, they need to experience the tangible, meaningful benefits it will produce. Positive experiences or mastery of activities facilitate appropriate health beliefs, self-efficacy, and behaviors. Management strategies that utilize active techniques with patient participation are vital (e.g., exercise programs) so that reliance on passive treatment techniques and the health professionals delivering them, is minimized. Successful completion of an exercise program represents controlled exposure to their fear-inducing stimulus. By exposing the individual to exercise (the person's fear) in a graded and controlled way, health providers can help desensitize the patient and then transfer these successes into the home and work environment. However, unsuccessful negative experiences, such as complex exercise regimens that require expensive, specialized equipment, facilities, and supervision, undermine self-efficacy and encourage passive coping strategies and dependency on others.

Practitioner Point 5: Psychological Theories

Successful behavior change is based on the understanding of certain psychological theories.

- **Behavior modification theory** involves the patient actively in the change process and has been successfully employed within cardiac rehabilitation programmes for several decades *(65)*.
- **Social-cognitive theory** provides insight into the interrelationships between beliefs, understanding, environment, and behavior *(51)*.
- **The transtheoretical or readiness to change theory** addresses the individual's ability to make permanent change based on their emotional and intellectual readiness to change. The stages of readiness to change are defined as precontemplation, contemplation, preparation, action, and maintenance *(66)*.

6. DISCONTINUING AN EXERCISE REGIMEN

Once an individual has reached an appropriate activity level that he or she is content with, continuing with that activity level will maintain his or her accomplishments. This requires the social support, encouragement, and positive feedback from spouses, family, friends, and health care professionals to maintain enthusiasm and motivation.

However, if the activity level is reduced, the benefits of exercise (i.e., strength and functional performance) will diminish *(32,53)*. This occurs relatively rapidly, for example, a 17% increase in knee strength achieved during a 24-week training period disappeared 12 weeks after the end of training in patients with RA *(52)*. The challenge for individuals and health professionals is to maintain motivation and the commitment to exercise over the long term.

7. EXERCISE MAINTENANCE

Long-term exercise participation, like other health-related behaviors (e.g., medication compliance) has a relatively high drop-out or attrition rate (50% or more people who begin exercising will cease within 1 year *(54)*). When attempting to address the issue of adherence to exercise, one must recognize that exercise is voluntary and time-consuming and therefore competes with other valued interests and activities. However, psychosocial variables, including the perception of the program, family lifestyle and support, and exercise self-efficacy, can all influence participation in habitual exercise *(55)*.

Enhancing exercise self-efficacy improves patient compliance and adherence with exercise programs *(56,57)*. To enhance self-efficacy for exercise, patients must believe in the benefits of an exercise regime, and believe they have the ability to perform the exercises effectively. This is best achieved by patients experiencing the benefits of a simple, practical exercise regime that can be performed conveniently at home or in community facilities.

Establishing achievable goals and making agreements or contracts with an individual, which can be monitored via exercise diaries recorded daily and cumulative exercise achievements, can influence adherence to exercise. Additionally, regular assessment of an individual's response to exercise (by reassessing some of the tests completed before exercise was initiated) may be carried out, as favorable changes can serve as powerful motivators for continued compliance with an exercise regimen.

The integration of activities into an individual's lifestyle and encouraging diversity of exercise types can increase the enjoyment and reduce the tedium of specific exercise sessions *(58)*. Furthermore, exercising with others can provide social support and an incentive to continue, as commitments made as part of a group tend to be stronger than those made independently *(59)*.

Providing written and visual information on the benefits of activity and the local opportunities in the community to be active or introducing novel educational tools (e.g., yoga classes for relaxation) can support long-term behavioral change *(58)*.

When combined with education on healthy living, self-management of disease, and strategies to maintain motivation and long-term adherence *(60)*, the long-term benefits of exercise are readily achievable for people with rheumatic diseases.

8. RECOMMENDATIONS

Exercise is essential for general health, and joint health in particular. It can be difficult to find the time and motivation to exercise regularly, but regular physical activity and exercise can be integrated into daily life and is essential to avoid the dangers of inactivity.

REFERENCES

1. Caspersen CJ, Powell KE, Christenson GM. Physical activity, exercise and physical fitness: definitions and distributions for health -related research. Public Health Rep 1985;100:126–130.
2. American College of Sports Medicine. American College of Sports Medicine's guidelines for exercise testing and prescription, 7th ed. Lippincott Williams and Wilkins, Philadelphia, PA, 2006.
3. Pate RR, Pratt M, Blair SN. Physical activity and public health. A recommendation from the Centers for Disease control and Prevention and the American College of Sports Medicine. JAMA 1995;273:402–407.
4. Minor MA, Hewett JE, Webel RR. Efficacy of physical conditioning exercise in patients with rheumatoid arthritis and osteoarthritis J Rheumatol 1989;15(6):905–111.
5. Ekdahl C, Broman G. Muscle strength, endurance and aerobic capacity in rheumatoid arthritis: a comparative study with health subjects. Ann Rheum Dis 1992;51:35–40.
6. Bearne LM, Scott DL, Hurley MV. Exercise can reverse quadriceps sensorimotor dysfunction caused by rheumatoid arthritis without exacerbating disease activity. Rheumatology 2002;41:157–166.
7. Harkcom TM, Lampman RM, Banwell BF, Castor CW. Therapeutic value of graded aerobic exercise training in rheumatoid arthritis. Arthritis Rheum 1985;28(1):32–39.
8. Munneke M, de Jong Z, Zwinderman AH, et al. Effect of a high-intensity weight-bearing exercise program on radiologic damage progression of the large joints in subgroups of patients with rheumatoid arthritis Arthritis Rheum 2005; 53(3):410–417.
9. Nordemar R, Ekblom B, Zachrisson L, Lundqvist K. Physical training in rheumatoid arthritis: a controlled long-term study. Scand J Rheumatol 1981;10(1):17–23.
10. Brosseau L, Wells GA, Tugwell P, Egan M. Ottawa panel evidence-based clinical practice guidelines for therapeutic exercises and manual therapy in the management of osteoarthritis. Phys Ther 2005;85(9):907–971.
11. EULAR. ASAS/EULAR recommendations for the management of ankylosing spondylitis. Ann Rheum Dis 2006; 65(4):442–452.
12. Folsom AR, Caspersen CJ, Gomez-Marin O, Knudsen J. Test-retest reliability of the Minnesota Leisure Time Physical Activity Questionnaire. J Chronic Dis 1986;39(7):505–511.
13. Topolski TD, LoGerfo J, Patrick DL, Williams B, Walwick J, Patrick MB. The Rapid Assessment of Physical Activity (RAPA) among older adults. Prev Chronic Dis 2006;3(4):A118.
14. American College of Sports Medicine. American College of Sports Medicine's Exercise management for people with chronic diseases and disabilities. Human Kinetics, Champaign, IL, 1997.
15. Terwee CB, Mokkink LB, Steultjens PM, Dekker J. Performance based methods for measuring the physical function of patients with osteoarthritis of the hip or the knee: a systematic review of measurement properties. Rheum Dis Clin North Am 2006;45:890–902.
16. Borg. G. Borg's Perceived Exertion and Pain Scales. Human Kinetics, Champaign, IL, 1998.
17. Borg GAV. Psychological basis of perceived exertion. Med Sci Sports Excer 1982;14:377–381.
18. Thompson PD. Exercise Prescription and Proscription for patients with Coronary artery disease. Circulation 2005;112:2354–2363.
19. James MJ, Cleland LG, Gaffney RD, Proudman SM, Chatterton BE. Effect of exercise on 99mTc-DTPA clearance from knees with effusions. J Rheum 1994;21:501–504.
20. Buckwalter JA. Osteoarthritis and articular cartilage use, disuse and abuse: Experiemental studies. J Rheumatol 1995;22(suppl 43):13–15.
21. Houlbrooke K, Vause K, Merrilees MJ. Effects of movement and weightbearing on the glucosaminoglycan content of sheep articular cartilage. Aust J Physiother 1990;36:88–91.

22. Suomi R, Lindauer S, Effectiveness of arthritis Foundation Aquatic Program on strength and ROM on women with arthritis. J Aging Phys Act 1997;5:341–351.
23. National Ankylosing Spondylitis Society. A Positive Response to Ankylosing Spondylitis—Guidebook for Patients The National Ankylosing Spondylitis Society, Surrey, UK, 2006.
24. Dagfinrud H, Kvien TK, Hagen K.B. The Cochrane review of physiotherapy interventions for ankylosing spondylitis. J Rheumatol 2005;32(10):1899–1906.
25. Brooke M, Kaplan H. Muscle pathology in rheumatoid arthritis, polymyalgia rheumatica and polymyositis. Arch Pathol 1972;94:101–118.
26. Edstrom L, Nordemar R. Differential changes in type 1 and 11 muscle fibres in rheumatoid arthritis. Scand J Rheumatol 1974;3:155–160.
27. McAlindon TE, Cooper C, Kirwan JR. Determinants of disability in osteoarthritis of the knee. Ann Rheum Dis 1993;52:258–262.
28. Hakkinen A, Hannonen P, Nyman K, Hakkinen K. Aerobic and neuromuscular capacity both in early and long-term rheumatoid arthritis compared to healthy controls. Scand J Rheumatol 2002;31: 345–350.
29. Hurley MV, Scott DL. Improvements in quadriceps sensoriomotor function and disability of patients with knee osteoarthritis following a clinically practicable exercise regime. Brit J Rheumatol 1998;37:1181–1187.
30. Nordemar R, Berg U, Ekblom B, Edstrom L. Changes in muscle fibre size and physical performance in patients with rheumatoid arthritis after 7 months physical training. Scand J Rheumatol 1976;5(4): 233–238.
31. Taylor NF, Dodd KJ, Damiano DL. Progressive resistance training in physical therapy: A summary of systematic reviews. Phys Ther 2005;85:1208–1223.
32. van den Ende CHM, Breedveld FC, le Cessie S, Dijkmans BAC, de Mug AW, Hazes JMW. Effect of intensive exercise on patients with active rheumatoid arthritis: a randomised clinical trial. Ann Rheum Dis 2000;59(8):615–621.
33. Hurley MV, Scott DL, Rees J, Newham DJ. Sensorimotor changes and functional performance in patients with knee osteoarthritis. Ann Rheum Dis 1997; 56(11):641–648.
34. Sharma L, Pai YC, Holtkamp K, Rymer WZ. Is knee joint proprioception worse in the arthritic knee versus the unaffected knee in unilateral knee osteoarthritis? Arthritis Rheum 1997;40(8):1518–1525.
35. Hurley MV, Dziedzic K, Bearne L, Sim J, Bury T. The clinical and cost effectiveness of physiotherapy in the management of older people with common rheumatological conditions. Chartered Society of Physiotherapy, London, UK, 2002.
36. Felson DT, Zhang Y, Anthony JM, Naimark A, Anderson JJ. Weight loss reduces the risk for symptomatic knee osteoarthritis in women. The Framlingham study. Ann Intern Med 1992;116: 535–539.
37. Jakicic JM. The role of physical activity in prevention and treatment of body weight gain in adults. J Nutr 2002;132(12):3826S–3829S
38. Manninen P, Riihimaki H, Heliovaara M, Suomalainen O. Physical exercise and risk of severe knee osteoarthritis requiring arthroplasty. Rheumatology 2001;;40(4):432–437.
39. Roubenoff R, Roubenoff R.A, Cannon J.G, et al. Rheumatoid cachexia: cytokine-driven hypermetabolism accompanying reduced body cell mass in chronic inflammation. J Clin Invest 1994;93(6):2379–2386.
40. Roubenoff R, Roubenoff RA, Ward LM, Holland SM, Hellmann DB. Rheumatoid cachexia: depletion of lean body mass in rheumatoid arthritis. Possible association with tumor necrosis factor. J Rheumatol 1992; 19(10):1505–1510.
41. Rall LC, Rosen CJ, Dolnikowski G, et al. Protein metabolism in rheumatoid arthritis and aging. Effects of muscle strength training and tumor necrosis factor alpha. Arthritis Rheum 1996;39 (7):1115–1124.
42. Ainsworth BE, Haskell WL, Leon AS. Compendium of physical activities: classification of energy costs of human physical activities. Med Sci Sport Exerc 1993;25:71–80.
43. Schilke JM, Johnson GD, Housh TJ. Effects of muscle strength training on the functional status of patients with osteoarthritis of the knee joint. Arthritis Rheum 1993;36:1207–1213
44. Tackson SJ, Krebs DE, Harris BA. Acetabular pressures during hip arthritis exercises. Arthritis Care Res 1997;10:308–319.

45. Voloshin D, Wosk J. Influence of artificial shock absorbers on human gait. Clin Orthop 1981;160: 52–56.
46. Waddell G. Volvo award in clinical sciences. A new clinical model for the treatment of low-back pain. Spine 1987;12(7):632–644.
47. Kendall NS. Guide to Assessing Psycho-Social Yellow Flags in Acute Low Back Pain: Risk Factors for Long-Term Disability and Work Loss. Accident and Compensation Commission of New Zealand and the National Health Committee, Wellington, New Zealand, 1997.
48. Crisson JE, Keefe FJ. The relationship of locus of control to pain coping strategies and psychological distress in chronic pain patients. Pain 1988;35(2):147–154.
49. Main CJ, Waddell G. A comparison of cognitive measures in low back pain: statistical structure and clinical validity at initial assessment. Pain 1991;46(3):287–298.
50. Waddell G. The Back Pain Revolution, 2nd ed. Butterworth Heinemann, Churchill Livingstone, Oxford, UK, 2004.
51. Bandura A. Self-efficacy: towards a unifying theory of behavior change. Psychol Rev 1977;84: 191–215.
52. Waddell G, Newton M, Henderson I, Somerville D, Main CJ. A Fear-Avoidance Beliefs Questionnaire (FABQ) and the role of fear-avoidance beliefs in chronic low back pain and disability. Pain 1993;52(2):157–168.
53. Hakkinen A, Malkia E, Hakkinen K, Jappinen I, Laitinen L, Hannonen P. Effects of detraining subsequent to strength training on neuromuscular function in patients with inflammatory arthritis. Br J Rheumatol 1997; 36(10):1075–1081.
54. Dishman R.K, Ickes W, Morgan W.P. Self motivation and adherence to habitual physical activity. J Appl Social Psychol 1980;10:115–132.
55. Gecht MR, Connell KJ, Sinacore JM. A survey of exercise beliefs and exercise habits among people with arthritis. Arth Care Res 1996;9:82–88.
56. McAuley E, Lox C, Duncan TE. Long-term maintenance of exercise, self-efficacy, and physiological change in older adults. J Gerontol (Psych Sci) 1993;48:218–224.
57. Rejeski WJ, Ettigner WH, Martin K. Treating disability in knee osteoarthritis with exercise: a central role for self-efficacy and pain . Arth Care Res 1998;11:94–101.
58. National Institute for Health and Clinical Excellence (NICE). Four Commonly Used Methods to Increase Physical Activity: Brief Interventions in Primary Care, Exercise Referral Schemes, Pedometers and Community-Based Exercise Programmes for Walking and Cycling. National Health Service, London, UK, 2006.
59. Massie JF, Shephard RJ. Physiological and psychological effects of training—a comparison of individual and gymnasium programs, with a characterization of the exercise "drop-outs." Med Sci Sports Excer 1971;3:110–117.
60. Lorig KR, Mazonson PD, Holman HR. Evidence suggesting that health education for self-management in patients with chronic arthritis has sustained health benefits while reducing health care costs. Arthritis Rheum 1993;36:439–446.
61. Price LG, Hewett JE, Kay DR. Five minute walking test of aerobic fitness for people with arthritis. Arthritis Care Res 1988;1:33–37.
62. Minor MA, Johnson JC. Reliability and validity of a submaximal treadmill test to estimate aerobic capacity in women with rheumatic disease J Rheumatol 1996;23(9):1517–1523.
63. MacSween A, Johnson NJ, Armstrong G, Bonn J. A validation of the 10-meter incremental shuttle walk test as a measure of aerobic power in cardiac and rheumatoid arthritis patients. Arch Phys Med Rehabil 2001; 82(6):807–810.
64. Moritani T, DeVries. Neural factors versus hypertrophy in the time course of muscle strength gain. Am J Phys Med 1979;58(3):115–131.
65. Nash J. Taking charge of your weight and well being. Bull Publishing, Palo Alto, CA, 1986.
66. Proclaska J, Di Clemente CC. Transtheoretical theory, towards a more integrative model of change. Psychol Theory Res Prac 1982;19:176–288.

6 Complementary and Alternative Therapies

Kevin Khaw and Sharon L. Kolasinski

Summary

- Complementary and alternative medicine encompasses a wide array of interventions, including diets, dietary supplements, and herbal products.
- Scientific evidence does not support a substantial role of special diets in the treatment of the majority of patients with rheumatic disease, but various dietary manipulations may be beneficial when combined with standard medical therapy.
- Long-term safety of dietary and herbal supplements is a legitimate concern and patients should always be cautioned about their use of these products.
- Observed benefits in disease activity owing to short-term trials may be more reflective of the natural history of rheumatic disease rather than true differences in long-term outcome.

Key Words: Alternative medicine; dietary supplements; herbal supplements; omega-3 fatty acids

1. INTRODUCTION

The use of complementary and alternative medicine (CAM) continues to grow. In 1990, 1 in 3 Americans used CAM, and in 1997, 4 in 10 Americans reported using CAM *(1,2)*. In 2004, the Centers for Disease Control and Prevention (CDC) reported that 62% of adults used some form of CAM therapy during the past 12 months, and 75% of adults have ever used CAM *(3)*. According to data published in 1997, the U.S. public spent more out-of-pocket fees for CAM health care providers than the amount spent on out-of-pocket fees for all hospitalizations *(2)*. The total U.S. expenditures for all CAM therapies were estimated to be between $36 and $47 billion in 1997 *(2)*. The federal government established the National Center of Complementary and Alternative Medicine (NCCAM) as part of the National Institutes of Health (NIH) in 1998. NCCAM first funded a research project in 1999 and that number has grown to more than 800 funded projects as of 2004 *(4)*.

NCCAM has defined CAM as a group of diverse medical and health care systems, therapies, and products that are not presently considered to be part of conventional medicine. The therapies are divided into five categories:

From: *Nutrition and Health: Nutrition and Rheumatic Disease*
Edited by: L. A. Coleman © Humana Press, Totowa, NJ

1. biologically based therapies such as dietary supplements, herbs, and foods;
2. alternative medicine systems such as homeopathy, naturopathy, traditional Chinese medicine and ayurvedic medicine;
3. manipulative and body-based therapies like chiropractic, osteopathy, and massage;
4. mind–body interventions such as meditation and prayer; and
5. energy therapies, such as qi gong, Reiki, and application of magnetic fields.

In one survey *(3)*, most individuals who used CAM said they did so because they felt that CAM combined with conventional medical treatments would help them. The most common conditions treated by CAM therapies were musculoskeletal disorders or conditions associated with chronic pain. Of adults in the survey, 19% used natural products, including herbal medicine, functional foods (garlic), and animal-based (fish oil) supplements *(3)*.

The array of CAM therapies continues to expand. The Institute of Medicine estimated that in 2004, 29,000 products were on the market with 1,000 new products being developed annually *(5)*. In 2002, annual sales of dietary supplements alone accounted for $19 billion *(5)*. Despite the dramatic increase in acceptance and research, the number of trials evaluating CAM is not keeping pace with the vast number of CAM therapies available on the market today. Furthermore, most of the trials have been relatively short term. The aim of this chapter is to discuss the role of CAM in rheumatic diseases, focusing on diets and dietary and herbal supplements.Attention will be given to those therapies for which well-designed trials provide some evidence-based data.

2. COMPLEMENTARY AND ALTERNATIVE MEDICINE IN RHEUMATIC DISEASES

Chronic pain and ailments involving the musculoskeletal system are among the leading reasons for patients to turn to CAM therapies. Patients with rheumatic conditions such as rheumatoid arthritis, fibromyalgia and osteoarthritis who use CAM often have inadequate pain control *(6)*. The most common types of CAM used in one study of patients with rheumatic arthritis were chiropractic care (31%), copper bracelets or magnets (29%), herbal therapies (28%), electrical stimulators (25%), vinegar preparations (25%), dietary supplements (22%), and special diets (20%). Half of those using dietary supplements were using glucosamine or chondroitin sulfate. Patients spend a significant amount of money for alternative care. In a population of patients with OA, the expenditures for alternative therapies averaged $1,127 per year per patient, compared with $1,148 for traditional therapies *(7)*.

3. DIETS AND DIETARY SUPPLEMENTS

Modifying the diet to treat illness has been practiced for many centuries across different ethnic groups and cultures. Much has been written about the possible relationship between diets and rheumatic diseases. Hippocrates postulated that changes in diet could ameliorate arthritis *(8)*. In modern times, the benefits of dietary manipulations to treat rheumatic conditions were reported in the early part of the 20th century *(9)*. Often, these reports were based on data that would not meet the rigors of current scientific standards, making conclusions difficult. To date, no specific food has been shown to cause or cure a rheumatic disease, but there have been observations of dietary modifications altering the symptoms of certain rheumatic conditions. For example, flares of gout are known to occur in relation to intake of particular kinds of food and drink. A weight loss of as little as 4.6 kg, in combination with exercise, improved symptoms and functioning in patients with OA of the knees *(10)*. There is a large amount of both clinical and basic science data that suggests some efficacy for glucosamine and chondrointin supplements in OA *(11)*. Fish- or plant-oil preparations have been reported to be effective in patients with RA.

3.1. Diets

In 1981, the Arthritis Foundation noted "the possible relationship between diet and arthritis has been thoroughly and scientifically studied. The simple proven fact is, no food has anything to do with causing arthritis and no food is effective in treating or 'curing' it" *(12)*. Despite this long held opinion within the rheumatology community, patients have often felt otherwise. Between 20 and 50% of patients with RA have tried dietary alterations in an attempt to relieve their symptoms *(13)*. There have been intriguing observations that diets could affect the course of rheumatic illnesses.

Some have postulated that some rheumatic diseases may at least in part be due to "sensitivity" to certain foods or that food allergens may worsen some patients' symptoms. In general, published reports showing possible association between specific foods and rheumatic diseases have been anecdotal at best *(14)* and no prospective clinical trials have been published. One early study focused on an elimination diet for RA. In a 6-week, single-blind, placebo-controlled trial, 53 patients with RA eliminated a variety of specific foods (including nuts, beef, pork, cheese, milk, eggs, wheat, and corn) from their diet. Significant improvements in the treatment group were seen in pain score on visual analog scale, duration of morning stiffness, grip strength, and number of painful joints. Symptoms recurred upon reintroduction of the offending foods *(15)*. This study suggested that certain foods could aggravate symptoms and that elimination of particular foods could improve symptoms at least in some patients who suffer from rheumatoid arthritis. However, this study does not meet current standards for trial design and reporting of results and cannot be used to defend the routine use of elimination diets for arthritis.

Various vegetarian diets have also been reported to improve clinical symptoms in RA and other arthritic conditions *(8,9,13)*. However, the trials have been of small size, short term, unblinded, and often hindered by high drop-out rates. Vegetarian diets are based on consumption of non-meat foods and generally fall into groups defined by the types of animal-derived foods that are consumed. For example, lacto-vegetarian diets include diary products, and lactoovovegetarian diets include diary products and eggs *(16)*. Vegan diets include only plant-based foods and are devoid of all foods from animals including meat, poultry, fish, eggs, milk, and cheese.

In a single-blind, placebo-controlled study, 27 patients with RA were placed on a vegan and lacto-vegetarian diet for 13 mo. Following an initial 7- to 10-day subtotal fast, the treatment group was placed on a vegan diet for 3.5 months, and then on a lactovegetarian diet for the remainder of the study. A control group of 26 matched patients ate a normal diet throughout the whole study. After 4 weeks, the treatment group showed improvement in number of tender joints, Ritchie articular index, number of swollen joints, pain score, duration of morning stiffness, grip strength, erythrocyte sedimentation rate (ESR), C-reactive protein (CRP), and Health Assessment Questionnaire (HAQ) score. These benefits were said to be sustained at 12 months *(17)*. The study was hindered by a 35% drop-out rate in the treatment group, including 22% because of disease flare. The study also lacked complete blinding of participants.

Another study evaluated the effects of a low-fat, vegan diet in patients with moderate to severe RA. Twenty-four patients in this uncontrolled study were maintained on a diet without animal products or added fats and oils of any kind for 4 weeks. At the end of this short trial, the participants had significant improvement in pain, function, tenderness, and swelling compared with their pretrial status. There was no difference in ESR, CRP, rheumatoid factor, or duration of stiffness *(9)*. This study was of short duration and was not controlled. Patients also had an average weight loss of 3 kg, which could have been a factor in reducing inflammation and associated symptoms.

Fasting can have short-term anti-inflammatory effects. Fasting for 7 to 10 days led to reductions in pain, stiffness, evidence of inflammation on physical examination and laboratory testing, and reduced medication requirements in one study of patients with RA *(8)*. The mechanisms by which fasting may result in reduced inflammation, are unclear. It has been proposed that a centrally mediated effect of calorie restriction activates endogenous steroid production leading to immunosuppression *(18)*. Fasting, however, is an impractical form of therapy at a minimum because it cannot be practiced on a long-term basis. Furthermore, poor nutrition may lead to other detrimental effects, particularly in patients who have chronic illnesses.

Based on the available evidence, it is clear that longer term, controlled studies are needed before conclusions can be made with certainty in regard to the effects of various diets and dietary manipulations in rheumatic diseases. Allergic reactions to food may occur in some individual patients who have rheumatic disease, but specialized diets such as fasting, elimination diets, and vegetarian diets do not have an established or specific therapeutic role in the care of patients with RA and other systemic inflammatory illnesses. Proper nutrition and a well-balanced diet are recommended as part of routine care for all patients.

3.2. Dietary Supplements

3.2.1. FISH OIL (OMEGA-3 POLYUNSATURATED FATTY ACIDS)

The first data to suggest the possible anti-inflammatory effects of omega-3 (n-3) fatty acids were derived from epidemiological studies of Greenland Eskimos. This group has seen noted to have a lower prevalence of chronic inflammatory diseases than inhabitants of most Western countries *(19)*. It was postulated that their seafood-rich diet containing high amounts of long-chain polyunsaturated fatty acids had an important role. There is currently a large amount of both biochemical and clinical data on these long-chain fatty acids. The beneficial effect of n-3 fatty acids in cardiovascular disease (CVD) has been established based on several randomized controlled clinical trials. The incidence and mortality from CVD is significantly reduced by n-3 fatty acids *(20)*. Beneficial effects in rheumatic diseases have also been reported. A number of investigators have reported that dietary fish-oil supplementation reduced symptoms in RA *(21–23)*.

The polyunsaturated fatty acids are categorized as n-3 or omega-6 (n-6) fatty acids based on the biochemical structure of the compounds, specifically, the location of the double bond proximal to the methyl terminus. Both n-3 and n-6 fatty acids are essential fatty acids that cannot be synthesized by the body and therefore must be obtained through the diet.

The n-3 fatty acids have anti-inflammatory and anti-thrombotic properties, whereas the n-6 fatty acids are proinflammatory and prothrombotic. Unfortunately, the modern human diet contains much more n-6 fatty acids as a result of consumption of vegetable oils high in n-6 fatty acids (such as corn, safflower, sunflower, and cottonseed oils) and meats from land animals. Fatty fish contain high amounts of n-3 fatty acids in the form of eicosapentaenoic acid (EPA) and docosahexaenoic acid (DHA). Cold water, oily species of fish contain the highest amounts of EPA and DHA (Table 1). In addition to fish, seeds, and oils (canola oil, flaxseed oil, walnut oil), green leafy vegetables, and beans contain n-3 fatty acid in the form of α-linolenic acid *(25)*.

The fatty acids play an important role in energy metabolism, cell membrane and tissue integrity, inflammation, and CVD. Dietary fat has several effects on inflammation. The n-6 fatty acid in the form of linoleic acid is converted to arachidonic acid, which is then metabolized by cyclooxygenase (COX) and 5-lipoxygenase to proinflammatory and prothrombotic n-6 prostaglandin PGE_2, thromboxane TXA_2, and leukotriene LTB_4 (Fig. 1).

In the form of α-linolenic acid, n-3 fatty acid is metabolized to form EPA and DHA, which are longer chain, physiologically active metabolites. EPA and DHA are precursors to a different group of anti-inflammatory and anti-thrombotic prostaglandins (PGE_3) and leukotrienes (LTB_5). EPA and DHA are competititve inhibitors of COX and subsequent arachidonic acid-derived proinflammatory prostaglandins and leukotrienes. A relative increase in n-6 fatty acids and reduction in n-3 fatty acids promote a proinflammatory state, including pain, swelling, warmth, redness, and loss of function.

Additional effects of n-3 fatty acids can result in a reduction of inflammation. These effects can reduce the function of antigen-presenting cells and, consequently, decrease pathogenic T cells mediating inflammation *(26)*. Interleukin (IL 1β) and tumor necrosis factor (TNF α) are cytokines that promote inflammation and tissue destruction. In several trials, dietary n-3 fatty acid supplementation in patients with RA and normal subjects led to reductions in TNF-α and IL-1β levels produced by stimulated peripheral blood mononuclear cells and macrophages *(27,28)*.

The n-3 fatty acids have also been shown to inhibit enzymes involved in chronic joint inflammation and cartilage destruction. For example, matrix metalloproteinases (MMPs) are stimulated by inflammatory cytokines IL-1β and TNF-α to destroy cartilage. The addition of n-3 fatty acids to *in vitro* assays of IL-1 stimulated bovine chondrocytes inhibited MMP expression and reduced proteoglycan degradation *(29)*. In human OA cartilage explants, n-3 fatty acids reduced colleganase and aggrecanase proteolytic activity *(30)*. These effects were not seen with other types of fatty acids.

3.2.1.1. Clinical Trials of Fish Oil in Rheumatoid Arthritis. In addition to the pharmacological and laboratory evidence, 14 randomized double-blind, controlled trials have reported beneficial effects of fish oil in RA *(13)*. However, all of the studies have involved relatively small number of subjects ($N = 16–67$). Patients with RA who took fish-oil supplements had improvement in outcome measures and required lower

Table 1
Amounts of EPA+DHA in Fish and Fish Oils and the Amount of Fish Consumption Required to Provide ~1 g of EPA+DHA per Day

	EPA+DHA Content g/3-oz Serving Fish (Edible Portion) or g/g Oil	Amount Required to Provide ~1 g of EPA+DHA per Day, oz (Fish) or g (Oil)
Fish		
Tuna		
Light, canned in water, drained	0.26	12
White, canned in water, drained	0.73	4
Fresh	0.24–1.28	2.5–12
Sardines	0.98–1.70	2–3
Salmon		
Chum	0.68	4.5
Sockeye	0.68	4.5
Pink	1.09	2.5
Chinook	1.48	2
Atlantic, farmed	1.09–1.83	1.5–2.5
Atlantic, wild	0.9–1.56	2–3.5
Mackerel	0.34–1.57	2–8.5
Herring		
Pacific	1.81	1.5
Atlantic	1.71	2
Trout, rainbow		
Farmed	0.98	3
Wild	0.84	3.5
Halibut	0.4–1.0	3–7.5
Cod		
Pacific	0.13	23
Atlantic	0.24	12.5
Haddock	0.2	15
Catfish		
Farmed	0.15	20
Wild	0.2	15
Flounder/Sole	0.42	7
Oyster		
Pacific	1.17	2.5
Eastern	0.47	6.5
Farmed	0.37	8
Lobster	0.07–0.41	7.5–42.5
Crab, Alaskan King	0.35	8.5
Shrimp, mixed species	0.27	11
Clam	0.24	12.5
Scallop	0.17	17.5
Capsules		
Cod liver oil*	0.19	5
Standard fish body oil	0.30	3
Omega-3 fatty acid concentrate	0.50	2
Omacor (Pronova Blocare)†	0.85	1

From reference 24

Metabolism of n-6 and n-3 Fatty Acids

Fatty Acid Family	n-6	n-3
18 carbon fatty acid	Linoleic acid (LA; 18:2n-6)	α-Linolenic acid (ALA; 18:3n-3)
Dietary sources	Sunflower, corn, and safflower oil	Flaxseed, canola, and rapeseed oil
Dietary intake	Large intake (7-8% dietary energy)[a]	Minor intake (0.3-1.0% dietary energy)[a]
Metabolism	↓	↓
20 carbon fatty acids		
Sources	Arachidonic acid (AA; 20:4n-6) Mainly synthesized from ingested linoleic acid	Eicosapentaenoic acid (EPA; 20:5n-3) Mainly from ingested EPA (fish, fish oil)
Metabolites of C20 fatty acid relevent to inflammation	Proinflammatory n-6 prostaglandins and leukotrienes (TXA$_2$, PGE$_2$, LTB$_4$)	Competitive inhibitors of n-6 prostaglandin and leukotriene formation
Effect on inflammatory cytokine production	Varied	Suppression IL-1β and TNF-α

Fig. 1. Metabolism of omega-6 (n-6) and omega-3 (n-3) fatty acids.

amount of long-term nonsteroidal anti-inflammatory drugs (NSAIDs *(31,32)*). Fish oil at dosages of at least 3 g per day (EPA plus DHA) significantly reduced the number of tender, swollen joints and morning stiffness *(27,33,34)*. The beneficial effects were not seen until 12 weeks after initiating fish oil. A combination diet of increased intake of n-3 fatty acids and decreased intake of n-6 fatty acids resulted in greater improvement than either supplement alone *(34)*, and allowed some patients with RA to reduce or discontinue use of NSAIDs *(31,32)*. A meta-analysis evaluating nine of the clinical trials and a personal communication showed that n-3 fatty acid taken for 3 months produced significant reduction in painful joint count and morning stiffness in patients with RA *(35)*. All of the trials in the meta-analysis were randomized, double-blind, placebo-controlled.

3.2.1.2. Cardiovascular Disease in RA and Role of n-3 Fatty Acids. CVD is a leading cause of mortality in patients with RA and evidence has been increasing that chronic inflammation is a risk factor for development of CVD. Prevention of CVD has become a key feature in the management of patients with RA and systemic lupus erythematosus (SLE). The American Heart Association recommends a daily intake of 1 g of EPA and DHA for cardioprotection in those with a history of coronary heart disease and consumption of two servings of fish per week for persons without a history of heart disease *(25,36)*. Thus, emphasis should be placed on the potential of fish-oil supplements to provide relief from arthritis as well as protection from CVD.

3.2.1.3. Potential Adverse Effects of Fish Oil. Although generally considered safe, fish oil may have some unwanted side effects. The most common are fishy aftertaste and gastrointestinal (GI) disturbances, both of which appear to be dose-related *(22)*. In two studies, GI upset was reported in 4.9% and 8% of patients taking 0.85 g daily and 6.9 g daily of n-3 fatty acids, respectively *(20)*.

Concern that certain other side effects might arise appears to be unfounded. Although n-3 fatty acids have anti-thrombotic effects, there have been no documented cases of abnormal bleeding caused by fish-oil supplementation even in combination with other anticoagulant medications *(38)*. Although there have been prior concerns of fish oil worsening hyperglycemia, a recent meta-analysis concluded that fish-oil supplements in the range of 3 g to 18 g per day had no statistically significant effect on glycemic control. Fish-oil supplements did not raise fasting glucose or hemoglobin A_{1C} levels *(39)*. The Food and Drug Administration (FDA) has ruled that intake of up to 3 g per day of fish oil in the form of EPA and DHA is generally recognized as safe and have categorized EPA and DHA n-3 fatty acids as dietary supplements *(40,41)*. Furthermore, fish-oil supplements are essentially free of mercury and other contaminants that may be present in fish *(42)*.

All fish species contain EPA and DHA, and consumption of fish has been promoted as a source of dietary n-3 fatty acids. However, fish and seafood are a major source of human exposure to methylmercury, polychlorinated biphenyls, dioxins, and other environmental contaminants. Larger, older, predatory fish tend to have higher concentrations of these contaminants. The Environmental Protection Agency and FDA recommend that women (potentially pregnant and breastfeeding mothers) and young children eliminate shark, swordfish, king mackerel, and tilefish from their diets, and limit to less than 12 ounces per week other fish that are lower in mercury *(43,44)*. Thus, it is important for consumers to be aware of both the advantages and risks of fish consumption, especially women and children who may be at increased risk of mercury intoxication.

In summary, there are a number of potential benefits of n-3 fatty acid supplements. These include relief from arthritis symptoms and reduction of NSAID use, thus, potentially avoiding their side effects. Furthermore, n-3 fatty acids have favorable cardiovascular benefits through anti-thrombotic properties. Finally, by virtue of their ability to block TNF-α and IL-1β, dietary n-3 fatty acid supplements can serve as a relatively safe and inexpensive adjunctive therapy to the high priced biological agents that are increasingly utilized in the treatment of inflammatory arthritis.

3.2.2. γ-LINOLENIC ACID

Essential fatty acids have immunomodulating effects through both pro- and anti-inflammatory pathways. As discussed in the fish-oil section, n-3 fatty acids are anti-inflammatory and n-6 fatty acids are for the most part pro-inflammatory. However, certain n-6 fatty acids derived from plant seed oils have predominantly anti-inflammatory effects. One such example is γ-linolenic acid (GLA), a polyunsaturated fatty acid found in the oils of evening primrose (*Oenothera biennis*) and borage seed (*Boragio officinalis*). This fatty acid is metabolized to form prostaglandin E_1 (PGE_1), an anti-inflammatory prostaglandin with immunoregulatory properties *(45)*. PGE_1 reduces polymorphonuclear leukocyte chemotaxis and inhibits lymphocyte function *(46)*. It also blocks metabolism of arachidonic acid to proinflammatory leukotriene LTB_4. Thus, increased intake of GLA may suppress inflammation through production of PGE_1 and competitive blockage of PGE_2 and LTB_4 production.

Clinical studies have shown that GLA was well tolerated and can be effective in treatment of RA *(45)*. In reports that showed benefit, the results became apparent after 3 to 4 months of supplementation. A 24-week, randomized, placebo-controlled trial of GLA supplementation (in the form of borage seed oil) in patients with RA showed a statistically significant reduction in signs and symptoms of disease activity compared with the placebo control group *(47)*. The study size was small with 19 subjects in the treatment group and 18 subjects in the placebo control group. The dose used was 1.4 g per day, a much higher amount than the usual preparation of evening primrose and borage seed oils that contain approximately 45 mg of GLA per capsule. Although no patients withdrew from the study because of adverse effects, a 28% withdrawal rate was observed in each group, perhaps because of the large number of capsules administered. Other studies using smaller doses of GLA (480–540 mg per day) did not show benefits *(47)*.

The efficacy of GLA in primary Sjogren's syndrome was evaluated in a 6-month, double-blind, placebo-controlled trial. Patients in the treatment group took 400 mg and 800 mg GLA supplements extracted from evening primrose oil. There was no statistically significant improvement in the primary end point of fatigue. Secondary end points of dry eyes, dry mouth, pain, results on Schirmer tear test, van Bijsterveld score, unstimulated whole sialometry, the use of artifical tears or analgesics did not improve significantly *(48)*.

Side effects of GLA are generally not severe and include headache, flatulence, constipation, and loose stools *(45,47,48)*. Consumption of borage seeds is not recommended during pregnancy and lactation due to potential contamination with liver-toxic pyrrolizidine alkaloids *(45)*. Overall, no definitive evidence exists to support the use of GLA in the routine care of patients with rheumatic diseases.

3.2.3. VITAMINS

Vitamins are organic compounds that are required in small amounts for normal metabolism. The human body does not synthesize vitamins, except for vitamin D; therefore, vitamins must be ingested in the diet. Various syndromes and diseases have been linked to vitamin deficiencies such as scurvy, osteoporosis, neuropathy, anemia, osteomalacia, and cancer. Therefore, vitamin supplementation has been promoted for good health and as a preventive measure against certain ailments. Vitamins are frequently used as supplements by patients *(3)*. The evidence for vitamin supplementation in rheumatic conditions is reviewed in the following section.

3.2.3.1. Vitamin D. The beneficial effect of vitamin D in bone health is well supported. The role of vitamin D in OA and RA is less clear. Epidemiological evidence suggests that vitamin D intake might be linked to OA. Results from the food-frequency questionnaires from the Framingham study and measurement of serum vitamin D levels showed that those with lowest intake and serum levels of vitamin D were three times more likely to have progression of established OA *(49)*. A second epidemiological study found that people with lower levels of vitamin D level were more likely to develop OA of the hip, defined by radiographic joint-space narrowing (JSN) *(50)*. The possible association between vitamin D intake and RA was evaluated in the Iowa Women's Health Study *(51)*. After 11 years of follow-up of a large cohort of women ($N = 29,368$), the investigators found that greater intake of vitamin D was associated with lower risk of RA in older women ages 55 to 69. These findings seem to suggest that vitamin D may play a role in both OA and RA, but the exact mechanisms are unknown, and no prospective treatment trials have been carried out.

3.2.3.2. Vitamin C. Vitamin C is important for the growth, development, and enzymatic reactions of bone and cartilage. Vitamin C acts as an antioxidant in facilitating the hydroxylation of proline and lysine to hydroxyproline and hydroxylysine in procollagen. These products are essential to the maturation of collagen molecules and, thus, to the construction of the extracellular matrix of cartilage. This mechanism has been explored in the guinea pig model of surgically induced or spontaneous OA. These animals, like humans, cannot synthesize ascorbic acid. Therefore, they must obtain vitamin C through the diet. In guinea pigs fed a diet poor in vitamin C, proteoglycan synthesis declines. This may be related to alterations in enzymatic activity or reductions in proline hydroxylation or both *(52)*. Early work on a surgically induced model of OA in the guinea pig showed that animals that received low-dose supplementation with vitamin C (a dose adequate to prevent scurvy) had more severe OA that those on high-dose supplementation (60 times as much) over a period of several weeks. It was hypothesized, because animals receiving higher doses had higher cartilages weights, that vitamin C protected against cartilage loss by stimulating collagen synthesis *(53)*.

However, more recent work has suggested that long-term exposure to vitamin C supplementation might have deleterious effects *(54)*. In these experiments, no surgical procedures were performed and the animals developed spontaneous OA. Guinea pigs were supplemented with low, medium, and high doses of vitamin C for 8 months. On subsequent histological evaluation, the animals that had received the medium and high doses had more severe histological changes, including the formation of osteophytes. The investigators hypothesized that the process of chondrophyte formation, with evolution into osteophytes, may have been facilitated by the enhanced collagen synthesis afforded by higher doses of ascorbic acid. On the basis of the most recent guinea pig data, it has been suggested that vitamin C supplementation above the currently recommended daily doses of 75 to 90 mg not be advised *(54)*.

No prospective data are yet available to offer guidance in this area. The only human data comes from an epidemiological investigation using the Framingham population *(55)*. In this study, vitamin C intake was measured by food-frequency questionnaire. The study compared 453 subjects without evidence of OA to 187 subjects with radiographic OA of the knee. The investigators found no correlation between vitamin C intake assessed at a single time point and the incidence of OA. However, they did identify a threefold reduction in the risk of OA (measured as radiographic evidence of cartilage loss) in the middle and highest tertiles of vitamin C intake. This observation suggests that further investigation is needed to clarify the role of vitamin C in human OA.

Whether or not additional mechanisms exist by which antioxidant supplements might be of benefit in OA is speculative *(56)* but interest in the use of antioxidants as therapeutic agents remains high among patients. The potential link between antioxidants in the diet other than vitamin C and OA was also investigated in the Framingham population *(55)*. Like vitamin C, β-carotene (odds ratio [OR] = 0.3) and vitamin E (OR = 0.7) intake were associated with a reduction in risk of OA progression. The role of β-carotene intake in the development or progression of OA has not been further investigated. Further work is available on vitamin E. Data from the Johnston County Osteoarthritis Project in North Carolina suggests that those with the highest ratios of serum α-tocopherol to γ-tocopherol had half the odds of developing radiographic OA of the knee *(57)*. This relationship was statistically significant in men and African Americans, but not for women or other ethnic groups among 400 participants studied. One prospective supplementation trial of vitamin E use for OA has been carried out. In this trial, 136 subjects were randomized to receive either vitamin E 500 IU or placebo for 2 years. Patients were followed with magnetic resonance imaging to measure tibial cartilage volume. There was no difference in medial or lateral tibial cartilage volume loss between the vitamin E-supplemented group and those who got placebo at the end of the trial. Furthermore, there was no relationship between dietary levels of antioxidants and cartilage volume loss. Taken together, these findings suggest that simple supplementation with vitamins is unlikely to be a straightforward treatment for OA.

3.2.3.3. **Vitamin K.** Vitamin K is an important regulator of bone and cartilage mineralization. It is an essential cofactor in the formation of skeletal matrix proteins containing the γ-carboxyglutamic acid residue. These proteins have high affinity for calcium and phosphate allowing for mineralization of skeletal tissue. Insufficient vitamin K can lead to abnormal chondrocyte differentiation and endochondral bone formation *(58,59)*. The vitamin-K dependent bone and cartilage proteins can inhibit excessive extracellular matrix calcifications believed to be responsible for abnormal osteophyte formation in osteoarthritis. Therefore, inadequate levels of vitamin K may lead to cartilage loss, JSN, and osteophyte formation. No clinical trials have been carried out to determine whether vitamin K supplementation can reduce OA. A recent analysis of vitamin K level in the Framingham Offspring Study cohort showed that low levels of vitamin K was associated with radiographic features of OA. The results of this study showed that as the plasma phylloquinone (the primary form of vitamin K) levels rose, the prevalence ratios of OA (defined by Kellgren/Lawrence grade 2 on greater on radiographs on a per-joint basis), osteophytes, and JSN significantly decreased. This statistically significant effect was seen in the radiographs of the hands and knees of a cohort of 672 subjects *(59)*.

3.2.3.4. **Glucosamine and Chondroitin.** The lay press and many in the medical community have advocated the dietary supplements glucosamine and chondroitin as effective and safe treatment options for OA. Both agents have been used for decades in the treatment of OA in Europe and more recently in the United States. Together, they are the most widely used dietary supplements for OA. Glucosamine and chondroitin are important constituents of normal joint tissue. Glucosamine is an aminomonosaccharide that is a component of glycoproteins, proteoglycans, and glycosaminoglycans. A number of laboratory and clinical studies have been carried out to investigate the potential efficacy of these agents in OA. The results, have been mixed and remain controversial. The following section reviews the laboratory evidence of the potential role of glucosamine and chondroitin in OA. A review and analysis of pertinent clinical studies follows.

Glucosamine and chondroitin levels are reduced or altered in osteoarthritic cartilage and synovial fluid *(61,62)*. Therefore, the notion of replenishing these agents through dietary intake in order to reduce joint symptoms has been proposed. A number of laboratory experiments have been carried out in an attempt to elucidate the action of these agents in OA. Orally administered glucosamine is detectable at low levels in the sera of human subjects, but there has been no direct demonstration that glucosamine is incorporated into cartilage *(63)*. In the subjects who took 1,500 mg of glucosamine sulfate mixed with water, the serum glucosamine levels reached a maximum of 4.8 µmol/L at a mean of 2 hours after ingestion. Based on the low serum levels achieved, the investigators concluded that it was unlikely that glucosamine contributed to proteoglycan synthesis *in vivo*.

Despite the fact that dietary supplementation of glucosamine and chondroitin has not been proven to raise levels of these compounds in the joints, numerous mechanisms of action have been proposed based on the assumption that they could. In addition to simply serving as building blocks of cartilage, glucosamine and chondrointin might affect the metabolism of cartilage constituents. It was shown in *in vitro* studies that glucosamine could stimulate proteoglycan synthesis by human chondrocytes and become incorporated into glycosaminoglycans *(62,64)*. However, whether this effect is seen *in vivo* is unknown.

Other laboratory studies have demonstrated that both glucosamine and chondroitin may have additional effects of countering the degradation process of cartilage in OA. In animal studies, glucosamine reduced cellular production of inflammatory mediators and inflammation *(65)*. Similarly, chondroitin can reduce collagen breakdown and MMP production by chondrocytes *(62,64)*.

A number of clinical trials have been carried out to study the efficacy of glucosamine and chondroitin in OA. Although the majority of earlier trials seem to suggest modest benefit in terms of pain relief as well as objective improvements, more recent meta-analyses of the studies indicated that the benefits might not be as great. Concerns of the scientific quality of the studies were also raised. One of the most widely cited clinical trials that showed benefits of glucosamine was carried out in Europe. In this study, 212 patients with OA of the knee were treated with oral glucosamine sulfate at a daily dose of 1,500 mg or placebo for 3 years. The Western Ontario and McMaster Universities Osteoarthritis Index (WOMAC) and weight-bearing anterioposterior view radiographs were used to evaluate the subjects. At the end of the trial, the subjects who were treated with glucosamine had an average of 11.7% improvement in WOMAC scores compared with baseline. WOMAC scores worsened by an average of 9.8% for those in the placebo group. Radiographs showed that the treatment group had a mean 0.06 mm of JSN compared with 0.31 mm of JSN in the placebo group *(66)*.

Another clinical trial contradicted these findings. In a discontinuation trial, 137 patients with OA of the knee who had felt improvement since starting glucosamine were randomized to receive either 1,500 mg of glucosamine sulfate or placebo for 6 months. Using WOMAC scores and an intention-to-treat analysis, 42% of the placebo group and 45% of the treatment group experienced disease flare. This result was not significant, suggesting that glucosamine did not prevent flares of OA *(67)*.

A recent meta-analysis to review glucosamine therapy in OA was reported by the Cochrane Collaboration. Twenty randomized controlled trials were reviewed. Overall, when compared with placebo, glucosamine showed a 28% improvement in pain and 21% improvement in function using the Lequesne Index. However, WOMAC scores did not show statistically significant differences. When the analysis was restricted to eight studies with the highest quality utilizing adequate allocation concealment, there was no improvement in pain or function *(68)*.

Clinical trials for chondroitin have also showed conflicting results. One study involved 120 subjects who took daily chondroitin in the form of 800 mg bovine chondroitin sulfate mixed in water or placebo for Months 0 to 3 and 6 to 9. The chondroitin-treated group had significantly greater improvements in the Lequesne Index, visual analog scale measurements for pain, and walking time than the placebo group. The treatment group also had less radiographic changes than the placebo group *(69)*.

Another trial of chondroitin did not show improvement in symptoms. In this randomized, double-blind, placebo-controlled trial, 300 participants with OA received either 800 mg chondroitin or placebo daily for 2 years. There was no significant difference in symptoms and function between the two groups as measured by the WOMAC scale. However, those who received chondroitin had less progression of JSN as measured on anteroposterior radiographs of the knee in flexion *(70)*.

In order to establish more definitive evidence of the role of these supplements in osteoarthritis, the NIH sponsored the Glucosamine/Chondroitin Arthritis Intervention Trial (GAIT). This was the first major multicenter clinical trial to rigorously evaluate the efficacy and safety of glucosamine, chondroitin, or the combination of the two in the treatment of OA. Patients with symptomatic OA of the knee were randomized into five groups receiving either 1500 mg of glucosamine hydrochloride daily, 1200 mg of chondroitin sulfate daily, a combination of the two, 200 mg of celecoxib (a COX-2 inhibitor), or placebo for 6 months. Overall, GAIT showed that glucosamine, chondroitin, and the combination of the two were no better at relieving OA symptoms than placebo as measured by WOMAC, patient and physician global assessments, and the HAQ. In subgroup analysis of subjects with moderate to severe pain, the combination of glucosamine and chondroitin, but neither alone, was better than placebo at relieving symptoms. This apparent benefit, however, must be interpreted with caution because the "positive control" group of patients treated with celecoxib did not show improvement. The study was hindered by several additional factors. There was a very high placebo-response rate of 60% and most of the patients had a mild degree of pain. Both of these effects may make it more difficult to detect differences between treatment arms. Other concerns raised included limitations induce the high attrition rate of 20% and the lack of sophisticated methodological analysis. Finally, the preparation of glucosamine used in the study was glucosamine hydrochloride rather than glucosamine sulfate. Glucosamine sulfate is the form that is widely available in the United States and has been the preparation used in other studies reporting efficacy *(11,71)*. The significance of using glucosamine hydrochloride preparation, rather than glucosamine sulfate, in this trial remains uncertain.

In summary, observations in laboratory and animal studies suggest mechanisms that support a possible beneficial role of glucosamine and chondroitin in the pathogenesis of OA. Early clinical trials seem to support the contention that these supplements can reduce the symptoms of OA and slow the progression of disease. But more recent high-quality studies do not show significant difference between these agents and placebo in the treatment of OA.

3.2.4. HERBAL SUPPLEMENTS

According to current U.S. regulations, herbal and dietary supplements are regulated differently than conventional medicines. The Dietary Supplement and Health Education Act of 1994 allowed for the sale of herbal and dietary supplements without the approval of the FDA. Normally, the FDA ensures that conventional drugs such as prescription or over-the-counter drugs contain the content and dosages listed on the label. Furthermore, the dosages are standardized based on rigorous efficacy and safety trials, and the manufacturers are required to collect and report their post-marketing experiences. No such standards apply to herbal and dietary supplements. Supplement preparations may or may not contain the correct dosages or even the advertised ingredients. Furthermore, contaminants such as lead, arsenic, as well as NSAIDs and wafarin, have been found in herbal medications *(72–74)*. Many of the herbal and dietary supplements have not undergone trials showing proof of efficacy or safety. Scientific studies to elucidate modes of action are lacking. Nonetheless, clinical trials have been carried out on several plant-based supplements. A review of some of these herbal medicines is provided in the following section.

3.2.4.1. Willow Bark (*Salix* **sp.**). Ground up willow bark has been used as an analgesic and antipyretic remedy since ancient times dating to Egyptian, Greek, and Roman civilizations. Willow bark contains salicin which, upon oxidation, yields salicylic acid. Aspirin (acetylsalicylic acid) is a refined product of the willow bark extract salicin. Clinical trials using willow bark as treatment have been carried out for low back pain and OA. In a 4-week randomized double-blind study, 210 patients with low back pain received low-dose (393 mg) or high-dose (786 mg) dry willow bark extract or placebo daily. The principle outcome measure was the number of patients who were pain-free and did not use a "rescue" analgesic for at least 5 days by the end of the study. After 6 months, both the high- and low-dose treatment groups (39 and 21%, respectively) were significantly less likely to have used the rescue analgesic than the placebo group (6%) *(75)*.

A second randomized, double-blind, placebo-controlled trial demonstrated efficacy of willow bark preparation for relieving OA knee and hip pain. In this study, 78 patients were randomized to receive two tablets of willow bark (240 mg salicin per day) or placebo for 2 weeks after a washout period of 4 to 6 days with placebo. All other medications for pain relief were not allowed during the study. At the end of the trial, there was a 14% reduction of the WOMAC pain score in the treatment group and a 2% increase in the placebo group *(76)*. The efficacy of this agent needs further confirmation especially in trials longer than 4 weeks.

3.2.4.2. Devil's Claw (*Harpagophytum procumbens*). The tubers of this perennial plant are used in African folk medicine for relief of pain caused by rheumatism. In a 4-week, double-blind study, 197 patients with chronic back pain received two daily doses of *Harpagophytum* extract, 600 mg daily and 1,200 mg daily, or placebo. Significantly higher numbers of patients were pain-free in the treated groups compared with the placebo group *(45)*. There have also been a handful of small, short-term trials that have shown efficacy of devil's claw extract in OA. Several double-blind studies showed that *Harpagophytum* can reduce pain and improve mobility in patients with OA. All of the trials have been short-term and devil's claw was well tolerated. Side effects included mild GI upset, likely because of its stimulatory effect on gastric secretions. Long-term studies on efficacy and side effects are needed.

3.2.4.3. Ginger (*Zingiber officinale*). Ginger has a long history of medicinal use in the Chinese and Ayurvedic traditions. Rhizomes of several ginger species, in both oral and topical forms, are used to treat a variety of inflammatory and arthritic conditions. Extracts of ginger have been reported to decrease joint pain and swelling in patients with arthritis. Anti-inflammatory effects have been shown in *in vitro* and animal model experiments *(77)*. Experimental studies have shown that ginger extract can inhibit prostaglandin and leukotrienes, inhibit the production of TNF-α gene expression in human OA synoviocytes and chondrocytes, and suppress proinflammatory chemokine expression in human synoviocytes *(77)*.

A study of 247 patients with OA of the knee showed that a ginger extract combination had a statistically significant effect in reducing knee pain *(78)*. The study was a double-blind, placebo-controlled clinical trial that spanned 6 weeks of treatment with ginger extract or placebo. The treatment group had greater improvement in primary outcome of reduction in knee pain on standing (63 vs 50%; $p = 0.048$). Secondary outcomes of mean reduction in pain after walking 50 ft and reduction in the WOMAC scores were statistically better in the treatment group. Patients who received the ginger extract had more gastrointestinal complaints (59 vs 21%), but the symptoms were mild.

Another trial was a 3-week randomized, double-blind, placebo-controlled, crossover study of ginger extract and ibuprofen in patients with OA of the hip or knee. The outcome measures were visual analog scale of pain and the Lequesne index. Based on these measurements the efficacy was ibuprofen → ginger extract → placebo. However, statistically significant effect of ginger extract was seen only by explorative statistical methods in the first period of treatment before crossover *(79)*.

3.2.4.4. Thunder God Vine (*Tripterygium wilfordii*). *Tripterygium wilfordii* is a perennial vine found in southern China. Its long history of use dates back to 16th-century China, when its roots, leaves, and flowers were used for medicinal purposes. The herb is also known as *Lei Gong Teng*, the Thunder God Vine. The modern-day medicinal form of the herb is derived from the root, not the flower or the vine *(45)*. Preparations of this herb have been used for various rheumatic disorders, including RA, SLE, Henoch-Schonlein purpura, Sweet's syndrome, systemic sclerosis, Behcet's syndrome, and psoriatic arthritis. The therapeutic and adverse effects are likely due to diterpenoid compounds with epoxide structures. These compounds have been shown to have immunosuppressive and anti-inflammatory effects in *in vitro* and *in vivo* studies. This herbal extract can inhibit proinflammatory cytokines IL-2 and interferon-γ, as well as PGE_2 and nitric oxide.

A randomized, double-blind, placebo-controlled study of *Tripterygium* in patients with long-standing RA who had failed conventional therapy showed some benefit. Patients were randomized to placebo, low-dose (180 mg per day), or high-dose (360 mg per day) of *Tripterygium* extract. Of the 35 patients who enrolled, 21 completed the 20-week study. A therapeutic effect as defined by American College of Rheumatology (ACR-20) was achieved in a significant number of patients treated with 360 mg per day of the herb extract when compared with the placebo group. Beneficial effect was also seen in the low-dose group when compared with the placebo group *(80)*. The number of patients who withdrew because of side effects was similar in both groups.

Considerable toxicity has been associated with the use of Thunder God Vine in anecdotal reports. Up to one-third of the patients experience GI side effects, which include diarrhea, nausea, vomiting, dry mouth, abdominal pain, gastritis, and oral ulcers. Reversible amenorrhea occurred in patients less than 40 years of age. However, in perimenopausal women, the amenorrhea can be irreversible *(45)*. Treatment-related deaths have occurred as a result of myocardial damage, renal failure, and severe GI side effects. This herb is not readily found in the United States, but is available in China.

3.2.4.5. Feverfew (*Tanacetum parthenium*). Feverfew plants grow widely in Europe and North America. This herb has been used as an antipyretic and anti-inflammatory folk remedy for centuries. Its use dates back to ancient Greek civilization when it was prescribed to treat "inflammations and hot swellings" *(45)*. The leaves can be chewed fresh or dried and made into tablets, which are available in the United States and Europe. The active component, parthenolide, has several anti-inflammatory effects. It inhibits, in a dose-dependent fashion, the production of prostaglandins and leukotrienes by human polymorphonuclear leukocytes. It can also suppress secretion of TNF-α and IL-1. Both crude feverfew extracts and purified parthenolide can inhibit adhesion molecule expression on rheumatoid synovial fibroblasts. Feverfew has an additional molecular mechanism of inhibiting the release of nuclear factor-κB, an important transcription factor in the expression of multiple genes involved in the inflammatory process *(45)*.

In a clinical trial of feverfew in patients with active RA, there was no benefit. The study was a 6-week, double-blind, placebo-controlled trial in which a powdered extract of *Tanacetum parthenium* or placebo was given to 41 women with active RA. The patients had no improvement in pain, stiffness, functional capacity, grip strength, CRP, or ESR *(81)*.

Feverfew may increase bleeding time, thus, it should be avoided in patients with coagulopathy or on warfarin. It can also cause GI disturbances. It should not be used in pregnant women due to the risk of spontaneous abortions. Individuals with allergies to ragweed should always avoid feverfew *(45)*.

3.2.4.6. Avocado and Soybean Unsaponifiables. Avocado and soybean unsaponifiables (ASU) are the fraction of avocado and soybean oil that, upon hydrolysis, does not produce soap. ASU is a mixture of one part avocado oil to two parts soybean oil. This compound has produced beneficial results in laboratory studies, as well as in clinical trials. In studies of human osteoarthritic chondrocyte cultures, ASU inhibited IL-1 and IL-1-induced activation of metalloproteinases, collagenase, PGE_2, IL-6, and IL-8 *(82)*. Furthermore, it may stimulate collagen synthesis. Another study showed the ASU prevented human osteoarthritic osteoblast-induced inhibition of cartilage matrix production, thus suggesting that it may promote cartilage repair in OA *(83)*.

A multicenter randomized, double-blind, placebo-controlled trial of 164 patients with OA of the hip and knee was carried out. Subjects were randomized to receive either 300 mg ASU or placebo capsules daily for 6 months. At the end of the trial, those treated with ASU had statistically better outcome as evidenced by improvements in pain and function (Lequesne index), and patients' and physicians' overall assessment on a 5-point scale *(84)*. There was also a reduction in NSAID requirement in the treated group, but this effect did not reach statistical significance. Side effects were comparable between the treated and placebo groups.

Another randomized study evaluated the effect of ASU in 260 patients with OA of the knee. The subjects were randomized into three groups. Group 1 received 600 mg ASU, group 2 received 300 mg ASU, and group 3 received placebo daily for 3 months. Significant improvements were seen in pain and functional parameters in the groups 1 and 2 compared with group 3, and there was a trend toward greater improvement with higher dose. NSAID and analgesic use decreased by more than 50 and 71% in patients receiving 300 mg per day and 600 mg per day, respectively whereas, the placebo group had a reduction of 36% in NSAID and analgesic use *(85)*.

One longer term study evaluated the structural effects of ASU on joint space loss in OA of the hip. In this trial, 163 patients with symptomatic OA of the hip and joint space of at least 1 mm were examined radiographically before and after treatment with 300 mg ASU daily for 2 years. No difference was detected between the treated and placebo groups. Further subgroup analysis divided the subjects into two groups based on baseline severity of radiographic joint disease. This analysis showed that in the patients with more severe disease, ASU was associated with less JSN compared with placebo. The two groups did not differ in Lequesne's functional index, NSAID/analgesic intake, pain, and functional assessments (visual analog scale), and patient's and physician's overall assessments or in adverse events *(86)*.

3.2.4.7. Turmeric (*Curuma longa*). Turmeric is a spice used commonly in India and other Eastern countries. It has also been used as a medicinal agent for centuries in these regions of the world. Curcumin is the principle curcuminoid compound that gives turmeric its yellow color and is considered the most active constituent. Curcumin has been shown to have anti-oxidant, anti-inflammatory, and anti-cancer activities. It blocked cyclooxygenase and lipoxygenase activities in cultured cells, reducing inflammatory mediators including prostaglandins, thromboxane, and leukotrienes *(87)*. An *in vitro* study was carried out to evaluate the effect of therapy with curcumin and the COX-2 inhibitor celecoxib *(88)*. Synovial fibroblast-like adherent cells were incubated with curcumin and celecoxib alone or in combination. The addition of curcumin to celecoxib augmented COX-2 inhibition as evident by a decrease of more than 95% in PGE_2 production. Curcumin also synergistically potentiated the growth inhibition and apoptosis of the synovial cells induced by celecoxib. Two small preliminary unblinded studies showed an anti-inflammatory effect of curcumin *(90,91)*. No large, double-blind, placebo-controlled studies have been performed to evaluate the clinical efficacy of this agent in rheumatic diseases.

A Phase I clinical trial of curcumin in patients with premalignant disease in Taiwan showed that curcumin is well tolerated even in doses up to 8 g per day *(89)*. No serious adverse effects have been reported in humans taking curcumin.

4. CONCLUSIONS

CAM encompasses a wide array of interventions. The overall impact of these therapies is great. Patient interest and use are high, as are the number of available products and practitioners, as well as the costs. The discussion in this chapter highlighted the evidence as it pertains to only a fraction of this vast topic: diets, dietary supplements, and herbal products and their role as therapies in rheumatic diseases.

Scientific evidence does not support a substantial role of special diets or dietary manipulations in the treatment of the majority of patients suffering from arthritis and rheumatic diseases. The level of available evidence has not yet risen to the standards expected for pharmacological interventions However, taken broadly, vegetarian diets and those high in n-3 fatty acids are more likely to be beneficial than the traditional American diet. Laboratory data indicate that long-chain fatty acids play a role in inflammation, suggesting a credible pathophysiological pathway through which beneficial effects in inflammatory diseases might be mediated.

Vitamins are necessary for normal health of bone and cartilage. However, the role of vitamin supplementation is not clear in the treatment of rheumatic diseases. There have not been adequate prospective observations to support the notion that vitamin supplementation beyond current federal recommendations is warranted in rheumatology patients.

A considerable amount of work has been published regarding the effects of glucosamine and chondroitin. The clinical data is mixed, but more recent clinical trials and meta-analyses do not show efficacy in OA.

A variety of small, short-term trials of a variety of herbal supplements have appeared in the literature. However, large, long-term, randomized, double-blind, placebo-controlled trials are lacking to show conclusive evidence to support the role of herbs in the treatment of rheumatic diseases. Long-term efficacy is important in rheumatic diseases such as OA and RA, which are chronic illnesses with variable progression over time. Results of short-term trials may only reflect fluctuations in natural disease activity rather than representing true differences in long-term outcome. Furthermore, long-term safety of dietary and herbal supplements is a legitimate concern especially in light of the current lack of FDA regulations.

REFERENCES

1. Eisenberg D, Kessler R, Foster C, et al. Unconventional medicine in the United States: prevalence, costs, and patterns of use. N Engl J Med 1993;328:246–252.
2. Eisenberg D, Davis R, Ettner S, et al. Trends in alternative medicine use in the United States, 1990–1997: results from a national survey. JAMA 1998;280:1569–1575.
3. Barnes P, Powell-Griner E, McFann K, Nahin R. Complementary and alternative medicine use among adults: united states, 2002. Advance Data From Vital and Health Statistics, Centers for Disease Control and Prevention 2004;343:1–20.
4. National Center for Complementary and Alternative Medicine. Available at: http://nccam.nih.gov/about/almanac/organization/NCCAM.htm.
5. Committee on the framework for evaluating the safety of dietary supplements. Dietary Supplement, a Framework for Evaluating Safety. National Academies Press, Washington, DC, The 2005.
6. Rao J, Mihaliak K, Kroenke K, et al. Use of complementary therapies for arthritis among patients of rheumatologists. Ann Intern Med 1999;131:409–416.
7. Ramsey S, Spencer A, Topolski T, et al. Use of alternative therapies by older adults with osteoarthritis. Arthritis Care Res 2001;45:222–227.
8. Henderson C, Panush R. Diets, dietary supplements, and nutritional therapies in rheumatic diseases. Rheum Dis Clin North Am 1999;25:937–968.
9. McDougall J, Bruce B, Spiller G, et al. Effects of very low-fat, vegan diet in subjects with rheumatoid arthritis. J Altern Complement Med 2002;8:71–75.
10. Felson D. Osteoarthritis of the knee. N Engl J Med 2006;354:841–848.
11. Clegg D, Reda D, Harris C, et al. Glucosamine, chondroitin sulfate and the two in combination for painful knee osteoarthritis.N Engl J Med 2006;354:795–808.
12. Arthritis Foundation. Arthritis: The Basic Facts.Arthritis Foundation, Atlanta, GA, 1981.
13. Stamp L, James M, Cleland L. Diet and rheumatoid arthritis: a review of the literature. Semin Arthritis Rheum 2005;35:77–94.
14. Panush R, Stroud R, Webster E. Food-induced (allergic) arthritis. Inflammatory arthritis exacerbated by milk. Arthritis Rheum 1986;29:220–226.
15. Darlington L, Ramsey N, Mansfield J. Placebo-controlled, blind study of dietary manipulation therapy in rheumatoid arthritis. Lancet 1986;1:237–239.

16. Vegetarian diet: a starter's guide to a plant based diet. Available at: http://mayoclinic.com/health/vegetarian-diet/HQ01596
17. Kjeldsen-Kragh J, Borchgrevink C, Mowinkel P, et al. Controlled trial of fasting and one-year vegetarian diet in rheumatoid arthritis. Lancet 1991;338:899–902.
18. Rhen T, Cidlowski, J. Antiinflammatory action of glucocorticoids—new mechanisms for old drugs. Arthritis Foundation 2005;353:1711–1723.
19. Kronmann N, Green A. Epidemiological studies in the Upernavik district, Greenland: incidence of some chronic diseases 1950–1974. Acta Med Scand 1980;208:401–406.
20. Gruppo Italiano per lo Studio Della Sopravvivenza nell'Infarto micocarico. Dietary supplementation with n-3 polyunsaturated fatty acids and vitamin E after myocardial infarction: results of the GISSI-Prevenzione trial.Lancet 1999;354:447–455.
21. Kremer J. n-3 Fatty acid supplements in rheumatoid arthritis. Am J Clin Nutr 2000;71:349S-351S.
22. Ariza-Ariza R, Mestanza-Peralta M, Cardiel M. Omega-3 fatty acids in rheumatoid arthritis: an overview. Semin Arthritis Rheum 1998;6:366–370.
23. Cleland L, James M, Proudman S. The role of fish oils in the treatment of rheumatoid arthritis. Drugs 2003;63:845–853.
24. Kris-Etherton P, Harris W, Appel L. Fish consumption, fish oil, omega-3 fatty acids, and cardiovascular disease. Circulation 2002;106:2747–2757.
25. Kris-Etherton P, Taylor D, Yu-Poth S, et al. Polyunsaturated fatty acids in the food chain in the United States. Am J Clin Nutr 2000;71:179S-188S.
26. Fujikawa M, Yamashita N, Yamazaki K, et al. Eicosapentaenoic acid inhibits antigen-presenting cell function of murine splenocytes. Immunology 1992;75:330–335.
27. Kremer J, Lawrence D, Jubiz W, et al. Effects of high-dose fish oil on rheumatoid arthritis after stopping non-steroidal anti-inflammatory drugs. Clinical and immune correlates. Arthritis Rheum 1995;38:1107–1114.
28. Endres S, Ghorbani R, Kelley V, et al. The effect of dietary supplementation with n-3 polyunsaturated fatty acids on the synthesis of interleukin-1 and tumor necrosis factor by mononuclear cells. N Engl J Med 1989;320:265–271.
29. Curtis C, Hughes C, Flannery C, et al. n-3 fatty acids specifically modulate catabolic factors involved in articular cartilage degradation. J Biol Chem 2000;275:721–724.
30. Curtis C, Rees S, Little C, et al. Pathological indicators of degradation and inflammation in human osteoarthritis cartilage are abrogated by exposure to n-3 fatty acids. Arthritis Rheum 2002;46:1544–1553.
31. Lau C, Morley K, Belch J. Effects of fish oil supplementation on non-steroidal anti-inflammatory requirement in patiens with mild rheumatoid arthritis—a double-blind placebo-controlled trial. Br J Rheumatol 1993;32:982–989.
32. Geusens P, Wouters C, Nijs J, et al. Long-term effect of omega-3 fatty acid supplementation in active rheumatoid arthritis. A 12-month, double-blind, controlled study. Arthritis Rheum 1994;37:824–829.
33. Kremer J, Lawrence D, Jubiz W, et al. Dietary fish oil and olive oil supplementation in patients with rheumatoid arthritis. Arthritis Rheum 1990;33:810–819.
34. Volker D, Firtzgerald P, Major G, et al.. Efficacy of fish oil concentrate in the treatment of rheumatoid arthritis. J Rheumatol 2000;27:2343–2346.
35. Fortin P, Lew R, Liang M, et al. Validation of a meta-analysis: the effects of fish oil in rheumatoid arthritis. J Clin Epidemiol 1995;48:1379–1390.
36. Burr M, Fehily A, Gilbert J, et al. Effects of changes in fat, fish, and fibre intakes on death and myocardial reinfarction: diet and reinfarction trial (DART). Lancet 1989;2:757–761.
37. Leaf A, Jorgensen M, Jacobs A, et al. Do fish oils prevent restenosis after coronary angioplasty? Circulation 1994;90:2248–2257.
38. Eritsland J, Arnesen H, Gronseth K, et al. Effect of dietary supplementation with n-3 fatty acids on coronary artery bypass graft patency. Am J Cardio 1996;77:31–36.
39. Montori V, Farmer A, Wollan P, et al. Fish oil supplementation in type 2 diabetes: a quantitative systematic review. Diabetes Care 2000;23:1217–1218.
40. Department of Health and Human Services, US Food and Drug Administration. Substances affirmed as generally recognized as safe: menhaden oil. Federal Register 1997;62:30751–30757.

Available at: http://frwebgate.access.gpo.gov/cgi-bin/getdoc.cgi?dbname=1997_register&docid=fr05jn97-5.
41. Office of Nutritional Products, Labeling, and Dietary Supplements, Center for Food Safety and Applied Nutrition, US Food and Drug Administration 2002. Available at: http://www.cfsan.fda.gov/~dms/ds-ltr28.html.
42. Harris, W, Ginsberg H, Arunakul N, et al. safety and efficacy of Omacor in severe hypertriglyceridemia. J Cardiovasc Risk 1997;4:385–391.
43. US Food and Drug Administration. What you need to know about mercury in fish and shellfish. FDA/CFSAN Consumer Advisory 2004. Available at: http://www.cfsan.fda.gov/~dms/admehg3.html.
44. Covington, M. Omega-3 fatty acids. Am Fam Physician 2004;70:133–140.
45. Setty A, Sigal L. Herbal medications commonly used in the practice of rheumatology: mechanisms of action, efficacy, and side effects. Semin Arthritis Rheum 2005;34:773–784.
46. Belch J, Hill A. Evening primrose oil and borage oil in rheumatologic conditions. Am J Clin Nutr 2000;71:352S-356S.
47. Leventhal L, Boyce E, Zurier R. Treatment of rheumatoid arthritis with gammalinolenic acid. Ann Int Med 1993;119:867–873.
48. Theander E, Horrobin D, Jacobsson L, et al. Gammalinolenic acid treatment of fatigue associated with primary Sjogren's syndrome. Scand J Rheumatol 2002;31:72–79.
49. McAlindon T, Felson D, Zhanf Y, et al. Relation of dietary intake and serum levels of vitamin D to progression of osteoarthritis of the knee among participants in the Framingham study. Ann Intern Med 1996;125:353–359.
50. Lane N, Gore L, Cummings S, et al. Serum vitamin D levels and incident changes of radiographic hip osteoarthritis. A longitudinal study. Arthritis Rheum 1999;42:854–860.
51. Merlino L, Curtis J, Mikuls T, et al. Vitamin D is inversely associated with rheumatoid arthritis: results from the Iowa Women's Health Study. Arthritis Rheum 2004;50:72–77.
52. Peterkosfsky B. Ascorbate requirement for hydroxylation and secretion of procollagen: relationship to inhibition of collagen synthesis in scurvy. Am J Clin Nutr 1991;54:1135S-1140S.
53. Schwartz E, Oh W, Leveille C. Experimentally induced osteoarthritis in guinea pigs: metabolic responses in articular cartilage to developing pathology. Arthritis Rheum 1981;24:1345–1355.
54. Kraus V, Huebner J, Stabler T, et al. Ascorbic acid increases the severity of spontaneous knee osteoarthritis in a guinea pig model. Arthritis Rheum 2004;50:1822–1831.
55. McAlindon T, Jacques P, Zhang Y, et al. Do antioxidant micronutrients protect against the development and progression of knee osteoarthritis? Arthris Rheum 1996;39:648–656.
56. Henrotin Y, Kurz G, Aigner T. Review: oxygen and reactive oxygen species in cartilage degradation: friend or foes? Osteoarthrtitis Cartilage 2005;13:643–654.
57. Jordan J, De Roos A, Renner J, et al. A case-control study of serum tocopherol levels and the alpha- to gamma-tocopherol ratio in radiographic knee osteoarthritis: the Johnston County Osteoarthritis Project. Am J Epidemiol 2004;159:968–977.
58. Newman B, Gigout L, Sudre L, et al. Coordinated expression of matrix Gla protein is required during endochondral ossification for chondrocyte survival. J Cell Biol 2001;154:659–666.
59. Neogi T, Booth S, Zhang Y, et al. Low vitamin K status is associated with osteoarthritis in the hand and knee. Arthritis Rheum 2006;54:1255–1261.
60. Kolata G. 2 Top-selling arthritis drugs are found to be ineffective. NY Times. Feb 23, 2006.
61. Lewis S, Crossman M, Flannelly J, et al. Chondroitin sulphation patterns in synovial fluid in osteoarthritis subset. Ann Rheum Dis 1999;58:441–445.
62. Kolasinski S. Glucosamine and Chondroitin: Update 2006. Alt Med Alert 2006;9:73–84.
63. Biggee B, Blinn C, McAlindon T, et al. Low levels of human serum glucosamine after ingestion of glucosamine sulphate relative to capability for peripheral effectiveness. Ann Rheum Dis 2006;65:222–226.
64. Bassleer C, Henrotin Y, Franchimont P. In vitro evaluation of drugs proposed as chondroprotective agents. Int J Tissue React 1992;14:231–240.
65. Neil K, Orth M, Coussens P, et al. Effects of glucosamine and chondroitin sulfate on mediators of osteoarthritis in cultured equine chondrocytes stimulated by use of recombinant equine interleukin-1b. Am J Vet Res 2005;66:1861–1869.

66. Reginster J, Deroisy R, Rovati L, et al. Long-term effects of glucosamine sulphate on osteoarthrtitis progression: a randomized, placebo-controlled clinical trial. Lancet 2001;357:251–256.
67. Cibere J, Kopee J, Thorne A, et al. Randomized, double-blind, placebo-controlled glucosamine discontinuation trial in knee osteoarthritis. Arthritis Rheum 2004;51:738–745.
68. Towheed T, Maxwell L, Anastassiades T, et al. Glucosamine therapy for treating osteoarthritis. The Cochrane Database of Systematic Reviews 2005;2:CD002946.
69. Uebelhart D, Malaise M, Marcolongo R, et al. Intermittent treatment of knee osteoarthritis with oral chondroitin sulfate: a one-year, randomized, double-blind multicenter study versus placebo. Osteoarthritis Cartilage 2004;12:269–276.
70. Michel B, Stucki G, Frey D, et al. Chondroitins 4 and 6 sulfate in osteoarthritis of the knee: a randomized, controlled trial. Arthritis Rheum 2005;52:779–786.
71. Hochberg M. Nutritional supplements for knee osteoarthritis-still no resolution. N Engl J Med 2006;52:858–860.
72. Weiger W, Smith M, Boon H, et al. Advising patients who seek complementary and alternative medical therapies for cancer. Ann Intern Med 2002;137:889–903.
73. Saper R, Kales S, Paquin J, et al. Heavy metal content of ayurvedic herbal medicine products. JAMA 2004;292:2868–2873.
74. Bent S, Ko R. Commonly used herbal medicines in the United States: a review. Am J Med 2004;116:478–485.
75. Chrubasik S, Eisenberg E, Balan E, et al. Treatment of low back pain exacerbations with willow bark extract: a randomized double-blind study. Am J Med 2000;109:9–14.
76. Schmid B, Ludtke R, Selbmann H, et al. Efficacy and tolerability of a standardized willow bark extract in patients with osteoarthritis: randomized placebo-controlled, double blind clinical trial. Phytother Res 2001;15:344–350.
77. Phan P, Sohrabi A, Polotsky A, et al. Ginger extract components suppress induction of chemokine expression in human synoviocytes. J Alt Complement Med 2005;11:149–154.
78. Altman R, Marcussen K. Effects of ginger extract on knee pain in patients with osteoarthritis. Arthritis Rheum 2001;44:2531–2538.
79. Bliddal H, Rosetzsky A, Schlichting P, et al. A randomized, placebo-controlled, cross-over study of ginger extracts and ibuprofen in osteoarthritis. Osteoarthritis Cartilage 2000;8:9–12.
80. Tao X, Younger J, Fan F, et al. Benefit of an extract of Tripterygium Wilfordii Hook F in patients with rheumatoid arthritis: a double-blind, placebo-controlled study. Arthritis Rheum 2002;46:1735–1743.
81. Pattrick M, Heptinstall S, Doherty M. Feverfew in rheumatoid arthritis: a double-blind, placebo controlled study. Ann Rheum Dis 1989;48:547–549.
82. Henrotin Y, Sanchez C, Deberg M, et al. Avocado/soybean unsaponifiables increase aggrecan synthesis and reduce catabolic and proinflammatory mediator production by human osteoarthritic chondrocytes. J Rheumatol 2003;30:1825–1834.
83. Henrotin Y, Deberg M, Cielaard J, et al. Avocado/soybean unsaponifiables prevent the inhibitory effect of osteoarthritic subchondral osteoblasts on aggrecan and type II collagen synthesis by chondrocytes. J Rheumatol 2006;33:1668–1678.
84. Maheu E, Mazieres B, Valat J-P, et al. Symptomatic efficacy of avocado/soybean unsaponifiables in the treatment of osteoarthritis of the knee and hip. Arthritis Rheum 1998;41:81–91.
85. Appelboom T, Schuermans J, Verbruggen G, et al. Symptoms modifying effect of avocado/soybean unsaponifiables (ASU) in knee osteoarthritis. Scan J Rheumatol 2001;30:242–247.
86. Lequesne M, Maheu E, Cadet C, et al. Structural effects of avocado/soybean unsaponifiables on joint-space loss in osteoarthritis of the hip. Arthritis Rheum 2002;47:50–58.
87. Hong J, Bose M, Ju J, et al. Modulation of arachidonic acid metabolism by curcumin and related b-diketone derivatives: effects on cytosolic phospholipase A2, cyclooxygenases and 5-lipoxygenase. Carcinogenesis 2004;25:1671–1679.
88. Lev-Ari S, Strier L, Kaznov D, et al. Curcumin synergistically potentiates the growth-inhibitory and pro-apoptotic effects of celecoxib in osteoarthritis synovial adherent cells. Rheumatology 2006;45:171–177.

89. Cheng A, Hsu C, Lin J, et al. Phase I clinical trial of curcumin, a chemopreventive agent, in patients with high-risk or pre-malignant lesions. Anticancer Res 2001;21:2895–2900.
90. Deodhar S, Sethi R, Srimal R. Preliminary study on antirheumatic activity of curcumin (diferuloyl methane). Indian J Med Res 1980;71:632–634.
91. Satoskar R, Shah S, Shenoy S. Evaluation of anti-inflammatory property of curcumin (diferuloyl methane) in patients with post-operative inflammation. Int J Clin PharmacolTher Toxicol 1986;24:651–654.

II Rheumatic Diseases

7 Rheumatoid Cachexia

Ronenn Roubenoff

Summary

- Rheumatoid cachexia is nearly universal in patients with established rheumatoid arthritis.
- Treatment that suppresses inflammation in rheumatoid arthritis does not reverse cachexia, although it will stop progressing. Reversal requires specific anabolic treatment, which is best done using resistance exercise.
- Micronutrient deficiencies—especially vitamin B_6 and antioxidants—are common in rheumatoid arthritis and should be treated judiciously.

Key Words: Cachexia; diet, exercise; metabolism; muscle; resistance training; rheumatoid arthritis

1. INTRODUCTION

Rheumatoid arthritis (RA) is the most common inflammatory disease of adults, affecting 1 to 2% of the population in developed countries *(1)*. RA is a multisystem illness that causes a symmetrical, additive polyarthritis of the small joints of the hands and feet; knees, hips, ankles, elbows, and shoulders tend to be involved later. Additionally, systemic inflammation is evinced by elevated serum acute phase reactants, such as C-reactive protein, fibrinogen, serum amyloid A, and so on. Extra-articular manifestations can involve the skin, vascular system, eyes, heart, intestines, tendons, and ligaments. Although no one dies of RA per se, mortality rates in patients with RA average twofold higher than healthy populations, and RA costs an average of 5 years of life to its victims *(2)*.

A characteristic of RA is that all patients develop some degree of muscle catabolism, which can often be profound. This phenomenon, called rheumatoid cachexia (RC), is a major contributor to the weakness, fatigue, and loss of daily functionality that is one of the major sequelae of RA. As outlined here, RC is driven largely by the inflammatory cytokines that are released in RA and must be treated using specific anabolic strategies—diet, exercise, and anti-inflammatory therapies—to reverse it. It is clear that the treatment of joint inflammation in RA is necessary but not sufficient for the reversal of RC, although it seems to prevent further deterioration in nutritional status.

From: *Nutrition and Health: Nutrition and Rheumatic Disease*
Edited by: L. A. Coleman © Humana Press, Totowa, NJ

In addition to the macronutrient deficiency that RC causes, several micronutrients are also altered by RA and its treatment. Most prominent among these are vitamin B_6, folic acid, and the antioxidants vitamins C and E. Specific dietary attention to these nutrients is necessary to maintain optimal nutritional status in patients with RA.

2. HISTORICAL PERSPECTIVE

RC was first described by Sir James Paget in the 19th century *(3)*, although this was in reference to regional muscle wasting he observed around tuberculous joints. Shortly after World War II, the discovery of corticosteroids revolutionized the treatment of RA *(4)*. In the 1950s, small studies described RC incidentally, and showed that muscle pathology was common in RA *(5)*. Furthermore, at least one study showed that androgen treatment could induce positive nitrogen balance and improve strength in RA *(6)*.

The next advance in the treatment of RC occurred in the early 1970s, when a series of papers from Sweden demonstrated the utility of exercise training in patients with RA to improve muscle mass and function *(7)*. However, this evidence did not gain wide attention in the United States. In 1988, we rediscovered negative nitrogen balance in RA, and found the prevalence of RC to be well over 50% using crude anthropometric measurements *(8)*. Subsequently, in the 1990s, we demonstrated the metabolic and functional impact of strength training on RC in larger, more systematic studies using modern methods of body composition and metabolic analysis *(9)*.

The discovery of low serum vitamin B_6 levels in RA was made by A. McKusick in 1964, and has been confirmed several times since *(10)*. In 1975, Schumacher showed that B_6 supplementation did not alter the clinical course of RA *(11)*. However, the question of whether low serum B_6 in RA represents true deficiency or an acute-phase redistribution to tissues was not clarified until studies by Chiang et al. in the past few years *(12)*. In the meantime, Weinblatt and others showed that methotrexate, an anti-folate medication originally developed for leukemia treatment, is a powerful disease-modifying anti-rheumatic drug (DMARD) at far lower doses than those needed for efficacy against cancer *(13)*. However, chronic methotrexate treatment can cause folate deficiency, which can be prevented with folic acid treatment, as shown by Morgan in 1987 *(14)*.

3. CLINICAL FEATURES

3.1. Signs and Symptoms of Rheumatoid Cachexia

There are few signs or symptoms of RC until it is very advanced. RA itself causes pain, fatigue, depression, and reduced physical activity. All of these, in addition to the direct catabolic effect of inflammation, contribute to loss of muscle mass, strength, "energy." and well-being. Experienced clinicians will recognize muscle wasting, especially around inflamed joints, in the thighs, shoulders, and hands. With more advanced RC, temporal wasting may be found.

Weight loss is not a common feature of RC, and its presence should raise the possibility of depression, vasculitis, or malignancy. In general, most patients lose muscle but their appetite is relatively intact and their physical activity is reduced, leading to gain in fat, which offsets the loss of lean mass (Fig. 1). Negative balances of nitrogen and calcium lead to muscle and bone loss, and osteoporosis is accelerated in RA. At the same time, the increase in fat mass, reduction in physical activity, systemic inflammation, and common use of corticosteroid medications increase the risk of atherosclerosis in RA *(15)*. In general, there is a dose–response relationship between the severity and duration of RA on the one hand and the severity of lean mass loss on the other (Fig. 2).

It is very unusual for cachexia in RA to be so severe as to cause a patient to be unable to rise from a chair or bed. Although such disability still occurs occasionally in RA, it is generally caused by the pain and joint deformities of the disease along with the muscle wasting, and it may be impossible to pinpoint to what extent the cachexia rather than the arthritis is responsible. However, these generally go hand in hand. Fortunately, the advent of more effective DMARDs has made such extremely severe RA rare in the developed countries.

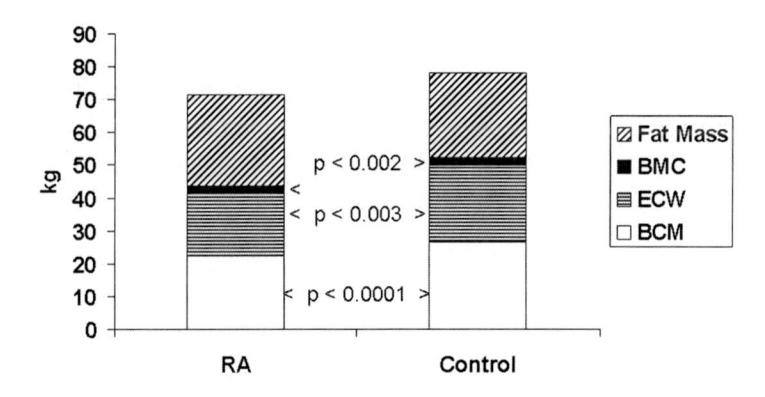

Fig. 1. Body composition of patients with rheumatoid arthritis (RA) and healthy controls matched on age, gender, race, and weight. (Modified from data in ref. *9*.)

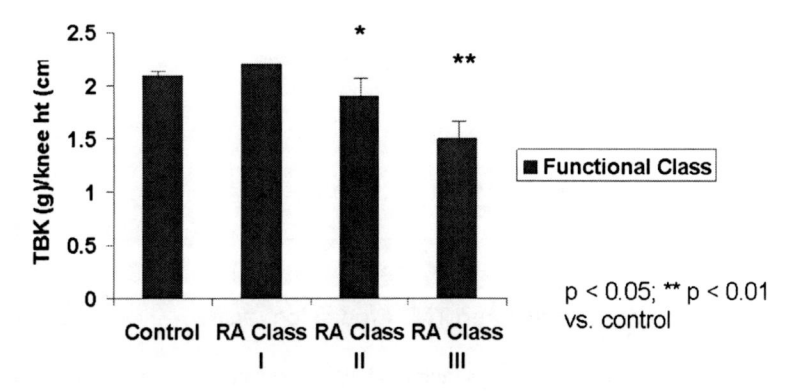

Fig. 2. The severity of rheumatoid cachexia correlates with the severity of rheumatoid arthritis. (Modified from ref. *9*.)

3.2. Pathophysiology of Rheumatoid Cachexia

3.2.1. INFLAMMATORY CYTOKINES

The inflammatory cytokines tumor necrosis factor (TNF)-α and interleukin (IL)-1β are thought to be centrally involved in the pathogenesis of RA. Both of these cytokines are produced primarily by monocytes and macrophages, but they are also produced by a variety of other cells, including B lymphocytes, T lymphocytes, and skeletal muscle *(16)*. Concentrations of TNF-α and IL-1β are high in patients with active RA *(9,17)*; these compounds act by stimulating the release of tissue-destroying matrix metalloproteinases, as well as by inhibiting the production of endogenous inhibitors of these metalloproteinases, the net result being joint damage *(18)*. Not only are TNF-α and IL-1β centrally involved in joint damage in RA, but these cytokines also exert a powerful influence on whole-body protein and energy metabolism (Fig. 3). The so-called sarcoactive (muscle-active) cytokines include, in addition to TNF-α and IL-1β, also, IL-6, interferon (IFN)-γ, transforming growth factor (TGF)-β and the transcription factor MyoD, mentioned in this context because of the integral role that MyoD has with TNF-α and TGF-β.

More than 20 years ago, researchers first demonstrated that circulating inflammatory cytokines such as TNF-α and IL-1β are released into the plasma by leukocytes and can stimulate protein degradation and whole-body protein wasting *(19)*. Although the specific mechanism by which TNF-α and IL-1β exert their catabolic effect is not known, we have shown that subjects with RA have higher rates of whole-body protein breakdown compared with young and elderly healthy subjects, and, furthermore, that

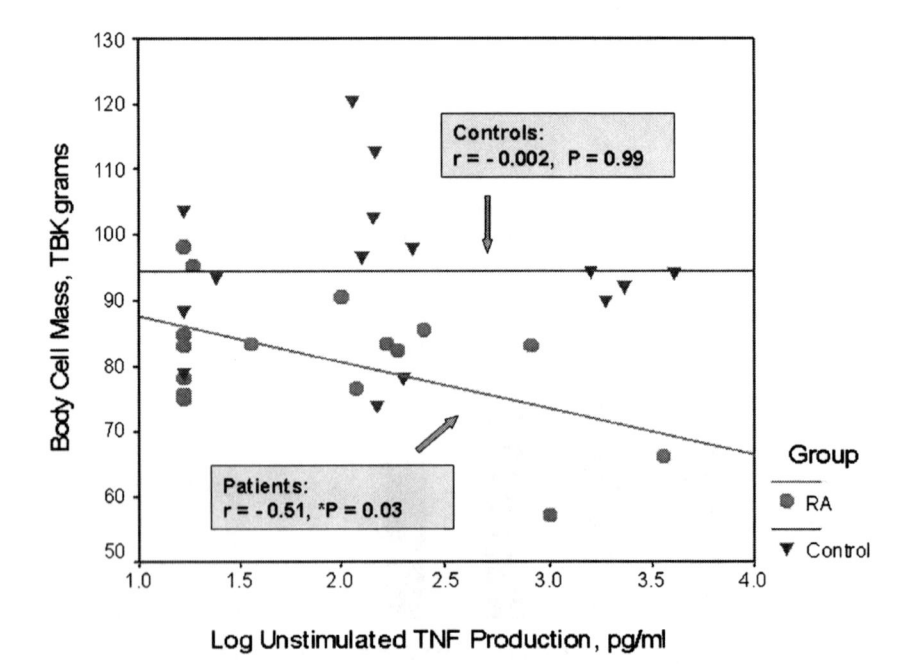

Fig. 3. Relationship between tumor necrosis factor (TNF)-α production by peripheral blood mononuclear cells (PBMC) and lean body mass (as total body potassium, TBK) in patients with rheumatoid arthritis (RA) and age- and body mass index-matched controls (From ref. *26*).

protein breakdown rates are directly associated with TNF-α production by peripheral blood mononuclear cells (PBMCs *(20)*).

Studies have also shown that skeletal muscle protein loss is dependent on the combined signaling activities of TNF-α and IFN-γ, and that nuclear factor-κB (NF-κB) activity is required for these cytokines to induce muscle damage *(18)*. Specifically, TNF-induced activation of NF-κB has been shown to inhibit skeletal muscle differentiation by suppressing MyoD mRNA at the post-transcriptional level *(21)*. MyoD regulates skeletal muscle differentiation and is essential for the repair of damaged tissue *(22)*. Recent additional work has suggested that protein kinase B and Smad3 proteins may also play a role in mediating the action of these sarcoactive cytokines by affecting the protection and vulnerability of cells against TGF-β1-induced apoptosis *(23)*.

3.2.2. ENERGY EXPENDITURE PROFILE

Early studies from our research group suggested that resting energy expenditure (REE) was elevated in patients with RA *(9)*. REE is only one component of total daily energy expenditure (TEE), however, the others being the energy expenditure of physical activity (EEPA) and the thermic effect of food (TEF), such that:

$$TEE = REE + EEPA + TEF.$$

Therefore, although REE may be elevated in RA, the net effect on TEE also depends on EEPA. We have recently examined this issue in women with RA and in age- and body mass index-matched controls, and found that TEE is actually significantly lower in patients with RA than in controls because of lower EEPA *(24)*. In fact, the magnitude of the difference in EEPA was quite large in this study: 257 kcal (1,034 KJ) per day (approx a 10% difference between RA and controls, *see* Fig. 4). Clearly, low EEPA predominates in determining TEE in patients with RA. Furthermore, in the years since we first showed that cachexia is common in RA, improvements in disease treatment

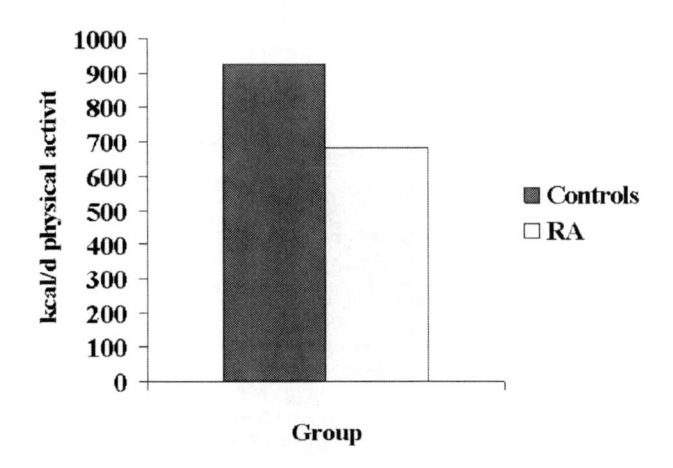

Fig. 4. Difference in daily energy expenditure of physical activity between patients with rheumatoid arthritis (RA) and age- and body mass index-matched controls. p <0.04 between groups. (From ref *24*.)

have made overt hypermetabolism (elevated REE) less common *(25)*. The implication of what is now known about energy metabolism in RA is that patients need to be cautioned to maintain a diet that is adequate—and not excessive—in terms of protein and calories in an attempt to maintain muscle but prevent fat gain.

3.2.3. WHOLE-BODY PROTEIN TURNOVER

We have consistently demonstrated that a loss of body cell mass (BCM) is common in patients with RA *(9,26)*. By definition, catabolism (negative protein balance) must occur in order for cachexia to develop, and, consistent with this, we have also found that adults with RA have increased whole-body protein breakdown rates (measured by ^{13}C-leucine infusion) *(20)*. Furthermore, Rall et al. observed a direct relationship between PBMC production of TNF-α and leucine flux—an indicator of whole-body protein breakdown in the fasting state—where higher TNF-α production was associated with higher rates of whole-body protein breakdown (Fig. 5 *(20)*).

At the same time that there is an increase in whole-body protein breakdown in RA, there is also a decline in the ability of skeletal muscle to synthesize new protein. Walsmith et al. found that skeletal muscle protein synthesis was approx 25% lower in adults with RA compared with controls ($p < 0.04$). Additionally, skeletal muscle quality (strength/mass) was approx 36% lower ($p < 0.03$), and correlated with the rate of muscle protein synthesis ($r = 0.65$; $p = 0.02$). These data suggest that the excess protein turnover in RA occurs in the immune system and visceral protein compartments, at the expense of the skeletal muscle *(26)*.

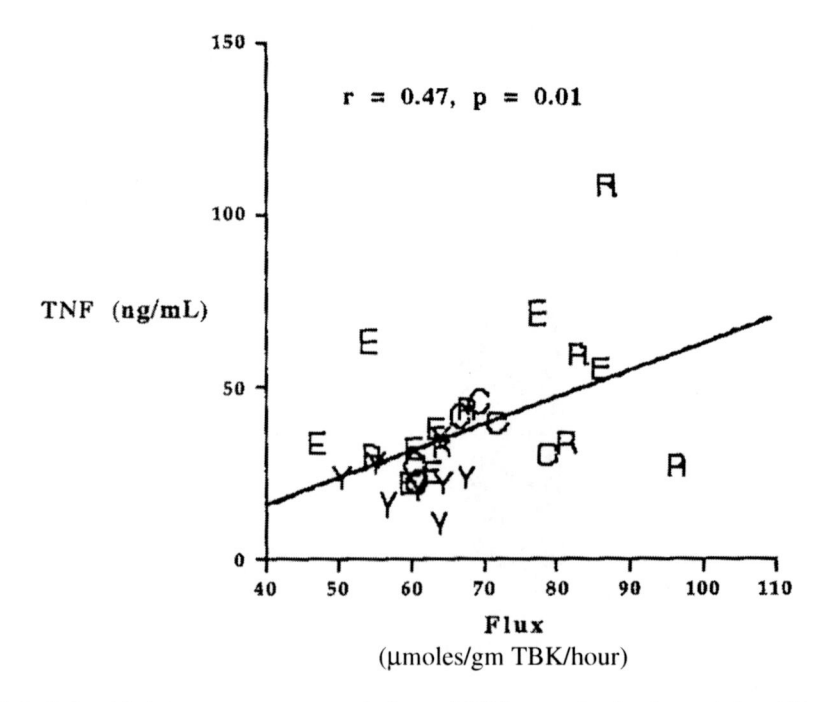

Fig. 5. Relationship between tumor necrosis factor (TNF)-α production by peripheral blood mononuclear cells and whole-body protein breakdown. E: Elderly; R: Rhenmatoid Arthritis; O: Old; Y: Young (From ref. *20*.)

3.2.4. PHYSICAL ACTIVITY

Patients with RA have low physical activity, averaging about 250 kcal per day less in middle-aged women *(8)*. This is a significant reduction in physical activity, given that an imbalance of as few as 10 kcal per day can lead to a 1 kg weight change in a year. Many factors contribute to reduced physical activity among patients with RA, including joint pain and stiffness, metabolic changes leading to loss of muscle mass and strength, and simple disuse, perhaps related to general caution with regard to physical activity.

3.2.5. HORMONES

3.2.5.1. Growth Hormone and Insulin-Like Growth Factor-I.
The loss of BCM that occurs in RA is similar to that which occurs in healthy aging. In the case of healthy aging, an association has been shown between this loss of lean mass and declining activity of the growth hormone (GH)–insulin-like growth factor (IGF)-I axis. This raises the question of whether GH is reduced in patients with RA, and whether a reduction in GH may contribute to some of the body composition changes observed in these patients. Evidence exists for abnormalities of various other hormones in RA *(27)*. However, a recent study measuring GH secretory kinetics by deconvolution analysis after 24-hour blood sampling found no differences between patients with RA and healthy control subjects after adjusting for differences in fat mass between the two groups, as fat is known to suppress GH secretion *(28)*. Patients with RA did, however, have significantly reduced BCM. These findings suggest that persistent GH deficiency does not appear to be the cause of RC. However, it should be noted that a trend toward lower serum IGF-I levels was found; these results have been supported by others, who observed significant reductions in circulating IGF-I *(28)*. It is thus possible that reduced IGF-I could contribute to RC.

3.2.5.2. Insulin.
Insulin acts to inhibit muscle protein degradation, thus making it a potent anabolic hormone. Several researchers have documented insulin resistance in inflammatory arthritis, although its effect on protein metabolism remains unknown*(29)*. We have hypothesized that the metabolic milieu created by a state of insulin resistance may be permissive to cytokine-driven muscle loss, although this hypothesis remains to be investigated *(30)*. The etiology of reduced peripheral insulin action in RA is not known, but TNF-α has been shown to interfere with insulin receptor signaling and may be a contributing factor *(31)*.

4. NUTRITIONAL STATUS

As the clinical section suggests, nutritional assessment of patients with RA should be multifactorial. Both macro and micronutrient status should be considered. For the former, it is important to ask the patient about weight loss, appetitie, strength and ability to rise from a chair and perform activities of daily living, and differentiation of limitations due to pain from those due to weakness.

On examination, the clinician should examine muscle mass in the thighs, upper arms, and temples. Additionally, one should examine the joints for signs of swelling, boggy joints, warmth, and redness, all indicative of active inflammation. Joint deformities should also be noted, as these indicate accumulated damage to joints and correlate closely with disability and (in the lower extremities) with increased energy requirements for ambulation.

The key laboratory tests for macronutrient status are assessments of lean body mass, fat mass, and bone mass. These can be done by a variety of methods *(32)*, many of which are difficult to obtain in the clinical setting. However, it is useful to include in each patient's evaluation a referral to a dietitian for anthropometric evaluation and diet history; calculation of body mass index (kg/m^2); evaluation of functional status using simple tests such as timed chair stands or 50-ft walk; and if possible, dual-energy X-ray absorptiometry to assess osteoporosis and (if financially feasible) to assess lean mass using a whole-body scan.

Micronutrient status in developed countries is generally assessed by blood tests. The micronutrients at greatest risk of deficiency in RA include:

- vitamin B$_6$ (measure serum vitamin B$_6$);
- folic acid (measure red blood cell folate and total plasma homocysteine);
- vitamin D (measure serum 25-hydroxyvitamin D$_3$ levels);
- antioxidants (although there is evidence that vitamins C and E may be low in RA, and that oxidative stress is increased, it is generally more cost-effective to prescribe a multivitamin containing the recommended daily intake of these vitamins rather than to measure levels, which may be difficult to interpret).

5. RECOMMENDATIONS FOR MANAGEMENT

Just as the pathophysiology of RC is complex and multifactorial (Fig. 6), the management of RC requires a multidisciplinary effort. First, there should be a comprehensive medical assessment and plan for anti-inflammatory treatment. It is crucial to discern whether there is active inflammation, which would respond to medication, or if all the damage is done and there is only end-stage joint degeneration that requires surgical intervention. Because patients with RA have such low physical activity, they are prone to obesity, and dietary prescription must find a balance between meeting protein, energy, and micronutrient needs on the one hand and overfeeding on the other. The most effective way to achieve this is to link the dietary prescription to an exercise prescription, and help patients find a physical therapist, exercise physiologist, or trainer who can work with them to improve muscle strength, mass, and endurance. Although some patients may be able to afford health club memberships and personal trainers, many will not. However, effective exercise can be performed at home with very little financial investment, as outlined in books for the general public *(33)*.

The goal of the dietary prescription should be about 1.5 g/kg protein, adequate energy intake for neutral caloric balance, and fat intake meeting the National Cholesterol Education Program Step 2 diet (25% of energy from fat, <8% from saturated fat). Increasing omega-3 fatty acids from fish makes sense, as there is a large literature indicating that these fats have immunomodulatory effects *(34)*. Simple sugars should be minimized as well, given the propensity for insulin resistance in inflammatory states such as RA.

The exercise prescription in RA should focus on strength training at first for several reasons. Progressive resistance training targets type II muscle fibers, which are the ones predominantly lost in RA and other inflammatory diseases and disuse syndromes *(35)*.

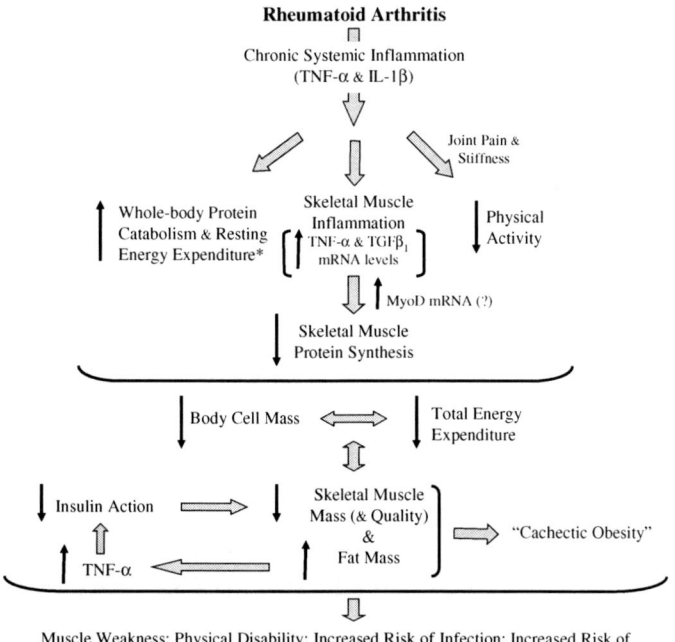

Fig. 6. Schematic view of interactions leading to rheumatoid cachexia.

Resistance training requires much less oxygen than endurance training, and is thus easier for sedentary patients to perform. A high-resistance, low-repetition program is the only known physiological way to increase muscle and bone mass and begin to address the muscle deficit of RC. Age is not a barrier to successful resistance training, nor is muscle wasting, but active joint inflammation is. The appropriate time to begin such a program is after successful suppression of joint swelling and pain using anti-inflammatory medications.

REFERENCES

1. Silman A, Hochberg M. Epidemiology of the Rheumatic Diseases. Oxford: Oxford University Press, 1993.
2. Wolfe F, Mitchell DM, Sibley JT, et al. The mortality of rheumatoid arthritis. Arthritis Rheum 1994;37(4):481–494.
3. Paget J. Nervous mimicry of organic diseases. Lancet 1873;2:727–729.
4. Hench P. The reversibility of certain rheumatic and nonrheumatic conditions by the use of cortisone or of the pituitary adrenocotropic hormone. Ann Intern Med 1952;36:1–38.
5. Traut E, Campione K. Histopathology of muscle in rheumatoid arthritis and other diseases. Arch Intern Med 1952;89(5):724–735.
6. Ruchelman H, Ford R. Inhibition of negative nitrogen balance by an anabolic agent (methandrostenolone) during corticosteroid therapy (dexamethasone) in rheumatoid arthritis. Metabolism 1962;11:524–529.
7. Ekblom B, Lovgren O, Alderin M, Fridstrom M, Satterstrom G. Effect of short-term training on patients with rheumatoid arthritis—I. Scand J Rheumatol 1975;4:80–86.

8. Roubenoff R, Roubenoff R, Ward L, Stevens M. Catabolic effects of high-dose corticosteroids persist despite therapeutic benefit in rheumatoid arthritis. Am J Clin Nutr 1990;52:1113–1117.
9. Roubenoff R, Roubenoff R, Cannon J, et al. Rheumatoid cachexia: cytokine-driven hypermetabolism accompanying reduced body cell mass in chronic inflammation. J Clin Invest 1994;93:2379–2386.
10. McKusick A, Sherwin R, Jones L, Hsu J. Urinary excretion of pyridoxine and 4-pyridoxic acid in rheumatoid arthritis. Arthritis Rheum 1964;7:636–653.
11. Schumacher H, Bernhart F, Gyorgy P. Vitamin B6 levels in rheumatoid arthritis: effect of treatment. Am J Clin Nutr 1975;28(11):1200–1203.
12. Chiang E-PI, Bagley P, Selhub J, Nadeau M, Roubenoff R. Abnormal vitamin B6 status is associated with severity of symptoms in patients with rheumatoid arthritis. Am J Med 2003;114:283–287.
13. Weinblatt M, Coblyn J, Fox D, et al. Efficacy of low dose methotrexate in rheumatoid arthritis. N Engl J Med 1985;312(13):818–822.
14. Morgan S, Baggott J, Altz-Smith M. Folate status of rheumatoid arthritis patients receiving long-term, low-dose methotrexate therapy. Arthritis Rheum 1987;30(12):1348–1356.
15. Tarqher G. Carotid atherosclerosis and rheumatoid arthritis. Ann Intern Med 2006;144(4):249–256.
16. Aggarwal B, Puri R. Human Cytokines: Their Role in Disease and Therapy. Blackwell Science, Cambridge, MA, 1995.
17. Eastgate J, Wood N, DiGiovine F, Symons J, Grinlinton F, Duff G. Correlation of plasma interleukin-1 levels with disease activity in rheumatoid arthritis. Lancet 1988;2:706–709.
18. Scott D, Kingsley G. Tumor necrosis factor inhibitors for rheumatoid arthritis. N Engl J Med 2006;355:704–712.
19. Baracos V, Rodemann H, Dinarello C, Goldberg A. Stimulation of muscle protein degradation and prostaglandin E2 release by leukocytic pyrogen (interleukin-1). N Engl J Med 1983;308:553–558.
20. Rall L, Rosen C, Dolnikowski G, et al. Protein metabolism in rheumatoid arthritis and aging: Effects of muscle strength training and tumor necrosis factor-alpha. Arthritis Rheum 1996;39:1115–1124.
21. Szalay K, Razga Z, Duda E. TNF inhibits myogenesis and downregulates the expression of regulatory factors myoD and myogenin. Eur J Cell Biol 1997;74(4):391–398.
22. Weintraub H, Davis R, Tapscott S, et al. The myoD gene family: nodal point during specification of muscle cell lineage. Science 1991;251(4995):761–766.
23. Liu D, Black B, Derynck R. TGF-beta inhibits muscle differentiation through functional repression of myogenic transcription factors by Smad3. Genes Dev 2001;15(22):2950–2966.
24. Roubenoff R, Walsmith J, Lundgren N, Dolnikowski G, Roberts S. Low physical activity reduces total energy expenditure in women with rheumatoid arthritis: Implications for dietary intake recommendations. Am J Clin Nutr 2002;76:774–779.
25. Roubenoff R, Roubenoff R, Ward L, Holland S, Hellmann D. Rheumatoid cachexia: depletion of lean body mass in rheumatoid arthritis. Possible association with tumor necrosis factor. J Rheumatol 1992;19:1505–1510.
26. Walsmith J, Abad L, Kehayias J, Roubenoff R. Tumor necrosis factor-alpha production is associated with less body cell mass in women with rheumatoid arthritis. J Rheumatol 2004;31:23–29.
27. Walsmith J, Roubenoff R. Cachexia in rheumatoid arthritis. Int J Cardiol 2002;85(1):89–99.
28. Rall L, Walsmith J, Snydman L, et al. Cachexia in rheumatoid arthritis is not explained by decreased growth hormone secretion. Arthritis Rheum 2002;46(10):2574–2577.
29. Svenson K, Lundqvist G, Wide L, Hallgren R. Impaired glucose handling in active rheumatoid arthritis: relationship to the secretion of insulin and counter-regulatory hormones. Metabolism 1987;36(10):940–943.
30. Roubenoff R. Inflammatory and hormonal mediators of cachexia. J Nutr 1997;127:1014S–1016S.
31. Hotamisligil G, Peraldi P, Budavari A, Ellis R, White M, Spiegelman B. IRS-1-mediated inhibition of insulin receptor tyrosine kinase activity in TNF-alpha- and obesity-induced insulin resistance. Science 1996;271(5249):665–668.
32. Roubenoff R, Kehayias J. The meaning and measurement of lean body mass. Nutr Rev 1991;46:163–175.
33. Nelson M, Baker K, Roubenoff R, Lindner L. Strong Women and Men Beat Arthritis. Putnam, New York, 2002.

34. Horstman J. The Arthritis Foundation's Guide to Alternative Therapies. Arthritis Foundation, Atlanta, GA, 1999.
35. Rall L, Meydani S, Kehayias J, Dawson-Hughes B, Roubenoff R. The effect of progressive resistance training in rheumatoid arthritis: increased strength without changes in energy balance or body composition. Arthritis Rheum 1996;39(415–426).

8 Nutrition and Nutritional Supplements and Osteoarthritis

Paola de Pablo, Grace Lo, and Timothy E. McAlindon

Summary

- There are numerous mechanisms by which micronutrients might be expected to influence the development or progression of osteoarthritis, but there has been insufficient research to draw definitive conclusions
- One observational study suggested a protective effect of vitamin C for progression of osteoarthritis of the knee. Intake of vitamin E and β-carotene bore no relationship to osteoarthritis incidence or progression in that study, suggesting that the mechanism of benefit of vitamin C may be mediated through nonantioxidant properties
- Clinical trials of vitamins E, C, and A and selenium have produced negative or inconsistent results
- Epidemiological data for vitamin D in the treatment of symptoms and structural progression of osteoarthritis are conflicting. A randomized controlled trial is currently underway to address the efficacy of vitamin D in both the treatment of symptoms and structural progression in osteoarthritis.
- Epidemiological data for vitamin K as a disease modifying micronutrient in osteoarthritis are conflicting. Randomized controlled trials are currently underway to address the efficacy of vitamin K in both the treatment of symptoms and structural progression in osteoarthritis.
- There have been numerous positive clinical trials of glucosamine and chondroitin products for OA that have shown them to be well tolerated; however, interpretation of these trials is clouded by issues of biological plausibility, heterogeneity, publication bias, inconsistent results and methodological problems.

Key Words: Antioxidant micronutrients; glucosamine and chondroitin products; nutritional supplements; osteoarthritis; vitamins

1. INTRODUCTION

There is a great public interest in the relationship between nutrition and arthritis. Patients often question their physicians about the influence of diet on osteoarthritis (OA). Speculative lay publications on this subject proliferate, and health food stores offer an excess of nutritional supplements represented as therapies for arthritis *(1)*. The over-the-counter consumption of such nutritional remedies is significant, with

From: *Nutrition and Health: Nutrition and Rheumatic Disease*
Edited by: L. A. Coleman © Humana Press, Totowa, NJ

glucosamine and chondroitin together ranking third among all top-selling nutritional products in the United States with annual sales amounting to $369 million *(2)*. Surveys suggest that 5 to 8% of adults in the United States have used at least one of these products at some time *(3)*.

2. HISTORICAL PERSPECTIVE

Previously thought to be a normal consequence of aging, OA results from the interplay of multiple factors, including genetics, local inflammation, mechanical forces, joint integrity, and cellular and biochemical processes. OA is one of the most prevalent chronic diseases affecting the elderly. OA is characterized by a progressive destruction of articular cartilage resulting in pain, impaired joint motion, and disability. The high prevalence of OA and the impact it has on activities of daily living represent an important public health problem.

The management of OA is largely palliative, focusing on symptom alleviation. Current therapy for OA consists of both nonpharmacological (weight loss, exercise, education programs) and pharmacological (analgesics, nonsteroidal anti-inflammatory drugs [NSAIDs], intra-articular corticosteroids) approaches. However, these modalities are often incompletely effective. Thus, there is a need for safe and effective alternative therapies as well as preventive strategies. Such interventions could be addressed by nutrition.

There are numerous biological mechanisms by which micronutrients might influence the pathophysiological processes in OA. Such processes include oxidative damage, cartilage matrix degradation and repair, and chondrocyte function and response in adjacent bone. However, it is surprising to find that there has been relatively little focus in scientific studies on the relationship between nutrition and OA given the situation in osteoporosis, a widespread age-related skeletal disorder, where numerous studies have demonstrated associations with dietary factors.

3. CLINICAL FEATURES

OA most commonly presents in persons older than age 40 years. The main symptom associated with OA is pain, which is typically exacerbated by activity and relieved by rest. With more advanced disease, pain may be noted with progressively less activity, eventually occurring at rest and at night. Pain in OA is not caused directly by cartilage damage because cartilage is aneural. Stiffness is also a common complaint in patients with OA. Morning stiffness typically resolves less than 30 minutes after a patient awakens, but may recur following periods of inactivity, a phenomenon termed *gelling*. OA commonly affects the cervical and lumbar spine, first carpometacarpal joint, proximal interphalangeal joint, distal interphalangeal joint, hip, knee, subtalar joint, first metarsophalangeal joint. Several objective findings may be present upon physical examination of the patient with OA: malalignment, tenderness to palpation of involved joints with or, more often, without associated signs of inflammation, crepitus, bony enlargement, and decreased range of motion. Crepitus is a common finding and is probably caused by the disruption of the normally smooth articulating surfaces of the joints. Osteophytes may be palpable as bony enlargements along the periphery of the joint. Joint effusions may be present, which typically exhibit a mild pleocytosis, normal viscosity, and modestly elevated protein. Radiographic features may include joint-space narrowing (JSN), subchondral sclerosis, marginal osteophytes, and subchondral cysts.

4. NUTRITIONAL STATUS AND DIETARY MANAGEMENT

4.1. Antioxidant Micronutrients

Reactive oxygen species (ROS) are chemicals with unpaired electrons, which are constantly formed in tissues via endogenous and some exogenous mechanisms *(4)*. About 1 to 2% of electrons leak from the mitochondrial respiratory chain-forming superoxide anions *(5)*. Other endogenous sources include release by phagocytes during the oxidative burst, generated by mixed function oxidase enzymes, and in hypoxia-reperfusion events *(6)*. ROS are capable of causing damage to many macromolecules including cell membranes, lipoproteins, proteins, and DNA *(7)*. ROS are implicated in the development of many common human diseases associated with aging *(4,8–10)*, including OA *(11)*.

Chondrocytes are potent sources of ROS. Oxidative damage to cartilage is physiologically important *(12–15)*, as superoxide anions can damage collagen structure, depolymerize synovial fluid hyaluronate, and damage mitochondria *(11,12,14,16,17)*, which probably also contributes to the age-related loss of chondrocyte function *(11)*. Evidence of oxidative damage owing to production of excessive amounts of nitric oxide (NO) and other ROS has been demonstrated in aging and osteoarthritic cartilage *(18)* and has been correlated with the extent of cartilage damage *(19)*. Subjects with chondral or meniscal lesions also have increased levels of ROS in their synovial fluid *(20)*.

The human body has an extensive multilayered antioxidant defense system *(4)*. Intracellular defense is provided primarily by antioxidant enzymes including superoxide dismutase, catalase, and peroxidases. In joints, hyaluronic acid may also have an antioxidant role *(21)*. Additionally, antioxidants may have an important function in the extracellular space where antioxidant enzymes are rare *(22)*. These include ascorbate (vitamin C), α-tocopherol (vitamin E), β-carotene (a vitamin A precursor), and other carotenoids. The serum concentrations of these antioxidants are primarily determined by dietary intake. However, when ROS are produced in increased amounts like in OA, the antioxidant capacity of cells and tissues can become insufficient to detoxify the ROS, which then contribute to cartilage degradation by inhibiting matrix synthesis, directly degrading matrix molecules, or activating matrix metalloproteinases (MMPs *(23)*). In such instances, micronutrient antioxidants might provide further defense against tissue injury. Thus, because of their antioxidant properties, vitamins could have beneficial effects in OA *(24,25)*. High dietary intake of these micronutrients may protect against age-related disorders. Because higher intake of dietary antioxidants appears beneficial with respect to outcomes such as cataract extraction and coronary artery disease *(8–10,26)*, it is plausible that they may confer similar benefits for OA.

4.2. Vitamin C

Vitamin C, also known as ascorbic acid or ascorbate, is a water-soluble antioxidant vitamin that is found naturally in citrus fruits, rose hips, blackcurrants, and strawberries, as well as in vegetables such as brussels sprouts, broccoli, peppers, cabbage, potatoes, and parsley.

Vitamin C plays several functions in the biosynthesis of cartilage molecules. Vitamin C is required for the post-translational hydroxylation of specific prolyl and lysyl residues in procollagen, through the vitamin C-dependent enzyme lysyl hydroxylase. This modification essential for stabilization of the mature collagen fibril *(8–10,26–28)*. Vitamin C also appears to stimulate collagen biosynthesis by pathways independent of hydroxylation, perhaps through lipid peroxidation *(29)*. Additionally, vitamin C participates in glycosaminoglycan (GAG) synthesis by acting as a carrier of sulfate groups *(30)*. Therefore, relative deficiency of vitamin C may impair not only the production of cartilage, but also its biomechanical quality.

Recent work on the impact of oxidative stress on cartilage has added insights into the biological mechanisms of OA progression. Yudoh et al. studied this from the viewpoint of genomic instability and replicative senescence in human chondrocytes *(19)*. They isolated chondrocytes from articular cartilage from patients with OA of the knee, looking to measure oxidative damage histologically by immunohistochemistry for nitrotyrosine (e.g., a maker of oxidative damage). They then assessed cellular replicative potential, telomere instability, and GAG production both under conditions of oxidative stress and in the presence of an antioxidant (ascorbic acid). Similarly, in the tissue cultures of the articular cartilage explants, they measured the presence of oxidative damage, chondrocyte telomere length and loss of GAGs in the presence or absence of ROS, or ascorbic acid.

They found lower anti-oxidative capacity and stronger staining of nitrotyrosine in osteoarthritic regions compared with normal regions within the same cartilage explants. Oxidative damage correlated with the severity of histological damage. During continuous culture of the chondrocytes, the telomere length, replicative capacity, and GAG production were all decreased in the presence of oxidative stress. In contrast, treatment of cultured chondrocytes with ascorbic acid resulted in greater telomere length and replicative life span of the cells. Similarly, in the tissue cultures of the cartilage explants, chondrocyte telomere length and GAG production in the cartilage tissue subjected to oxidative stress were lower in than in the control groups, whereas those treated with ascorbic acid exhibited a tendency to maintain the chondrocyte telomere length and GAG production. These results suggest that oxidative stress induces chondrocyte telomere instability and catabolic changes in cartilage matrix structure and composition. This process may contribute to the development and/or progression of OA.

The results of *in vitro* and *in vivo* studies support this hypothesis. Peterkovsky et al. observed decreased synthesis of cartilage collagen and proteoglycan molecules, in guinea pigs deprived of vitamin C. Moreover, addition of ascorbate to tissue cultures of adult bovine chondrocytes resulted in decreased levels of degradative enzymes, and increased synthesis of type II collagen and proteoglycans *(30,31)*. Yudoh et al. also demonstrated greater telomere length and replicative life span of human chondrocytes in culture medium treated with ascorbate *(19)*. Schwartz et al. and Meacock et al. found that vitamin C supplementation in a guinea pig model of surgically induced OA reduced the extent of joint damage *(32,33)*.

Epidemiological data from the Framingham OA cohort also suggest that higher intake of vitamin C may reduce progression of OA *(34)*. In that study, participants had knee X-rays taken at a baseline and at follow-up approx 8 years later. OA of the knee was classified using the Kellgren and Lawrence (K/L) grading system *(35)*. Nutrient intake, including supplement use, was calculated from dietary habits reported at the mid-point of the study using a food-frequency questionnaire (FFQ). In the analyses, micronutrient intakes were ranked into gender-specific tertiles and tested to see if higher intakes of vitamins C and E and β-carotene, compared with a panel of nonantioxidant "control" micronutrients, were associated with reduced incidence and reduced progression of OA of the knee. All analyses presented were adjusted for age, gender, body mass index (BMI), physical activity, and total energy intake. Assessments were completed for 640 participants (mean age 70.3 years). There were no significant associations with vitamin C and incident radiographic OA of the knee. However, with respect to *progression* of radiographic OA of the knee, there was a threefold reduction in risk for those in the middle and highest tertiles compared with those in the lowest tertile of vitamin C intake (adjusted odds ratio [OR] 0.3; 95% confidence [CI], 0.1–0.6). Those in the highest tertile for vitamin C intake also had reduced risk of developing knee pain (OR 0.3; 95% CI, 0.1–0.9). Reduction in risk of progression was also seen for -carotene (OR 0.4; 95% CI, 0.2–0.9) and vitamin E (OR 0.7; 95% CI, 0.3–1.6) but these findings were less compelling, in that the β-carotene association diminished substantially after adjustment for vitamin C, and the vitamin E effect was seen only in men (OR 0.07; 95% CI, 0.07–0.6).

Vitamin C is a water-soluble compound with a broad spectrum of antioxidant activity owing to its ability to react with numerous aqueous free radicals and ROS *(4)*. The extracellular nature of ROS-mediated damage in joints, and the aqueous intra-articular environment, may favor a role for a water-soluble agent such as vitamin C, rather than fat-soluble molecules like -carotene or vitamin E. Additionally, it has been suggested that vitamin C may "regenerate" vitamin E at the water-lipid interface by reducing -tocopherol radical back to -tocopherol. Whether this occurs *in vivo*, however, is controversial. An alternative explanation is that the protective effects of vitamin C relate to its biochemical participation in the biosynthesis of cartilage collagen fibrils and proteoglycan molecules, rather than its antioxidant properties. No significant associations were observed for any of the micronutrients among alleged nonantioxidants.

Baker and colleagues investigated the relationship of vitamin C intake (evaluated using an FFQ) and knee pain over a 30-month period among 324 (mostly men) participants in the Boston Osteoarthritis of the Knee Study (BOKS), a natural history study of knee osteoarthritis *(36)*. In this cross-sectional analysis, pain score was computed as an average of Western Ontario and McMaster Universities osteoarthritis index (WOMAC) pain scores reported at all visits. Vitamin C status was based on the average vitamin C level from all visits. Individuals with in the lowest tertile of vitamin C intake had more knee pain after adjusting for age, BMI, and energy intake compared with those in the middle and highest tertiles of vitamin C intake with the relation being stronger in men than in women.

There are numerous reasons to expect that vitamin C might have beneficial effects in OA, so the results of a recent study of the effects of ascorbic acid supplementation on the expression of spontaneous osteoarthritis in the Hartley guinea pig are surprising *(37)*. This rigorous investigation tested the effects of three doses of ascorbic acid on the *in vivo* development of histological OA of the knee. The low dose represented the minimum amount needed to prevent scurvy. The medium dose was the amount present in standard laboratory guinea pig chow and resulted in plasma levels comparable with those achieved in a person consuming five fruits and vegetables daily. The high dose was the amount shown in a previous study of the guinea pig to slow the progression of surgically induced OA *(33)*.

A positive association between ascorbic acid supplementation and the severity of spontaneous OA was observed with a higher dose of vitamin C being associated with greater severity of arthritis. A dose-dependent increase in all elements of the knee joint histological scores was seen across the three arms of the study. There was a significant correlation of histological severity score with plasma ascorbate concentration ($r = 0.38$; $p = 0.01$). Of note, there was evidence of active transforming growth factor (TGF) in the guinea pigs in this study, predominantly expressed in marginal osteophytes where as little was seen in the extracellular matrix (ECM) of the articular cartilage, remote from osteophytes *(37)*. TGF has been implicated in the pathophysiology of OA *(38–40)*, and ascorbate may function on an activator of this cytokine *(41)*. The presence of TGF in osteophytes supports a role of this cytokine in the effects of vitamin C on histological severity.

Although these findings are provocative, it remains uncertain to what extent they can be generalized to humans. The model of spontaneous OA used in this study may not reflect the same pathology as OA in humans. Furthermore, it is difficult to extrapolate the concentrations of vitamin C considered pathological in guinea pigs to humans. Nonetheless, it is paradoxical that an apparently beneficial effect of dietary vitamin C was found in the Framingham cohort study *(34)* and in the BOKS. Thus, the current knowledge predicates a need for further studies of vitamin C in humans.

One multicenter, randomized, double-blind, placebo-controlled case-crossover study of 133 patients with radiographic OA of the hip and/or knee evaluated the effectiveness of 1 g of oral calcium ascorbate *(42)*. Each participant received vitamin C for 14 days and placebo for 14 days, separated by a 7-day washout period. The participants were randomized to the sequence of administration of vitamin C and placebo. The primary outcome was pain on visual analog scale (VAS) in a preselected joint. Using intent-to-treat (ITT) analysis, treatment with vitamin C resulted in a greater improvement in pain compared with placebo with a mean difference of 4.6 mm ($p = 0.0078$).

These results are exciting and support the possibility that vitamin C is effective in improving symptoms related to OA of the knee and/or hip. However, there are several limitations to this study preventing vitamin C from being hailed as a treatment for symptomatic OA. First, the dosage of vitamin C used in this trial was more than 10 times that of the recommended dietary allowances of 60 to 200 mg per day, although it has been reported that oral doses up to 3 g daily are unlikely to cause adverse reactions. The long-term safety of such high doses of vitamin C in elderly patients with OA needs further evaluation, and efficacy needs to be confirmed by longer studies. Also, this trial was relatively small and it included participants with OA of the knee and/or hip, likely a heterogenous population. Finally, it is unclear whether a mean difference of 4.6 mm on VAS is a meaningful difference, although the duration of action of vitamin C is unclear and treatments with a prolonged duration of action potentially will have apparently diluted out effects in studies with a case-crossover design, biasing the results toward the null. Thus, the presence of even a small effect of vitamin C may still be very meaningful.

4.3. Vitamin D

Vitamin D, also known as calciferol, is a broad term inclusive of a collection of steroid-like substances such as vitamin D_2 (ergocalciferol) and vitamin D_3 (cholecalciferol). Vitamin D is only found in animal sources and can be produced by the body with exposure to ultraviolet radiation.

Normal bone metabolism requires the presence of vitamin D. Suboptimal vitamin D levels may have adverse effects on calcium metabolism, osteoblast activity, matrix ossification, and bone density *(43,44)*. Hence, low tissue levels of vitamin D may impair the ability of bone to respond optimally to pathophysiological processes in OA, and predispose to disease progression.

Reactive changes in the bone underlying, and adjacent to, damaged cartilage are an integral part of the osteoarthritic process *(45–51)*. Sclerosis of the underlying bone, trabecular micro-fracturing, attrition, and cyst formation are all likely to accelerate the degenerative process as a result of adverse biomechanical changes *(52,53)*. Other phenomena, such as osteophyte (bony spur) formation may be attempts to repair or stabilize the process *(54,55)*. It has also been suggested that bone mineral density (BMD) may influence the skeletal expression of the disease with a more erosive form occurring in individuals with "softer" bone *(56)*. Although some cross-sectional studies have suggested a modest inverse relationship between presence of OA and osteoporosis, recent prospective studies have suggested that individuals with lower BMD are at increased risk for OA progression *(57)*. The idea that the nature of bony response in OA may determine outcome has been further advanced by the demonstration that patients with bone scan abnormalities adjacent to an osteoarthritic knee have a higher rate of progression than those without such changes *(58)*.

Animal studies suggest that vitamin D might also have direct effects on chondrocytes in osteoarthritic cartilage. They suggest that vitamin D might exert an effect on the development or progression of OA through cartilage as well as bone. Although these findings emanate from animal studies, they serve as preliminary data that these relationships may also exist in humans. During bone growth, vitamin D regulates the transition in the growth plate from cartilage to bone. It had been assumed that chondrocytes in developing bone lose their vitamin D receptors with the attainment of skeletal maturity. Corvol et al., however, found that chondrocytes isolated from mature rabbit growth plate cartilage were able to transform 25-hydroxycholecalciferol to 24,25-dihydroxycholecalciferol *(59,60)*. They also observed that 24,25-dihydroxycholecalciferol could stimulate proteoglycan synthesis by mature chondrocytes, and that it increased DNA polymerase activity in chondrocytes during cell division. Additionally, they demonstrated the presence of nuclear receptors for 24,25-dihydroxy-cholecalciferol in chondrocytes *(59)*.

Tetlow and Woolley were able to demonstrate a regional association of (VDR) expression with MMP expression in osteoarthritic human chondrocytes, a phenomenon virtually absent in normal cartilage *(61)*. In further analyses using chondrocyte culture systems, they found that 1,25-dihydroxyvitamin D3 (1-25[OH]2D3) could upregulate expression of matrix MMP-3, yet suppress phorbol 12-myristate 13-acetate-induced production of MMP-9 and prostaglandin (PG)E2. Thus, *in vitro* vitamin D has both enhancing and suppressive roles in the regulation of chondrocyte products. Because these could have differential effects on cartilage, and the net overall effect is unknown, Tetlow et al. (broadly) concluded that the disparate modulatory effects of 1,25(OH)2D3 might be of relevance to the chondrolytic processes that occur in OA, and that further research is needed.

Additionally, vitamin D deficiency could also affect other elements of disease in OA, including pain and muscle weakness. Bischoff et al. investigated the in situ expression of 1,25(OH)2D3 receptor in human skeletal muscle tissue *(62)*. Intraoperative periarticular muscle biopsies were obtained from 20 female patients receiving total hip arthroplasty as a result of OA of the hip or an osteoporotic hip fracture or back surgery. The immunohistological distribution of the VDR was investigated using a monoclonal rat antibody to the receptor. The receptor-positive nuclei were quantified by counting 500 nuclei per biopsy. Strong intranuclear immunostaining of the VDR was detected in human muscle cells. Biopsies of hip patients had significantly fewer receptor-positive nuclei compared with those of back surgery patients ($p = 0.002$). VDR expression was significantly correlated with age (correlation coefficient = 0.46; $p = 0.005$), but not with vitamin D levels. The data demonstrated presence of nuclear 1,25(OH)2D3 receptor in human skeletal muscle.

In a subsequent study, Bischoff et al studied whether VDR expression in vivo is related to age or vitamin D status, or whether VDR expression differs between skeletal muscle groups *(63)*. They investigated these factors and their relation to 1,25(OH)2D3 (VDR) expression in muscle. Intranuclear immunostaining of the VDR was present in muscle biopsy specimens of all orthopedic patients undergoing total hip arthroplasty or spinal surgery. Older age was significantly associated with decreased VDR expression ($\beta = -2.56$; $p = 0.047$), independent of biopsy location and serum 25-hydroxyvitamin D(25[OH]D) levels.

Additionally, higher BMD *(57,64)* has been found to be associated with a decrease in disease progression in persons with OA of the knee. Zhang et al., in a prospective analysis, found that high BMD as well as BMD gain decreased the risk of progression of radiographic OA of the knee in the Framingham cohort *(57)*. Furthermore, a significant positive association between serum 25(OH)D and BMD in individuals with primary OA of the knee, was observed in the Framingham study, independent of gender, age, BMI, knee pain, physical activity, and disease severity *(65)*, suggesting that vitamin D supplementation may enhance BMD in persons with OA.

McAlindon et al. tested the association of vitamin D status on the incidence and progression of OA of the knee among the Framingham OA Cohort Study participants *(66)*. This study included both a dietary assessment and a serum assay of 25(OH) D. Dietary intake of vitamin D and serum 25(OH)D levels were unrelated to OA incidence. Risk of progression over 8 yr, however, was three- to fourfold higher for participants in the middle and lower tertiles of both vitamin D intake (OR for lowest vs highest tertile 4.0, 95% CI, 1.4–11.6) and serum level (OR 2.9; 95% CI, 1.0–8.2).

Low serum vitamin D level also predicted cartilage loss, assessed by loss of joint space (OR 2.3; 95% CI, 0.9–5.5) and osteophyte growth (OR 3.1; 95% CI, 1.3–7.5).

Lane et al. tested the relationship of serum 25-and 1,25-(OH)D with the development of radiographic OA of the hip among elderly white women participating in the Study of Osteoporotic Fractures *(67)*. They measured serum vitamin D levels in 237 subjects randomly selected from 6,051 women who had pelvic radiographs taken at both the baseline examination and after 8 years of follow-up. They analyzed the association of vitamin D levels with the occurrence of JSN and with the development of osteophytes, and with changes in the mean joint space width and individual radiographic feature scores during the study period. The risk of incident OA of the hip, defined as the development of definite JSN, was increased for subjects who were in the middle (OR 3.21; 95% CI, 1.06–9.68) and lowest (OR 3.34; 95% CI, 1.13–9.86) tertiles for vitamin D compared with those in the highest tertile. Vitamin D levels were not associated with incident OA of the hip, defined as the development of definite osteophytes or new disease. No association between serum vitamin D and changes in radiographic OA of the hip was found.

Recently, Felson et al. evaluated the relationship between vitamin D status and cartilage loss in OA *(68)*. They measured 25(OH)D levels by radioimmunoassay in participants from two longitudinal cohort studies, the Framingham Osteoarthritis Study and the BOKS. The Framingham Osteoarthritis study included individuals without OA of the knee (87% of knees had a K/L ≤ 1), whereas participants in BOKS had symptomatic OA of the knee at baseline (21% of knees had a K/L score ≤ 1). In both studies, worsening was defined by radiographic tibiofemoral joint-space loss. Additionally, the BOKS also obtained magnetic resonance imaging (MRI) of the knee at baseline and at 15 and 30 months, of which 26% had a K/L score of 1 or less at baseline. The mean vitamin D level was 20 ng/mL at baseline in both studies, and about 20% of knees exhibited joint-space loss during the observation periods. The investigators found no association of baseline vitamin D levels with radiographic worsening or cartilage loss measured on MRI. In the BOKS, 57% of knees with MRI showed progressive cartilage loss on follow-up MRI (≥ 1 cartilage plate). In this cohort, the risk of cartilage loss was lower for subjects with vitamin D deficiency (25(OH)D <20 ng/mL) compared with those with sufficient vitamin D levels (25(OH)D ≥ 20 ng/mL), adjusting for age, gender, BMI and baseline cartilage score (OR 0.74; 95% CI, 0.50–1.09). However, the analyses did not distinguish between incidence of radiographic OA and progression. Also, as noted by the authors, MRIs were not acquired in a way that permits evaluation of change in cartilage volume.

Carbone et al. tested the relationship of antiresorptive drug use to structural findings and symptoms of OA of the knee *(70)* in the Women in the Health, Aging and Body Composition Study. They found associations of use of alendronate and/or estrogen with lower structural lesion and lower pain scores *(70)*. However, as pointed out by DeMarco *(71)*[7], the original report did not account for potential influence of vitamin D on these associations. Carbone et al., therefore, re-analyzed their results to adjust for a possible effect of vitamin D supplement use *(72)*. Of the participants in this study, 16% used vitamin D supplements at any dosage. Vitamin D supplements use was not associated with structural changes of OA or pain severity, nor did its inclusion as a covariate in the statistical models change the formerly observed associations.

Thus, the epidemiological evidence on the relationship of vitamin D to OA—and OA progression—is conflicting. Clearly, it is a public health priority to establish whether vitamin D has disease-modifying properties for OA. Therefore, we are currently involved in conducting a randomized, double-blind, placebo-controlled trial evaluating longitudinal structural progression and symptom effects of vitamin D supplementation on OA.

4.4. Vitamin E

Vitamin E comprises eight fat-soluble compounds, tocopherols (derivatives of tocol), α-, β-, γ-, and δ-tocopherol and α-, β-, γ-, and δ-tocotrienol, produced solely by plants. Some of the richest sources of vitamin E include vegetable and nut oils, safflower, nuts, sunflower seeds, and whole grains. The most common and biologically active form is α-tocopherol (5,7,8 tri-methyltocol). Synthetic α-tocopherols and their esters also exist. α-Tocopherylacetate is often used commercially because vitamin E esterification protects it from oxidation. In the human body, the ester is rapidly cleaved by cellular esterases making natural vitamin E available.

Vitamin E has diverse influences on the metabolism of arachadonic acid, a proinflammatory fatty acid found in all cell membranes. Vitamin E blocks formation of arachidonic acid (AA) from phospholipids and inhibits lipoxygenase activity, without having much effect on cyclooxygenase (COX (73)). It is, therefore, possible that vitamin E reduces the modest synovial inflammation that may accompany OA.

In vitro effects of vitamin E on chondrocytes have been investigated. Tiku et al. showed that vitamin E reduced the catabolism of collagen by preventing the protein oxidation mediated by aldehydic down products of lipid peroxidation when chondrocytes were submitted to an oxidative burst (74). Vitamin E strongly increased the sulfate incorporation while slightly reducing the glucosamine incorporation (75), suggesting that it increased GAG sulfatation or that it increased GAG synthesis while reducing glycoproteins or glycolipids synthesis. Like vitamin C, vitamin E affected the activities of lysosomal enzymes: It decreased the activities of arylsulfatase A and of acid phosphatase in cultures of human articular chondrocytes (75). However, vitamin E did not affect the lipopolysaccharide-induced catabolism of GAGs (76) and did not prevent synoviocyte apoptosis induced by superoxide anions(77).

Previous studies suggest that vitamin E may enhance chondrocyte growth via protection against ROS and ultimately modulate the development of OA (15,78). In the Framingham OA Cohort, men with higher vitamin E levels were less likely to have OA of the knee progression compared with those with lower levels (34).

Benefit from vitamin E therapy has been suggested by several small human studies of OA (79–(82)). In a 6-week double-blind, placebo-controlled trial of 400 mg α-tocopherol (vitamin E) in 56 patients with OA (83), vitamin E-treated participants experienced greater improvement in every efficacy measure including pain at rest (69% better in vitamin E vs 34% better in placebo, p <0.05), pain on movement (62% better on vitamin E vs 27% on placebo, p <0.01), and use of analgesics (52% less on vitamin E; 24% less on placebo, p <0.01). The rapid response in symptoms observed in this study suggests that vitamin E does not exert a structural effect in OA; instead, perhaps the beneficial effect results from some metabolic action such as inhibition of AA metabolism.

Two trials concluded that vitamin E was more efficient than placebo in decreasing pain. In a small 10-day crossover trial on spondylosis, 600 mg of vitamin E per day was superior to placebo as assessed by a patient questionnaire *(84)*. One trial suggested that vitamin E was no less efficient than diclofenac in decreasing pain. In a 3-week randomized controlled trial (RCT), no significant difference was found between 544 mg of α-tocopherylacetate three times a day and 50 mg diclofenac three times a day on VAS of pain *(85)*. However, the two most recent trials failed to show any benefit over placebo on OA of the knee. Vitamin E (500 IU per day) showed no symptomatic benefit over placebo as assessed by WOMAC in a 6-month RCT *(86)*.

Results from a 2-year double-blind, placebo-controlled trial among 136 patients with OA of the knee do not support a chondroprotective effect of vitamin E. Wluka et al. tested whether vitamin E (500 IU) affects cartilage volume loss in patients with OA of the knee *(87)*. The primary outcome was change in tibial cartilage volume from baseline to 2 years follow-up measured by MRI. Secondary outcomes included pain, stiffness, function, and total WOMAC scores as well as the Short Form-36. The study was completed by 117 participants, for a loss to follow-up rate of 14%. Loss of medial and lateral tibial cartilage was similar in subjects treated with vitamin E and placebo (e.g., mean loss in the medial compartment 157 vs 187 μm^3, $p = 0.5$). There were no significant differences between the vitamin E- and placebo-treated groups in improvement of symptoms from baseline. The authors concluded that vitamin E does not appear to benefit cartilage volume loss in OA.

However, there are limitations that should be considered in the interpretation of these results. First, this study was powered to detect a 50% reduction in the rate of cartilage loss in the treatment arm. This effect size likely was an over-estimate of any effect that could have been expected from vitamin E over a 2-year follow-up period. Second, the structural outcome measure evaluated in this study was cartilage volume assessed on MRI. This is problematic because cartilage volume uncorrected for surface area lacks construct validity *(88)*. Furthermore, cartilage volume has not been tested for sensitivity to change, thus it is unclear whether a real change in cartilage volume within a given individual can be distinguished from measurement error. Cartilage volume needs to be comprehensively validated and evaluated for reliability before it should replace JSN on plain radiograph as the structural outcome measure recommended in OA clinical trials *(89)*. In this study, cartilage volume was the only structural outcome measured.

A recent systematic review observed that although three out of the five RCTs concluded that vitamin E decreased pain, the two longest, largest, and highest quality trials failed to detect any symptomatic or structural effects in OA of the knee, suggesting that, at least for this condition, vitamin E alone has no medium-term beneficial effect. According to the best-evidence synthesis, the authors concluded that there is no evidence of symptom-modifying efficacy for vitamin E and some evidence of inefficacy regarding structure-modifying effects *(90)*.

4.5. Vitamin K

The primary form of vitamin K, a fat-soluble vitamin, in the diet is phylloquinone (vitamin K_1), which is concentrated in dark green leafy vegetables and vegetable oils. Although there is some endogenous production of vitamin K, a subclinical deficiency can develop by limiting dietary intake of phylloquinone. Low dietary intake of vitamin K is common, and studies evaluating biochemical measures of vitamin K status suggest that inadequate intake of vitamin K is widespread among adults in the United States and the United Kingdom *(91,92)*.

Although it is not known to have anti-oxidant effects, vitamin K does have bone and cartilage effects, which may be relevant for osteoarthritis. Post-translational γ-carboxylation of glutamic acid residues to form γ-carboxyglutamic acid (Gla) residues confers functionality to these "Gla" proteins *(93)*. Vitamin K is an essential cofactor for this process *(93)*. Multiple coagulation, bone, and cartilage proteins are dependent on vitamin K because the Gla residues are required for these proteins to function appropriately. Bone and cartilage Gla proteins include growth arrest-specific protein 6 (Gas-6), and the skeletally expressed ECM proteins, osteocalcin and matrix Gla protein (MGP *(93–96)*).

The vitamin K-dependent γ-carboxylation of these bone and cartilage proteins is important for their normal functioning. Gas-6, through its interactions with the Axl tyrosine kinase receptor, prevents chondrocyte apoptosis and is involved in chondrocyte growth and development *(94)*. Low levels of vitamin K could lead to inadequate levels of functional Gas-6, contributing to increased chondrocyte apoptosis and attendant mineralization. Another Gla protein is osteocalcin, the most abundant noncollagenous protein in bone, and a potent inhibitor of hydroxyapatite mineralization. MGP, a protein that plays a role in chondrocyte development and maturation, is associated with mineralization in hypertrophic chondrocytes and endochondral ossification, the same process through which osteophytes form *(97,98)*. Also, MGP may inhibit mineralization via its interaction with bone morphogenetic protein-2 (BMP-2). BMP-2 is a known inducer of chondrocyte and osteoblast differentiation that signals through Smad1, together enhancing bone formation. Interference by MGP leads to diminished bone-forming capacity *(99)*, and conversely, under-carboxylated MGP could lead to increased bone-forming capacity.

Beyond being a necessary co-factor for γ-carboxylation, vitamin K compounds also exhibit anti-inflammatory properties, reducing PGE_2 and interleukin (IL)-6 production and inhibiting IL-1 and PGE_2-mediated bone resorption *(100,101)*.

The effects of inadequately functioning vitamin K-dependent proteins has been seen in warfarin (vitamin K antagonist) embryopathy, Keutel syndrome (a genetic disorder where MGP is deficient), and an MGP knock-out mouse model, all of which exhibit growth-plate cartilage abnormalities *(102–104)*. These abnormalities may reflect a process similar to osteophyte formation because both cartilage plate abnormalities and osteophyte formation involve endochondral ossification. Thus, vitamin K is an important regulator of bone and cartilage mineralization and function, and may play a role in OA.

Neogi et al. investigated the potential association between vitamin K and OA in the Framingham Osteoarthritis cohort. In their first assessment, they examined the relationship between dietary vitamin K intake (evaluated using an FFQ) and radiographic evidence of osteophytes *(105)*. They demonstrated an association between higher vitamin K intake and lower osteophyte prevalence, but the association was not significant with prevalence ratios of osteophytes from lowest to highest vitamin K intake quartiles of 1.0 (reference), 1.1, 0.8, 0.9 (p for trend = 0.2). In a follow-up study,

Neogi et al. subsequently measured vitamin K levels using plasma vitamin levels *(106)*. In this study, they showed an association between plasma phylloquinone and severity of radiographic OA, particularly of osteophytes, in the hand and knee, after adjusting for age, gender, BMI, femoral neck BMD, total energy intake, and plasma vitamin D. The prevalence of hand and knee osteophytes in those in the highest plasma phylloquinone quartile was 40% lower than in those in the lowest quartile. No significant associations were noted for control nutrients, vitamins B_1 and B_2, suggesting that a healthy lifestyle does not account for these results.

If a relationship between vitamin K and osteophytes does exist, the public health benefits could potentially be enormous. However, based on these two observational studies, it is unclear whether there is an association between vitamin K and OA. It seems reasonable to expect that plasma levels of micronutrients are more accurate measures compared with dietary intake measures, lending more credibility to the latter study supporting an association between vitamin K and osteophytes.

The data is suggestive that vitamin K deficiency is associated with features of OA and OA severity, thus vitamin K supplementation has the potential of being classified as a modifying OA drug. To address this possibility, Neogi and others are currently involved in conducting a randomized, double-blind, placebo-controlled trial evaluating longitudinal structural and symptom effects of vitamin K supplementation on OA.

4.6. Selenium and Iodine: Studies of Kashin-Beck Disease

Selenium is an integral component of iodothyronine deiodinase as well as glutathione peroxidase. Kashin-Beck disease is an osteoarthropathy of children and adolescents, which occurs in geographic areas of China in which deficiencies of both selenium and iodine are endemic. Strong epidemiological evidence supports the environmental nature of this disease *(107)*. Although the clinical and radiological characteristics of Kashin-Beck disease differ from OA, its existence raises the possibility that environmental factors also play a role in OA.

Selenium deficiency together with pro-oxidative products of organic matter in drinking water (mainly fulvic acid) and contamination of grain by fungi have been proposed as environmental causes for Kashin-Beck disease. The efficacy of selenium supplementation in preventing the disorder, however, is controversial. Moreno-Reyes et al. studied iodine and selenium metabolism in 11 villages in Tibet in which Kashin-Beck disease was endemic and 1 village in which is was not *(108)*. They found iodine deficiency to be the main determinant of Kashin-Beck disease in these villages. It should be noted, however, in the three groups—those with disease in villages with Kashin-Beck disease, those without disease in villages with Kashin-Beck disease and those in the control group without Kashin-Beck disease—all had selenium levels that were very low and those in the latter group had the lowest levels. In an accompanying editorial, Utiger inferred that Kashin-Beck disease probably results from a combination of deficiencies of both of these elements, and speculated that growth-plate cartilage is both dependent on locally produced triiodothyronine and sensitive to oxidative damage *(107)*. It should be noted that there is little evidence, if any, to suggest that Kashin-Beck disease has any similarities with adult-onset spontaneous OA.

Jordan et al. evaluated the relationship between selenium and OA of the knee in an observational community-based population, the Johnston County Osteoarthritis

Project *(109)*, in which 940 participants submitted toenail clippings for a selenium assessment by Instrumental Neutron Activation Analysis. Radiographic OA of the knee was scored using a definition of K/L grade of 2 or more. Mean selenium levels were 0.76 parts per million (ppm; ±0.12). Compared with those in the lowest tertile of selenium, those in the highest tertile had an OR of 0.62 (95% CI, 0.37–1.02) for having prevalent OA of the knee and an OR of 0.56 (95% CI, 0.31–0.97) for having bilateral OA of the knee. Based on these findings, low selenium levels appear to be associated with prevalent OA of the knee, particularly bilateral disease.

Although results from this study are provocative, there are several limitations to it. First, although the measurement of selenium via toenail clippings has been used in the past, the duration of exposure to different selenium levels cannot be ascertained using this measurement. Second, given that Kashin-Beck disease was the model from which selenium deficiency was hypothesized to be associated with OA, information on iodine status would have been of interest in this study. Admittedly, the supplementation of iodine in salt within the United States makes it less likely to find people severely deficient in iodine. However, if iodine status were predictive of OA in participants with low selenium levels as has been seen in Kashin-Beck disease, it would be important in enhancing our understanding of the role of selenium in OA pathophysiology. Finally, it is possible that selenium concentration could be the surrogate for another unmeasured micronutrient. An RCT of selenium supplementation (perhaps in factorial design with iodine supplementation) is needed to evaluate whether it would be effective as a disease-modifying OA drug.

There is little research evaluating the efficacy of selenium in treating OA symptoms. There is one small published clinical trial of supplemental selenium in which Hill and Bird conducted a 6-mo double-blind, placebo-controlled study of selenium-ACE, a proprietary nutritional supplement in the United Kingdom, among 30 patients with either primary or secondary OA of the knee or hip *(110)*. The "active" treatment contained on average 144 µg of selenium as well as 450 µg, 90 mg, and 30 mg of vitamins A, C, and E, respectively. In fact, the placebo also contained 2.9 µg of selenium. Pain and stiffness scores remained similar for the two groups at both 3 and 6 months of follow-up. The authors concluded that their data did not support efficacy for selenium-ACE in relieving OA symptoms.

It is unlikely that the aforementioned clinical trial will provide any insight regarding the efficacy of selenium in the treatment of symptoms in OA. With just 30 participants in the trial, it is too small to detect even a moderate effect of selenium. Even if investigators would have found an effect of the active treatment, it would have been impossible to attribute the effects to selenium as the active treatment also contained moderate-high doses of vitamins A, C, and E. A larger randomized, placebo-controlled, clinical trial evaluating selenium supplementation should be conducted to evaluate its efficacy in the treatment of symptoms related to OA.

4.7. Glucosamine and Chondroitin Sulfate

Glucosamine and chondroitin sulfate are cartilage ECM components that have been widely promulgated as dietary supplements that have potential benefit in reducing pain and slowing the progression of OA on the basis that they might provide a substrate for matrix synthesis and repair. However, their mechanisms of action remain unclear.

Glucosamine, an amino monosaccharide found in chitin, glycoproteins, and GAGs, is also known as 2-amino-2-deoxyglucose or 2-amino-2-deoxy-β-D-glucopyranose. Glucosamine is available as a nutritional supplement in three forms, glucosamine sulfate, glucosamine hydrochloride, and *N*-acetyl-glucosamine.

According to our understanding of the metabolic pathways involved, glucosamine, as an amino sugar, should be rapidly degraded by the liver during first-pass metabolism. Early pharmacodynamic studies assessed absorption of the compounds only indirectly *(111,112)*. A recent pharmacokinetic study in dogs, using a refined high-performance liquid chromatographic assay, demonstrated that glucosamine hydrochloride is absorbed with a bioavailability of approx 10 to 12% from single or multiple doses *(113)*. Furthermore, laboratory work in rats has suggested that glucosamine is substantially degraded in the lumen of the gastrointestinal tract *(114)*. To evaluate the absorption of glucosamine sulfate in humans, Biggee et al. performed a small study evaluating 10 participants with OA, measuring serum levels of glucosamine every 15 to 30 minutes over 3 hours after ingestion of the recommended 1,500 mg of oral glucosamine sulfate *(115)*. Of the 10 subjects, 9 had detectable serum glucosamine beginning to rise at 30 to 45 minutes and peaking at 90 to 180 minutes. The mean maximal serum level was 12 μmoles/L. This would provide less than 2% of ingested glucosamine to blood and interstitial fluid combined. Based on the very small serum levels seen in this study, the authors concluded that ingestion of standard glucosamine sulfate is unlikely to stimulate cartilage chondroitin synthesis. Persiani et al. evaluated both serum and synovial fluid levels of glucosamine in five people with OA of the knee before and after administration of daily oral glucosamine for 2 weeks and found similar increase in serum synovial fluid glucosamine concentrations of 7.9 micromoles/L and 7.2 micromoles/L, respectively *(116)*.

In addition to the fact that serum levels of glucosamine are very low, the notion that exogenous glucosamine might be incorporated into the structure of hyaluronan or cartilage proteoglycans is also problematic because while glucosamine can enter the GAG biosynthetic pathway after its conversion to uridine diphosphate-*N*-galactosamine, glucose is a much more abundant substrate. Recent *in vitro* and *in vivo* studies in animals, have shown increases in proteoglycan synthesis by chondrocytes after addition of glucosamine to the culture medium, suggesting instead of providing substrate for hyaluronan or cartilage proteoglycans, glucosamine sulfate's mechanism of action may be an anti-inflammatory effect *(111,112)*.

A potential adverse effect of glucosamine that was recently highlighted in a report from the Institute of Medicine *(117)*. Glucosamine may lead to an increase in insulin dysregulation among individuals predisposed to such problems. These concerns are based on the known ability of glucosamine to bypass the glutamine:fructose-6-phosphate amidotransferase step of hexosamine biosynthesis and desensitize glucose transport *(118)*. Insulin dysregulation is of particular interest to individuals with OA because high BMI is a risk factor for OA, insulin resistance, and diabetes mellitus. Although the effects of glucosamine have been well documented in animal models, less is known about its effects on glucose metabolism in humans. Preliminary studies have been reassuring; however, their interpretation has been limited by the considerable variability in measures and small numbers of participants *(119,120)*.

Chondroitin sulfate is a GAG composed of linear repeating units of D-galactosamine and D-glucuronic acid. This compound is the predominant GAG found in articular cartilage. In humans it is also found in bone, cartilage, cornea, skin, and the arterial wall. Chondroitin sulfate comes in three forms, A, B, and C. The two most common found in chondroitin sulfate nutritional supplements are types A (chondroitin 4-sulfate) and C (chondroitin 6-sulfate). Chondroitin sulfate is found primarily in fish cartilage as well as cartilaginous rings of bovine trachea and pig ears and snouts.

The biologic fate of orally administered chondroitin sulfate is less clear, but some evidence exists to suggest that the compound may be absorbed following oral administration, possibly as a result of pinocytosis *(121)*. Chondroitin sulfate is able to cause an increase in RNA synthesis by chondrocytes *(122)* that appears to correlate with an increase in the production of proteoglycans and collagens *(123–126)*. Additionally, there is evidence that chondroitin sulfate partially inhibits leukocyte elastase and may, therefore, reduce the degradation of cartilage collagen and proteoglycans, which is prominent in the OA process *(127–130)*.

Recently, Jackson et al. conducted a study to delineate the pharmacokinetics of glucosamine and chondroitin sulfate. Based on the Glucosamine/chondroitin Arthritis Interventon Trial (GAIT) dosing schedule and dosages, 33 subjects (11 per treatment arm) were randomized to receive glucosamine 1,500 mg, chondroitin sulfate 1,200 mg, or a combination of both glucosamine and chondroitin sulfate for 12 weeks. The results of this study have been reported in abstract form at the time of this publication *(131)*. Nine blood samples per subject were subsequently obtained over 36 h and plasma concentrations of glucosamine and chondroitin sulfate were measured in duplicate. Similar to the previously reported oral single-dose pharmacokinetics, plasma glucosamine levels in both the glucosamine and combination treatment groups achieved peak concentrations 2 to 3 hours post-dose with a terminal elimination half-life of approx 3 hours. The mean maximal plasma concentration was 211.1 ng/mL for glucosamine and 216.6 ng/mL for chondroitin sulfate. Area under the concentration-time curve (AUC) was slightly decreased in the combination group compared with glucosamine alone, whereas C_{max} was roughly equal. The data for both groups was well fit to a one-compartment open model including first-order absorption. Compared to oral single-dose pharmacokinetics, both AUC and C_{max} for glucosamine were lower following multiple-dose ingestion. No appreciable change in plasma chondroitin sulfate from baseline was detected following multiple-dose oral administration of either chondroitin sulfate alone or combination. The authors concluded that glucosamine is substantially absorbed and rapidly eliminated following multiple-dose oral administration of glucosamine alone and combination in humans whereas no change in basal plasma chondroitin sulfate concentration can be detected with similar administration of chondroitin sulfate alone or in combination. Compared to single-dose ingestion, a decrease in AUC and C_{max} for glucosamine was observed following multiple-dose administration possibly reflecting a change in absorption, cellular utilization or elimination with sustained oral use.

4.7.1. SULFATE

Cartilage proteoglycans are highly sulfated. The amount of sulfate made available to cells is an important factor in the degree of proteoglycan sulfation *(132,133)*. *In vitro* experiments on cultured cells suggest that increases in serum sulfate concentration enhance GAG synthesis *(134)*. It has also been found that the rate of sulfated GAG synthesis in human articular cartilage is sensitive to small deviations from physiologic sulfate concentrations *(135)*. Additionally, sulfate pools in humans are among the smallest of all species *(136)*, making them especially susceptible to physiologically relevant small changes. In humans, sulfate balance is poorly understood and may vary on dietary factors or on dietary supplements. One study measured human urinary sulfate excretion after ingestion of methionine or chondroitin sulfate supplements in the setting of high- or low-protein diets. The authors observed that more sulfate was excreted in the urine in those with a background of high-protein diets compared with those on low-protein diets. This suggests that in the low-protein state, the body increased sulfate retention from supplements *(137)*. These observations raise the possibility that sulfate supplementation may have a beneficial role in cartilage health.

Also, low sulphate levels in blood may contribute to OA by decreasing cartilage chondroitin sulphation. A recent study measured serum levels of sulphate during 3 hours of fasting or glucose ingestion after overnight fasts to determine how much sulphate lowering may occur during this period. Sera samples of 14 patients with OA who fasted overnight were obtained every 15 to 30 minutes during 3 hours of continued fasting and during 3 hours after ingestion of 75 g of glucose. Continuation of overnight fasting for 3 hours resulted in a near-linear 3-hour decrease in levels for all 14 patients ranging from 3 to 20% with a mean drop of 9.3%, whereas the 3-hour decrease after glucose ingestion ranged from 10 to 33% with a mean drop of 18.9%. The authors concluded that a 3-hour continuation of fasting caused a marked reduction in serum sulphate levels, whereas ingestion of 75 g of glucose in the absence of protein resulted in doubling the reduction, suggesting that fasting and ingestion of protein-free calories may produce periods of chondroitin under-sulphation that could affect OA *(138)*.

4.7.2. EFFICACY FOR PAIN AND FUNCTION

Glucosamine and chondroitin sulfate had been the subject of numerous clinical trials in Europe and Asia, all of which (until recently) had demonstrated favorable effects *(139–153)*. In 2000, McAlindon performed a meta-analysis and quality assessment of 15 eligible double-blind, placebo-controlled clinical trials of glucosamine and chondroitin *(154)*, noting that most of the trials were sponsored by a manufacturer of the product, all reported positive results. The results suggested publication bias and highlighted methodological problems. The aggregated effect sizes (standardized mean differences [SMDs]) were 0.44 (95% CI, 0.24–0.64) for glucosamine and 0.78 (95% CI, 0.60–0.95) for chondroitin. Results were similar when including only pain as an outcome. As a reference, 0.2 is considered a small effect, 0.5 a moderate effect, and 0.8 a large effect *(155)*.

Towheed et al. also performed a systematic review of RCTs of glucosamine, which they recently updated *(166)*. They found an SMD for pain and function of 0.61 (95% CI, 0.28–0.95), consistent with a moderate effect of glucosamine. However, when the analysis was restricted to the eight higher quality studies, no benefit of glucosamine was seen (SMD = 0.19; 95% CI, –0.11–0.50). In the subset of trials that tested the Rotta preparation of glucosamine sulfate (N=10), a surprisingly large effect on pain was seen (1.31; 95% CI, 0.64–1.99 *(166)*). This SMD (1.3) is as large as the effect of a total joint replacement.

Regarding chondroitin sulfate, a meta-analysis performed by Leeb et al. included seven double-blind, RCTs evaluating 703 patients *(159)*. The estimated pooled effect sizes were 0.9 (95% CI, ~0.8–1.0) for pain and 0.74 (95% CI, ~0.650.85) for function. The authors concluded that chondroitin sulfate might be useful in OA. However, they acknowledged several major problems in interpreting the data including small numbers of participants in the eligible trials and the fact that no study was evaluated using ITT analysis. They also estimated that the evident publication bias in this review could lead to a relative error of 30% *(159)*.

Reichenbach et al. also conducted a meta-analysis of 18 randomized trials of chondroitin for pain owing to OA of the hip or knee *(160)*. The pooled effect size was –0.67 (95% CI, –0.91 to –0.43) but there was considerable heterogeneity (I^2= 86%; p <0.001, and greater effects in small trials (p = 0.002) and those without an ITT analysis (p = 0.01). After pooling the two large trials that had performed an ITT analysis (N = 931), the effect size was 0.00 (95% CI, –0.13–0.13) and there was no between-trial heterogeneity (I^2= 0%, p = 0.67). Thus, these authors found no robust evidence for an effect of chondroitin on pain.

The body of evidence concerning the efficacy of glucosamine and chondroitin has been altered by the publication of recent independently funded clinical trials, some of which had completely null results *(161–164)*. The first of these enrolled 114 patients with OA of the knee who were naïve to glucosamine and chondroitin, and randomized them into a 2-month placebo-controlled trial of 500 mg divided in three doses per day of glucosamine sulfate *(164)*. They found no difference in pain outcomes between the two groups after either 30 or 60 days of treatment.

Hughes and Carr performed a double-blind, placebo-controlled RCT of glucosamine sulfate (1.5 g per day) in participants with relatively severe OA of the knee; 23% had a K/L grade of 4 and a mean WOMAC score of 9.2 (SD = 3.5 *(163)*). No significant between-group differences were found in the primary endpoint (VAS overall assessment of pain in the affected knee) or any of the secondary pain assessments in this study at 6, 12, and 24 weeks of follow-up.

Cibere et al. performed a glucosamine withdrawal trial in 137 people with OA of the knee who were already using the product with at least moderate benefit *(161)*. The design was a 6-month, randomized, placebo-controlled glucosamine discontinuation trial in which enrollees were randomly assigned to placebo or to the treatment, where participants continued taking glucosamine sulfate. The primary outcome was the proportion of disease flares. Ultimately, disease flares occurred in 42% of the placebo arm and 45% of the glucosamine arm (difference –3%, 95% CI, –19–14). In the multivariate regression analysis, time-to-disease flare was not significantly different between the glucosamine and the placebo group (hazard ratio of flare = 0.8; p = 0.4). No differences were found in severity of disease flare or other secondary outcomes between placebo and patients taking glucosamine. Cibere et al. also analyzed samples for type II collagen degradation biomarkers as a proxy for OA progression *(165)*. However, they found no statistically significant effect of glucosamine sulfate on type II collagen fragment levels, with the primary outcome being the ratio of C1, C2 epitope/C2C epitope in the urine and serum at baseline, at 4, 12, and 24 weeks of follow-up.

The Glucosamine Unum in Die Efficacy trial *(167)*, tested glucosamine sulfate among 318 patients with OA of the knee, randomized to 1,500 mgonce a day, or acetaminophen 1 g thrice a day (3 g per day total), or placebo, for 6 months. The rescue medication was ibuprofen 400 mg. The primary end point was the 6-months change in the Lequesne index in the ITT population. The effect of glucosamine sulfate was significant on all parameters, for example, Lequesne difference −1.2 (95% CI, −2.3 to −0.8; WOMAC difference −4.7 (95% CI, −9.1 to −0.2), and Osteoarthritis Research Society International-A responders 39.6 versus 21.2% ($p = 0.007$). Acetaminophen had more responders than placebo, but it failed to reach a significant difference on the Lequesne ($p = 0.18$) and WOMAC ($p = 0.077$) indexes. The authors concluded that glucosamine sulfate at the oral once-daily dose of 1,500 mg is an effective symptomatic medication in treatment of OA of the knee.

As an attempt to settle the question of the efficacy of glucosamine and chondroitin sulfate in symptomatic improvement in OA, the National Institutes of Health sponsored the GAIT, the largest comparative trial of these treatments (168). Participants (N = 1,583) were randomized to one of five arms: placebo, celecoxib 200 mg daily, glucosamine hydrochloride 1,500 mg daily, chondroitin sulfate 1,200 mg daily, or the combination of glucosamine hydrochloride and chondroitin sulfate. The primary outcome in this study was treatment response, defined as a 20% improvement in knee pain. The respective response rates were 60.1, 70.1, 64, 65.4, and 66.6%. The difference between combination treatment and placebo was reported as near statistically significant ($p = 0.09$). In a subgroup analysis of participants with a higher WOMAC score at baseline, the response rates were 54.3, 69.4, 65.7, 61.4, and 79.2. In this analysis, the combination treatment was significantly different from placebo ($p = 0.002$). The authors concluded that glucosamine and chondroitin sulfate alone or in combination did not reduce pain effectively in the overall group. The combination therapy may be effective in treating moderate to severe knee pain resulting from OA.

The study was limited by an attrition rate of at least 20% in each group, as well as unusually high response rates in the placebo group. Furthermore, the analyses did not incorporate data from all time points, as study participants were also evaluated at 4, 8, 16, and 24 weeks. Also, although not explicitly stated, the subgroup analysis looking at those with higher baseline pain scores appeared to be a post-hoc analysis where the placebo response rate was slightly lower and the combination treatment response rate was slightly higher. Also, the trial tested glucosamine hydrochloride and not glucosamine sulfate.

4.7.3. EFFICACY AS DISEASE-MODIFYING AGENTS

Rotta Pharmaceuticals sponsored two large multicenter RCTs to examine the possibility that glucosamine might reduce rate of loss of articular cartilage (169,170). These enrolled approx 200 outpatients with primary OA of the knee into 3-year RCTs comparing 1.5 g of Rotta glucosamine sulfate, taken once daily, with placebo. The primary outcome in each trial was based on joint-space measurements obtained from conventional, extended-view, standing anteroposterior knee radiographs, a recommended radiographic approach at that time. Both trials showed quantitatively similar benefits in the glucosamine-treatment arms, with respect to the rate of loss of joint-space width and symptoms.

Unfortunately, the approach that was used to estimate joint-space width in these RCTs has proved to be problematic, although it was the recommended technique at the inception of the trials *(89)*. Precise measurement of this variable is contingent on highly reproducible radio-anatomic positioning of the joint, and may be biased by the presence of pain. If those in the glucosamine group had less pain at their follow-up X-ray, they may have stood with the knee more fully extended, a nonphysiological position that may be associated with the femur riding up on the tibial edge, giving the appearance of a better preserved joint space. What appeared to have been a slower rate of joint space loss may have reflected between-group differences in the degree of knee extension at the follow-up radiograph.

Michel et al. reported the results of a 2-year randomized, double-blind, controlled trial of 800 mg chondroitin sulfate or placebo once daily among 300 patients with OA of the knee *(171)*. The primary outcome was joint-space loss over 2 years as assessed by a posteroanterior radiograph of the knee in mild flexion, a better validated technique *(172)*. Secondary outcomes included pain and function. The participants in the placebo arm exhibited significant joint-space loss with a mean cumulative joint-space loss of 0.14 mm (±0.61) at 2 years of follow-up compared with no change in the chondroitin arm, 0.00 mm (±0.53). In the ITT analysis, the between-group difference in mean joint-space loss was 0.14±0.57 mm; $p = 0.04$. In contrast, the differences in the symptom outcomes between the groups were trivial and nonsignificant. However, chondroitin was well tolerated, with no significant differences in rates of adverse events between the two groups. Although the authors focused on the results providing evidence of structure damage modification by chondroitin, important questions remain about the internal validity of joint-space width as a measure of cartilage loss, and its relevance to the clinical state of the patient with OA of the knee—especially in the absence of any overt impact on symptomatic outcomes. Of note, the lack of symptomatic improvement of chondroitin sulfate in this moderate to large intervention trial further highlights the likely overestimation of effect sizes of symptoms as an outcome reported in the two meta-analyses of this treatment.

Similarly, Reginster et al. recently conducted the multicenter STudy on Osteoarthritis Progression Prevention assessing the effect of chondroitin sulfate on the structural progression of OA of the knee, comparing orally administered chondroitin 4&6 sulfate, 800 mg and placebo over 24 months in 622 patients with OA of the knee. The results of this study have been presented in abstract form at the time of this publication *(173)*. The primary outcome was the minimal JSN measured over 2 years, on digitalized radiographs (Lyon schuss view). Secondary outcomes included pain. The study groups were balanced at baseline with respect to demographic and clinical variables, including severity of OA. Ninety-three patients (30.1%) from the chondroitin sulfate group and 80 patients (25.6%) from the placebo group dropped out. The ITT analysis showed a mean (SE) JSN of 0.24 (±0.03) mm at 2 years in the placebo group, which was significantly reduced in the chondroitin sulfate group (0.10±0.03 mm; $p <0.01$). The per protocol analysis confirmed the results obtained in the ITT analysis. The interaction time × treatment showed a statistically significant difference in pain VAS and WOMAC ($p <0.01$) in favor of chondroitin sulfate. The authors concluded that chondroitin 4&6 sulfate significantly reduced progression of JSN compared with placebo in patients with OA of the knee.

4.8. Diacerein

Diacerein is metabolized to rhein, which has analgesic and anti-inflammatory properties *(174)*. *In vitro*, rhein induced the synthesis of PGE_2 and inhibited the production IL-1β by cultured chondrocytes *(175–177)*. A systematic review of seven trials including 2,069 participants with osteoarthritis using a VAS for pain, noted a modest benefit of diacerein compared with placebo (difference –5.16 mm; 95% CI, –9.75 to –0.57*(178)*). The efficacy for pain was similar for OA of the knee and hip. Of those taking diacerein, 42% reported diarrhea.

A clinical trial comparing diacerein 50 mg thrice daily with placebo over 3 years among 507 participants with OA of the hip observed that the rate of JSN was significantly lower for those receiving diacerein on weight-bearing pelvic radiographs obtained with patients standing at 1 m from the X-ray source, with a 20° internal foot rotation (0.18 vs. 0.22 mm per year for the placebo group *(179)*).

However, a clinical trial with three arms comparing intra-articular hyaluronate plus oral placebo, intra-articular saline plus oral placebo, and intra-articular saline plus diacerein, among 301 participants with OA of the knee found no differences in pain at any time during 1 year of treatment when comparing 50 mg of diacerein thrice daily with placebo *(180)*. With regards to radiographic progression, the mean decrease in joint-space width was similar in all treatment arms (0.09 mm per year). Although a modest short-term benefit on pain has been noted, long-term studies on the potential of diacerein as a disease-modifying agent are lacking.

4.9. *Polyunsaturated Fatty Acids*

Polyunsaturated fatty acid (PUFA) classification is based on the position of the last double bond along the fatty acid chain. PUFAs are classified as omega-3 (n-3), omega-6 (n-6), or omega-9 (n-9). The main dietary PUFAs are n-3 (i.e., eicosapentenoic acid [EPA] and linolenic acid) and n-6 (i.e., AA and linoleic acid). Omega-3 is found in fish and canola oils, as well as in flaxseeds, soybean, and walnuts. Omega-6 is found in sunflower oil, soybean, safflower, corn, and meat. These PUFAS are metabolized by COX and lipooxygenases (LOX) into different eicosanoids. The n-6-derived eicosanoids tend to be proinflammatory, whereas the n-3-derived eicosanoids tend to be anti-inflammatory.

The n-3s have a range of potentially favorable effects on chondrocytes, including decreased expression of aggrecanase, COX-2, 5-LOX, FLAP (5-LOX-activating protein), IL-1a, and TNF-a, and MMP-3 and MMP-13 *(192–194)*. Overall, these results indicate that n-3 PUFAs have anticatabolic and anti-inflammatory properties. However, a low n-6:n-3 ratio might also be detrimental. A dietary intervention study in rats showed that low intake of n-6 induced cartilage surface irregularities and localized proteoglycan depletion *(195)*.

The utility of n-3 for OA was tested in a 24-week, double-blind, placebo-controlled trial of cod liver oil (10 mL containing 786 mg of EPA) as an adjunct to NSAIDs in 86 patients with OA. Participants were assessed at 4-week intervals for joint pain/inflammation and disability. There was no significant benefit for the patients taking cod liver oil compared with placebo *(195)*. Further studies are needed to determine whether these are of benefit for OA.

4.10. *Avocado/Soybean Unsaponifiables*

Avocado and soybean unsaponifiables (ASUs) have anabolic, anticatabolic, and anti-inflammatory effects on chondrocytes *in vitro*. ASUs increase collagen synthesis *(181)*, inhibit collagenase activity *(182,183)*, increase the basal synthesis of aggrecan, reverse the IL-1β- induced aggrecan synthesis inhibition *(184)*, decrease the production of MMP-3, IL-6 and 8, and PGE$_2$, while weakly reversing the IL-1β-induced decrease in tissue inhibiting metalloproteinase-1 production *(181,183,184)*. ASUs decrease the spontaneous production of NO and macrophage inflammatory protein-1β *(184)* while stimulating the expression of TGF-β and plasminogen activator inhibitor (PAI)-1*(185)*.

Piascledine (Pharmascience, Inc), composed of one-third avocado and two-thirds soybean unsaponifiables *(183)*, is the most frequently investigated lipid combination. In sheep with lateral meniscectomy, 900 mg once a day for 6 months reduced the loss of toluidine blue stain in cartilage and prevented subchondral sclerosis in the inner zone of the lateral tibial plateau but not focal cartilage lesions *(186)*.

Four trials were pooled in a meta-analysis that had positive results *(187)*. ASUs were evaluated on OA of the knee and hip in four double-blind, randomized, placebo-controlled trials *(187–191)*. In two 3-month RCTs, one on OA of the knee and hip *(188)* and one on OA of the knee *(190)*, 300 mg once a day decreased NSAID intake. There was no difference between 300 and 600 mg per day *(190)*. In a 6-month RCT on OA of the knee and hip, 300 mg once a day resulted in an improved Lequesne functional index compared with placebo *(189)*. ASUs had a 2-month delayed onset of action as well as residual symptomatic effects 2 months after the end of treatment. In a 2-year RCT on OA of the hip, 300 mg once a day did not have an effect on JSN *(191)*, or any of the secondary end points (pain, function, and patient global assessment). However, a post-hoc analysis suggested that ASUs might decrease JSN in patients with severe OA of the hip.

Recently, Ameye and Chee concluded based on a best-evidence synthesis, that good evidence is provided by ASUs for symptom-modifying effects in OA of the knee and hip but there is some evidence of absence of structure-modifying effects *(90)*. ASUs seem to have symptom-modifying effects on OA of the knee and hip over the medium term, however, their symptom-modifying effects in the long term have not been confirmed.

4.11. Other Nutritional Products

There appears to be an increasing number of nutritional remedies being promulgated for purported benefits in arthritis. Trials of *S*-adenosylmethionine also have had apparently positive results, albeit somewhat limited by adverse effects and high drop-out rates *(198–203)*. A ginger-derived product has also been tested in a trial that had moderately positive results *(204)*.

5. WEIGHT LOSS

Epidemiological data indicate that overweight people are at considerably increased risk for the development of OA of the knee, and may also be more susceptible to OA of both the hip and the hand *(205)*. Because overweight individuals do not necessarily have increased load across their hand joints, investigators have wondered whether systemic factors, such as dietary factors or other metabolic consequences of obesity, may mediate part of this relationship. Early laboratory studies using strains of mice and rats suggested that there is an interaction between body weight, genetic factors, and diet, although attempts to demonstrate a direct effect of dietary fat intake have proved inconclusive *(206,207)*. The fact that adipose cells share a common stem cell precursor with connective tissue cells such as osteoblasts and chondrocytes has prompted investigation into the possibility that their phenotypic differentiation might be influenced by the metabolic milieu *(208)*. Indeed, fat and fatty acids can influence prostaglandin and collagen synthesis *in vitro* and have been associated with osteoarthritic changes in joints *(196,208)*. Preliminary evidence also suggests that leptin, an adipose tissue-derived hormone, may have anabolic effects in osteoarthritic cartilage *(209)*.

Based on these observations, weight loss is considered a priority in the management of overweight individuals with OA. However, there have been relatively few rigorous studies testing weight loss as a therapeutic intervention to reduce symptoms, prevent disability, or delay disease progression. The recent Arthritis, Diet, and Activity Promotion Trial is, thus, significant in examining whether long-term exercise and dietary weight loss are effective interventions for functional impairment, pain, and mobility in older overweight individuals with OA of the knee *(210)*. The results that suggest diet- and exercise-induced weight loss are independently effective but that the combination of the two is additive and more effective than either alone. Furthermore, only the combination treatment consistently showed a significant effect.

In this trial, 316 adults with OA of the knee and a BMI of at least 28 kg/m^2 were recruited and randomized to one of four interventions: healthy lifestyle (i.e., participants met monthly for 1 hour for 3 months to listen to a lecturer or to watch a videotape on topics concerning OA, obesity, and exercise), diet only, exercise only, and diet plus exercise. The primary outcome was self-reported physical function as measured with the WOMAC. Secondary outcomes included weight loss, 6-minute walk distance, stair-climb time, and WOMAC pain and stiffness scores. Of the participants, 80% completed the 18-month study. Adherence ranged from 60% (exercise only) to 73% (healthy lifestyle). The main finding of the trial was that the diet intervention led to significant benefits at 18 months of follow-up (Δ –4.23; 95% CI, –1.27 to –7.19), with the effect being larger with the addition of exercise (Δ –5.73; 95% CI, –2.63 to –8.83). The reduction in WOMAC physical function at 18 months follow-up in the combination group and the diet-only group were both significantly different (<0.05) as compared with healthy lifestyle. The diet and exercise group lost more weight than the diet-only group (5.7 vs 4.9%). This suggests that the improvement in symptoms is likely related to the amount of weight that is lost, irrespective of the means by which weight loss is achieved.

In contrast, a more recent study by Christensen et al. *(211)* differs with the Arthritis, Diet, and Activity Promotion Trial both in design and conclusions. On the basis that weight loss might relieve symptoms of OA of the knee both through biomechanical effects and influences on body fat *(212)*, they tested the effectiveness of a rapid diet-induced weight-loss intervention on overweight individuals with OA of the knee, enrolling 96 persons (mostly women) with OA of the knee into a comparison of a low-energy diet (LED) intervention (3.4 MJ per day ~800 kcal per day) with a control diet (5 MJ per day ~1,200 kcal per day). The LED intervention consisted of a nutrition powder taken as six daily meals that met the recommendations for a daily intake of high-quality protein such that 37% of the energy provided from the powder was from soy protein. The control intervention (i.e., "hypoenergetic diet") consisted of a traditional low-calorie high-protein diet taken in the form of ordinary foods individually chosen by participants based on recommendations from a 2-hour nutritional advice session. The LED group also had weekly dietary sessions, whereas the control group was given a booklet describing weight-loss practices. The primary outcome was self-reported pain and physical function limitation measured by the WOMAC index. Changes in body weight and body composition as independent predictors of changes in symptoms of OA of the knee were also examined.

There were nine drop outs, mainly because of noncompliance. However, this appeared to be nondifferential, so the authors performed an analysis based on completers. The LED group lost considerably more weight than the controls (11.1 vs. 4.3%) with a mean difference of 6.8% (95% CI, 5.5–8.1%). The LED group also lost 2.2% more body fat (95% CI, 1.5–3.0%). There were substantially greater falls in WOMAC scores among the LED intervention group. The mean between-group difference for the total WOMAC index was 219.3 mm ($p = 0.005$). Oddly, this was not reflected in the Lequesne Index assessment, which detected no between-group difference. In subsidiary analyses they estimated that the number needed to treat to obtain an improvement in WOMAC score of 50% or greater in at least one patient was 3.4. They also found that the changes in WOMAC score were best predicted by reduction of body fat, with a 9.4% improvement in WOMAC score for each percent of body fat reduced ($p = 0.0005$).

These results indicate that rapid and substantial weight loss may, by itself, translate into reduced pain and improved function in overweight patients with OA of the knee. However, some caution needs to be exerted in interpreting these results. The long-term effectiveness of this short-term intervention is uncertain. The participants were very heavy (mean BMI 36 kg/m^2), and the results may not be generalizable to a less overweight population. Although the authors assert that the groups were balanced, the effect of censoring from the analysis the participants who discontinued the intervention is uncertain. The higher WOMAC scores at baseline in the LED group compared with the control group provides further evidence that the groups were not balanced at baseline. This difference makes it difficult to attribute the differences seen in the two arms at follow-up to effect of either intervention. The greater effect of LED as measured by a greater change in WOMAC may have resulted from a stronger tendency for regression to the mean in the LED group. Support for this hypothesis is that the Lequesne Index was equal in both groups at baseline and this measure was not different in the two groups at 8 weeks of follow-up. Another issue regarding this study is that the LED group preferentially received more attention with weekly sessions for 8 weeks with the dietician to encourage a high degree of compliance, whereas the hypoenergetic group only met with the dietician once at the beginning of the study, a difference that was not controlled for in their analyses. Finally, the study was also essentially unblinded, which may also have led to between-group biases. Nevertheless, the results are of considerable interest and underscore a need for further research into potential benefits from more extreme weight-reduction interventions. For instance, preliminary results from a study of musculoskeletal complaints among morbidly obese patients undertaking gastric bypass surgery showed a 52% reduction in the number of symptomatic sites, and an approx 50% reduction in WOMAC score, 6 to 12 months following the procedure *(213)*.

6. CONCLUSIONS AND RECOMMENDATIONS

There are numerous mechanisms by which micronutrients might be expected to influence the development or progression of osteoarthritis. Such micronutrients include vitamins C and D and possibly vitamins E and K, and selenium. However, robust nutritional epidemiological studies of OA are few in number and far from conclusive. Elucidation of simple and safe interventions for OA is clearly a public health priority. Therefore, further studies, including clinical trials where appropriate, are needed to identify potential nutritional interventions for OA.

Of all the supplements of interest, glucosamine and chondroitin have been the most frequently studied. However, the question of efficacy of these treatments with respect to symptomatic improvement and structural progression still remains. Additional nonindustry-sponsored clinical trials evaluating the efficacy of these treatments are underway. Hopefully, the results of these trials will bring us closer to clarifying the efficacy of these treatments in OA.

Studies evaluating diet and exercise interventions for OA symptoms suggest that treatment with the combination is more effective than either intervention alone.

REFERENCES

1. Theodosakis J, Adderly B, Fox B. The Arthritis Cure. St. Martin's Press. St. Martin's Press, 1997.
2. Marra J. The state of dietary suplements—even slight increases in growth are better than no growth at all. Nutraceuticals World 2002:32–40.
3. Anonymous. U.S. nutrition industry: top 70 supplements 1997–2001. Nutr Bus J 2001;Chart 14.
4. Frei B. Reactive oxygen species and antioxidant vitamins: mechanisms of action. Am J Med 1994;97(suppl 3A):5S–13S.
5. Boveris A, Oshino N, Chance B. The cellular production of hydrogen peroxide. Biochem J 1972;128:617–630.
6. Blake DR, Unsworth J, Outhwaite JM, et al. Hypoxic-reperfusion injury in the inflamed human. Lancet 1989;11:290–293.
7. Ames BN, Shigenaga MK, Hagen TM. Oxidants, antioxidants and the degenerative diseases of aging. Proc Natl Acad Sci U S A 1993;90:7915–7922.
8. Jacques PF, Chylack LT, Taylor A. Relationships between natural antioxidants and cataract formation. In: Frei B, ed. Natural Antioxidants in Human Health and Disease. Academic Press, San Diego, CA, 1994, pp. 515–533.
9. Gaziano JM. Antioxidant vitamins and coronary artery disease risk. Am J Med 1994;97(suppl 3A):18S–21S.
10. Hennekens CH. Antioxidant vitamins and cancer. Am J Med 1994;97(suppl 3A):2S–4S.
11. Martin JA, Buckwalter JA. Aging, articular cartilage chondrocyte senescence and osteoarthritis. Biogerontology 2002;3(5):257–264.
12. Henrotin Y, Deby-Dupont G, Deby C, De Bruyn M, Lamy M, Franchimont P. Production of active oxygen species by isolated human chondrocytes. Br J Rheumatol 1993;32(7):562–567.
13. Henrotin Y, Deby-Dupont G, Deby C, Franchimont P, Emerit I. Active oxygen species, articular inflammation, and cartilage damage. EXS 1992;62:308–322.
14. Rathakrishnan C, Tiku K, Raghavan A, Tiku ML. Release of oxygen radicals by articular chondrocytes: A study of luminol-dependent chemoluminescence and hydrogen peroxide secretion. J Bone Miner Res 1992;7:1139–1148.
15. 15. Tiku ML, Allison GT, Naik K, Karry SK. Malondialdehyde oxidation of cartilage collagen by chondrocytes. Osteoarthritis Cartilage 2003;11(3):159–166.
16. Greenwald RA, Moy WW. Inhibition of collagen gelation by action of the superoxide radical. Arthritis Rheum 1979;22(3):251–259.

17. McCord JM. Free radicals and inflammation: protection of synovial fluid by superoxide dismutase. Science 1974;185:529–530.
18. Loeser RF, Carlson CS, Del Carlo M, Cole A. Detection of nitrotyrosine in aging and osteoarthritic cartilage: Correlation of oxidative damage with the presence of interleukin-1beta and with chondrocyte resistance to insulin-like growth factor 1. Arthritis Rheum 2002;46(9):2349–2357.
19. Yudoh K, Nguyen T, Nakamura H, Hongo-Masuko K, Kato T, Nishioka K. Potential involvement of oxidative stress in cartilage senescence and development of osteoarthritis: oxidative stress induces chondrocyte telomere instability and downregulation of chondrocyte function. Arthritis Res Ther 2005;7(2):R380–R391.
20. Haklar U, Yuksel M, Velioglu A, Turkmen M, Haklar G, Yalcin AS. Oxygen radicals and nitric oxide levels in chondral or meniscal lesions or both. Clin Orthop 2002(403):135–142.
21. Sato H, Takahashi T, Ide H, et al. Antioxidant activity of synovial fluid, hyaluronic acid, and two subcomponents of hyaluronic acid. Synovial fluid scavenging effect is enhanced in rheumatoid arthritis patients. Arthritis Rheum 1988;31(1):63–71.
22. Briviba K, Seis H. Non-enzymatic antioxidant defense systems. In: Frei B, ed. Natural Antioxidants in Human Health and Disease. Academic Press, San Diego, CA, 1994, pp. 107–128.
23. Henrotin Y, Kurz B, Aigner T. Oxygen and reactive oxygen species in cartilage degradation: friends or foes? Osteoarthritis Cartilage 2005;13(8):643–654.
24. McAlindon T, Felson DT. Nutrition: risk factors for osteoarthritis. Ann Rheum Dis 1997;56(7):397–400.
25. Sowers M, Lachance L. Vitamins and arthritis. The roles of vitamins A, C, D, and E. Rheum Dis Clin North Am 1999;25(2):315–332.
26. Hankinson SE, Stampfer MJ, Seddon JM, et al. Nutrient intake and cataract extraction in women: a prospective study. BMJ 1992;305(6849):335–339.
27. Peterkofsky B. Ascorbate requirement for hydroxylation and secretion of procollagen: relationship to inhibition of collagen synthesis in scurvy. AM J Clin Nutr 1991;54:1135S–1140S.
28. Spanheimer RG, Bird TA, Peterkofsky B. Regulation of collagen synthesis and mRNA levels in articular cartilage of scorbutic guinea pigs. Arch Biochem Biophys 1986;246:33–41.
29. Houglum KP, Brenner DA, Chijkier M. Ascorbic acid stimulation of collagen biosynthesis independent of hydroxylation. Am J Clin Nutr 1991;54:1141S–1143S.
30. Schwartz ER, Adamy L. Effect of ascorbic acid on arylsulfatase activities and sulfated proteoglycan metabolism in chondrocyte cultures. J Clin Invest 1977;60(1):96–106.
31. Sandell LJ, Daniel LC. Effects of ascorbic acid on collagen mRNA levels in short-term chondrocyte cultures. Connect Tiss Res 1988;17:11–22.
32. Meacock SCR, Bodmer JL, Billingham MEJ. Experimental OA in guinea pigs. J Exp Path 1990;71:279–293.
33. Schwartz ER, Oh WH, Leveille CR. Experimentally induced osteoarthritis in guinea pigs: metabolic responses in articular cartilage to developing pathology. Arthritis Rheum 1981;24(11):1345–1355.
34. McAlindon TE, Jacques P, Zhang Y, et al. Do antioxidant micronutrients protect against the development and progression of knee osteoarthritis? Arthritis Rheum 1996;39(4):648–656.
35. Kellgren J, Lawrence JS. The Epidemiology of Chronic Rheumatism: Atlas of Standard Radiographs, Vol 2. Blackwell Scientific, Oxford, 1963.
36. Baker K, Niu J, Goggins J, Clancy M, Felson D. The effects of vitamin C intake on pain in knee osteoarthritis (OA). Arthritis Rheum 2003;48(9):S422.
37. Kraus VB, Huebner JL, Stabler T, et al. Ascorbic acid increases the severity of spontaneous knee osteoarthritis in a guinea pig model. Arthritis Rheum 2004;50(6):1822–1831.
38. Bakker AC, van de Loo FA, van Beuningen HM, et al. Overexpression of active TGF-beta-1 in the murine knee joint: evidence for synovial-layer-dependent chondro-osteophyte formation. Osteoarthritis Cartilage 2001;9(2):128–136.
39. Scharstuhl A, Glansbeek HL, van Beuningen HM, Vitters EL, van der Kraan PM, van den Berg WB. Inhibition of endogenous TGF-beta during experimental osteoarthritis prevents osteophyte formation and impairs cartilage repair. J Immunol 2002;169(1):507–514.
40. van Beuningen HM, Glansbeek HL, van der Kraan PM, van den Berg WB. Osteoarthritis-like changes in the murine knee joint resulting from intra-articular transforming growth factor-beta injections. Osteoarthritis Cartilage 2000;8(1):25–33.

41. Barcellos-Hoff MH, Dix TA. Redox-mediated activation of latent transforming growth factor-beta 1. Mol Endocrinol 1996;10(9):1077–1083.
42. Jensen NH. [Reduced pain from osteoarthritis in hip joint or knee joint during treatment with calcium ascorbate. A randomized, placebo-controlled cross-over trial in general practice]. Ugeskr Laeger 2003;165(25):2563–2566.
43. Kiel DP. Vitamin D, calcium and bone: descriptive epidemiology. In: Rosenberg IH, ed. Nutritional Assessment of Elderly Populations: Measurement and Function. Raven, New York, 1995, pp. 277–290.
44. Parfitt AM, Gallagher JC, Heaney RP, Neer R, Whedon GD. Vitamin D and bone health in the elderly. AM J Clin Nutr 1982;36:1014–1031.
45. Radin EL, Paul IL, Tolkoff MJ. Subchondral changes in patients with early degenerative joint disease. Arthritis Rheum 1970;13:400–405.
46. Layton MW, Goldstein SA, Goulet RW, Feldkamp LA, Kubinski DJ, Bole GG. Examination of subchondral bone architecture in experimental osteoarthritis by microscopic computed axial tomography. Arthritis Rheum 1988;31(11):1400–1405.
47. Milgram JW. Morphological alterations of the subchondral bone in advanced degenerative arthritis. Clin Orthop Rel Res 1983;173:293–312.
48. Kellgren JH, Lawrence JS. The Epidemiology of Chronic Rheumatism: Atlas of Standard Radiographs.Blackwell Scientific, Oxford, UK, 1962.
49. Anonymous. Cartilage and bone in osteoarthrosis. Brit Med J 1976;2:4–5.
50. Dequecker J, Mokassa L, Aerssens J. Bone density and osteoarthritis. J Rheumatol 1995;22(suppl 43):98–100.
51. Dedrick DK, Goldstein SA, Brandt KD, O'Connor BL, Goulet RW, Albrecht M. A longitudinal study of subchondral plate and trabecular bone in cruciate-deficient dogs with osteoarthritis followed up for 54 months. Arthritis Rheum 1993;36:1460–1467.
52. Ledingham J, Dawson S, Preston B, Milligan G, Doherty M. Radiographic progression of hospital-referred osteoarthritis of the hip. Ann Rheum Dis 1993;52:263–267.
53. Radin EL, Rose RM. Role of subchondral bone in the initiation and progression of cartilage damage. Clin Orthop Rel Res 1986;213:34–40.
54. Pottenger LA, Phillips FM, Draganich LF. The effect of marginal osteophytes on reduction of varus-valgus instability in osteoarthritic knees. Arthritis Rheum 1990;33(6):853–858.
55. Perry GH, Smith MJG, Whiteside CG. Spontaneous recovery of the joint space in degenerative hip disease. Ann Rheum Dis 1972;31:440–448.
56. Smythe SA. Osteoarthritis, insulin and bone density. J Rheumatol 1987;14(suppl):91–93.
57. Zhang Y, Hannan MT, Chaisson CE, et al. Bone mineral density and risk of incident and progressive radiographic knee osteoarthritis in women: the Framingham Study. J Rheumatol 2000;27(4): 1032–1037.
58. Dieppe P, Cushnaghan J, Young P, Kirwan J. Prediction of the progression of joint space narrowing in osteoarthritis of the knee by bone scintigraphy. Ann Rheum Dis 1993;52:557–563.
59. Corvol MT. Hormonal control of cartilage metabolism. Bull Schweiz Akad Med Wiss 1981:205–209.
60. Corvol MT, Dumontier MF, Tsagris L, Lang F, Bourguignon J. [Cartilage and vitamin D in vitro (author's transl)]. Ann Endocrinol (Paris) 1981;42(4–5):482–487.
61. Tetlow LC, Woolley DE. Expression of vitamin D receptors and matrix metalloproteinases in osteoarthritic cartilage and human articular chondrocytes in vitro. Osteoarthritis Cartilage 2001;9(5):423–431.
62. Bischoff HA, Borchers M, Gudat F, et al. In situ detection of 1,25-dihydroxyvitamin D3 receptor in human skeletal muscle tissue. Histochem J 2001;33(1):19–24.
63. Bischoff-Ferrari HA, Borchers M, Gudat F, Durmuller U, Stahelin HB, Dick W. Vitamin D receptor expression in human muscle tissue decreases with age. J Bone Miner Res 2004;19(2):265–269.
64. Hart DJ, Cronin C, Daniels M, Worthy T, Doyle DV, Spector TD. The relationship of bone density and fracture to incident and progressive radiographic osteoarthritis of the knee: the Chingford Study. Arthritis Rheum 2002;46(1):92–99.
65. Bischoff-Ferrari HA, Zhang Y, Kiel DP, Felson DT. Positive association between serum 25-hydroxyvitamin D level and bone density in osteoarthritis. Arthritis Rheum 2005;53(6):821–826.

66. McAlindon TE, Felson DT, Zhang Y, et al. Relation of dietary intake and serum levels of vitamin D to progression of osteoarthritis of the knee among participants in the Framingham Study. Ann Intern Med 1996;125(5):353–359.
67. Lane NE, Gore LR, Cummings SR, et al. Serum vitamin D levels and incident changes of radiographic hip osteoarthritis: a longitudinal study. Study of Osteoporotic Fractures Research Group. Arthritis Rheum 1999;42(5):854–860.
68. Felson DT, Niu J, Clancy M, et al. Low levels of vitamin D and worsening of knee osteoarthritis: Results of two longitudinal studies. Arthritis Rheum 2006;56(1):129–136.
69. McLaughlin S, Jacques P, Goggins J, et al. Effect of 25-hydroxyvitamin D and parathyroid hormone on progression of radiographic knee osteoarthritis. Arthritis Rheum 2002;46(9 suppl):S299.
70. Carbone LD, Nevitt MC, Wildy K, et al. The relationship of antiresorptive drug use to structural findings and symptoms of knee osteoarthritis. Arthritis Rheum 2004;50(11):3516–3525.
71. Demarco PJ, Constantinescu F. Does vitamin D supplementation contribute to the modulation of osteoarthritis by bisphosphonates? Comment on the article by Carbone et al. Arthritis Rheum 2005;52(5):1622–1623.
72. Carbone LD, Barrow KD, Nevitt MC. Reply. Arthritis Rheum 2005;52(5):1623.
73. Panganamala RV, Cornwell DG. The effects of vitamin E on arachidonic acid metabolism. Ann N Y Acad Sci 1982;393:376–391.
74. Tiku ML, Shah R, Allison GT. Evidence linking chondrocyte lipid peroxidation to cartilage matrix protein degradation. Possible role in cartilage aging and the pathogenesis of osteoarthritis. J Biol Chem 2000;275(26):20069–20076.
75. Schwartz ER. Effect of vitamins C and E on sulfated proteoglycan metabolism and sulfatase and phosphatase activities in organ cultures of human cartilage. Calcif Tissue Int 1979;28(3):201–208.
76. Tiku ML, Gupta S, Deshmukh DR. Aggrecan degradation in chondrocytes is mediated by reactive oxygen species and protected by antioxidants. Free Radic Res 1999;30(5):395–405.
77. Galleron S, Borderie D, Ponteziere C, et al. Reactive oxygen species induce apoptosis of synoviocytes in vitro. Alpha-tocopherol provides no protection. Cell Biol Int 1999;23(9):637–642.
78. Kaiki G, Tsuji H, Yonezawa T, et al. Osteoarthrosis induced by intra-articular hydrogen peroxide injection and running load. J Orthop Res 1990;8(5):731–740.
79. Hirohata K, Yao S, Imura S, Harada H. Treatment of osteoarthritis of the knee joint at the state of hydroarthrosis. Kobe Med Sci 1965;11(suppl):65–66.
80. Doumerg C. Etude clinique experimentale de l'alpha-tocopheryle-quinone en rheumatologie et en reeducation. Therapeutique 1969;45:676–678.
81. Machetey I, Quaknine L. Tocopherol in osteoarthritis: a controlled pilot study. J Am Ger Soc 1978;26:328–330.
82. Scherak O, Kolarz G, Schodl C, Blankenhorn G. Hochdosierte vitamin-E-therapie bei patienten mit aktivierter arthrose. Z Rheumatol 1990;49:369–373.
83. Blankenhorn G. Clinical efficacy of spondyvit (vitamin E) in activated arthroses. A multicenter, placebo-controlled, double-blind study. Z Orthop 1986;124:340–343.
84. Machtey I, Ouaknine L. Tocopherol in Osteoarthritis: a controlled pilot study. J Am Geriatr Soc 1978;26(7):328–330.
85. Scherak O, Kolarz G, Schodl C, Blankenhorn G. [High dosage vitamin E therapy in patients with activated arthrosis]. Z Rheumatol 1990;49(6):369–373.
86. Brand C, Snaddon J, Bailey M, Cicuttini F. Vitamin E is ineffective for symptomatic relief of knee osteoarthritis: a six month double blind, randomised, placebo controlled study. Ann Rheum Dis 2001;60(10):946–949.
87. Wluka AE, Stuckey S, Brand C, Cicuttini FM. Supplementary vitamin E does not affect the loss of cartilage volume in knee osteoarthritis: a 2 year double blind randomized placebo controlled study. J Rheumatol 2002;29(12):2585–2591.
88. Hunter DJ, Niu J, Zhang Y, et al. Cartilage Volume Must be Normalized to Bone Surface Area in Order to Provide Satisfactory Construct Validity: The Framingham Study. Osteoarthritis Cartilage 2004;12(suppl B):Abstract M4.

89. Altman R, Brandt K, Hochberg M, et al. Design and conduct of clinical trials in patients with osteoarthritis: recommendations from a task force of the Osteoarthritis Research Society. Results from a workshop. Osteoarthritis Cartilage 1996;4(4):217–243.
90. Ameye LG, Chee WS. Osteoarthritis and nutrition. From nutraceuticals to functional foods: a systematic review of the scientific evidence. Arthritis Res Ther 2006;8(4):R127.
91. Thane CW, Paul AA, Bates CJ, Bolton-Smith C, Prentice A, Shearer MJ. Intake and sources of phylloquinone (vitamin K1): variation with socio-demographic and lifestyle factors in a national sample of British elderly people. Br J Nutr 2002;87(6):605–613.
92. Booth SL, Suttie JW. Dietary intake and adequacy of vitamin K. J Nutr 1998;128(5):785–788.
93. Furie B, Bouchard BA, Furie BC. Vitamin K-dependent biosynthesis of gamma-carboxyglutamic acid. Blood 1999;93(6):1798–1808.
94. Loeser RF, Varnum BC, Carlson CS, et al. Human chondrocyte expression of growth-arrest-specific gene 6 and the tyrosine kinase receptor axl: potential role in autocrine signaling in cartilage. Arthritis Rheum 1997;40(8):1455–1465.
95. Hale JE, Fraser JD, Price PA. The identification of matrix Gla protein in cartilage. J Biol Chem 1988;263(12):5820–5824.
96. Price PA. Gla-containing proteins of bone. Connect Tissue Res 1989;21(1–4):51–57; discussion 57–60.
97. Newman B, Gigout LI, Sudre L, Grant ME, Wallis GA. Coordinated expression of matrix Gla protein is required during endochondral ossification for chondrocyte survival. J Cell Biol 2001;154(3): 659–666.
98. Yagami K, Suh JY, Enomoto-Iwamoto M, et al. Matrix GLA protein is a developmental regulator of chondrocyte mineralization and, when constitutively expressed, blocks endochondral and intramembranous ossification in the limb. J Cell Biol 1999;147(5):1097–1108.
99. Zebboudj AF, Imura M, Bostrom K. Matrix GLA protein, a regulatory protein for bone morphogenetic protein– 2. J Biol Chem 2002;277(6):4388–4394.
100. Hara K, Akiyama Y, Tajima T, Shiraki M. Menatetrenone inhibits bone resorption partly through inhibition of PGE2 synthesis in vitro. J Bone Miner Res 1993;8(5):535–542.
101. Reddi K, Henderson B, Meghji S, et al. Interleukin 6 production by lipopolysaccharide-stimulated human fibroblasts is potently inhibited by naphthoquinone (vitamin K) compounds. Cytokine 1995;7(3):287–290.
102. Neuropathic joints. Degenerative joint disease. Arthritis Rheum 1970;13(5):571–578.
103. Hall JG, Pauli RM, Wilson KM. Maternal and fetal sequelae of anticoagulation during pregnancy. Am J Med 1980;68(1):122–140.
104. Luo G, Ducy P, McKee MD, et al. Spontaneous calcification of arteries and cartilage in mice lacking matrix GLA protein. Nature 1997;386(6620):78–81.
105. Neogi T, Zhang Y, Booth S, Jacques PF, Terkeltaub R, Felson DT. Is there an association between osteophytes and vitamin K intake? Arthritis Rheum 2004;50(9):S350.
106. Neogi T, Booth SL, Zhang YQ, et al. Low vitamin K status is associated with osteoarthritis in the hand and knee. Arthritis Rheum 2006;54(4):1255–1261.
107. Utiger RD. Kashin-Beck disease–expanding the spectrum of iodine-deficiency disorders [editorial; comment]. N Engl J Med 1998;339(16):1156–1158.
108. Moreno-Reyes R, Suetens C, Mathieu F, et al. Kashin-Beck osteoarthropathy in rural Tibet in relation to selenium and iodine status [see comments]. N Engl J Med 1998;339(16):1112–1120.
109. Jordan JM, Fang F, Arab L, et al. Low Selenium Levels are Associated with Increased Risk for Osteoarthritis of the Knee. Arthritis and Rheumatism 2005;52(9 suppl):Abstract 1189.
110. Hill J, Bird HA. Failure of selenium-ace to improve osteoarthritis. Br J Rheumatol 1990;29(3):211–213.
111. Setnikar I, Ralumbo R, Canali S, Zanolo G. Pharmacokinetics of glucosamine in man. Drug Res 1993;43:1109–1113.
112. Setnikar I, Giachetti C, Zanolo G. Absorption, distribution and excretion of radio-activity after a single I.V. or oral administration of [14C]glucosamine to the rat. Pharmatheceutica 1984;3:358.
113. Adebowale A, Du J, Liang Z, Leslie JL, Eddington ND. The bioavailability and pharmacokinetics of glucosamine hydrochloride and low molecular weight chondroitin sulfate after single and multiple doses to beagle dogs. Biopharm Drug Dispos 2002;23(6):217–225.

114. Aghazadeh-Habashi A, Sattari S, Pasutto F, Jamali F. Single dose pharmacokinetics and bioavailability of glucosamine in the rat. J Pharm Pharm Sci 2002;5(2):181–184.
115. Biggee BA, Blinn C, McAlindon T, Nuite M, Silbert J. Human serum glucosamine and sulfate levels after ingestion of glucosamine sulfate. Arthritis Rheum 2004;50(9 suppl):S657.
116. Persiani S, Rovati L, Foschini V, Giacovelli G, Locatelli M, Roda A. Oral bioavailability and dose-proportionality of crystalline glucosamine sulfate in man. Arthritis Rheum 2004;50(9suppl):S146.
117. Academies IoMNRCotN. Glucosamine: Prototype Monograph Summary. In: Dietary Supplements: A Framework for Evaluating Safety. National Academies Press, Washington DC, 2005, pp. 363–364.
118. Marshall S, Yamasaki K, Okuyama R. Glucosamine induces rapid desensitization of glucose transport in isolated adipocytes by increasing GlcN-6-P levels. Biochem Biophys Res Commun 2005;329(3):1155–1161.
119. Tannis AJ, Barban J, Conquer JA. Effect of glucosamine supplementation on fasting and non-fasting plasma glucose and serum insulin concentrations in healthy individuals. Osteoarthritis Cartilage 2004;12(6):506–511.
120. Yu JG, Boies SM, Olefsky JM. The effect of oral glucosamine sulfate on insulin sensitivity in human subjects. Diabetes Care 2003;26(6):1941–1942.
121. Theodore G. Untrsuchung von 35 arhrosefallen, behandelt mit chondroitin schwefelsaure. Schweiz Rundschaue Med Praxis 1977;66.
122. Vach J, Pesakova V, Krajickova J, Adam M. Efect of glycosaminoglycan polysulfate on the metabolism of cartilage RNA. Arzneim Forsch/Drur Res 1984;34:607–609.
123. Ali SY. The degrdation of cartilage matrix by an intracellular protease. Biochem J 1964;93:611.
124. Hamerman D, Smith C, Keiser HD, Craig R. Glycosaminoglycans produced by human synovial cell cultures collagen. Rel Res 1982;2:313.
125. Lilja S, Barrach HJ. Normally sulfated and highly sulfated glycosaminoglycans affecting fibrilloge-nesis on type I and type II collage in vitro. Exp Pathol 1983;23:173–181.
126. Knanfelt A. Synthesis of articular cartilage proteoglycans by isolated bovine chondrocytes. Agents Actions 1984;14:58–62.
127. Baici A, Salgam P, Fehr K, Boni A. Inhibition of human elastase from polymorphonuclear leucocytes by gold sodium thiomalate and pentosan polysulfate (SP-54). Biochem Pharmacol 1981;30(7):703–708.
128. Baici A. Interactions between human leucocytes elastase and chondroitin sulfate. Chem Biol Interactions 1984;51:11.
129. Marossy K. Interaction of the antitrypsin and elastase-like enzyme of the human granulocyte with glycosaminoglycans. Biochim Biophys Acta 1981;659:351–361.
130. De Gennaro F, Piccioni PD, Caporali R, Luisetti M, Contecucco C. Effet du traitement par le sulfate de galactosaminoglucuronoglycane sur l'estase granulocytaire synovial de patients atteints d'osteoarthrose. Litera Rhumatologica 1992;14:53–60.
131. Jackson CG, Plaas AH, Barnhill JG, Harris CL, Hua C, Clegg DO. The multiple-dose pharmacokinetics of orally administered glucosamine and chondroitin sulfate in humans. Arthritis Rheum 2006:S1681.
132. Humphries DE, Silbert CK, Silbert JE. Glycosaminoglycan production by bovine aortic endothelial cells cultured in sulfate-depleted medium. J Biol Chem 1986;261(20):9122–9127.
133. Silbert CK, Humphries DE, Palmer ME, Silbert JE. Effects of sulfate deprivation on the production of chondroitin/dermatan sulfate by cultures of skin fibroblasts from normal and diabetic individuals. Arch Biochem Biophys 1991;285(1):137–141.
134. Silbert JE, Sugumaran G, Cogburn JN. Sulphation of proteochondroitin and 4-methylumbelliferyl beta-D-xyloside-chondroitin formed by mouse mastocytoma cells cultured in sulphate-deficient medium. Biochem J 1993;296 (Pt 1):119–126.
135. van der Kraan PM, Vitters EL, de Vries BJ, van den Berg WB. High susceptibility of human articular cartilage glycosaminoglycan synthesis to changes in inorganic sulfate availability. J Orthop Res 1990;8(4):565–571.
136. Morris ME, Levy G. Serum concentration and renal excretion by normal adults of inorganic sulfate after acetaminophen, ascorbic acid, or sodium sulfate. Clin Pharmacol Ther 1983;33(4):529–536.
137. Cordoba F, Nimni ME. Chondroitin sulfate and other sulfate containing chondroprotective agents may exhibit their effects by overcoming a deficiency of sulfur amino acids. Osteoarthritis Cartilage 2003;11(3):228–230.

138. Blinn CM, Biggee BA, McAlindon TE, Nuite M, Silbert JE. Sulphate and osteoarthritis: decrease of serum sulphate levels by an additional 3-h fast and a 3-h glucose tolerance test after an overnight fast. Ann Rheum Dis 2006;65(9):1223–1225.
139. D'Ambrosio E, Casa B, Bompani R, Scali G, Scali M. Glucosamine sulphate: a controlled clinical investigation in arthrosis. Pharmatherapeutica 1981;2(8):504–508.
140. Crolle G, D'Este E. Glucosamine sulphate for the management of arthrosis: a controlled clinical investigation. Curr Med Res Opin 1980;7(2):104–109.
141. Drovanti A, Bignamini AA, Rovati AL. Therapeutic activity of oral glucosamine sulfate in osteoarthrosis: a placebo-controlled double-blind investigation. Clin Ther 1980;3(4):260–272.
142. Noack W, Fsicher M, Forster KK, Rovatis LC, Senikar I. Glucosamine sulfate in osteoarthitis of the knee. Osteoarthritis Cart 1994;2:51–59.
143. Pujalte JM, Llavore EP, Ylescupidez FR. Double-blind clinical evaluation of oral glucosamine sulphate in the basic treatment of osteoarthrosis. Curr Med Res Opin 1980;7(2):110–114.
144. Reichelt A, Forster KK, Fischer M, Rovati LC, Setnikar I. Efficacy and safety of intramuscular glucosamine sulfate in osteoarthritis of the knee: A randomized, placebo-controlled, double-blind study. Drug Res 1994;44:75–80.
145. Vaz AL. Double-blind clinical evaluation of the relative efficacy of ibuprofen and glucosamine sulphate in the management of osteoarthrosis of the knee in out-patients. Curr Med Res Opin 1982;8:145–149.
146. Vajaradul Y. Double-blind clinical evaluation of intra-articular glucosamine in outpatients with gonarthrosis. Clin Ther 1981;3(5):336–343.
147. Tapadinhas MJ, Rivera IC, Bignamini AA. Oral glucosamine sulphate in the management of arthosis: Report on a multi-centre open investigation in Portugal. Pharmatherapeutica 1982;3(3):157–168.
148. Vetter VG. Glukosamine in der therapie des degenerativen rheumatismus. Duet Med J 1965;16:446–449.
149. L'Hirondel JL. Klinische doppelblind-studie mit oral verabreichtem chondroitinsulfat gegen placebo bei der tibiofemoralen gonarthrose (125 patienten). Litera Rhumatologica 1992;14:77–84.
150. Kerzberg EM, Roldan EJ, Castelli G, Huberman ED. Combination of glycosaminoglycans and acetylsalicylic acid in knee osteoarthrosis. Scand J Rheumatol 1987;16(5):377–380.
151. Mazieres B, Loyau G, Menkes CJ, et al. [Chondroitin sulfate in the treatment of gonarthrosis and coxarthrosis. 5-months result of a multicenter double-blind controlled prospective study using placebo]. Rev Rhum Mal Osteoartic 1992;59(7–8):466–472.
152. Rovetta G. Galactosaminoglycuronoglycan sulfate (matrix) in therapy of tibiofibular osteoarthritis of the knee. Drugs Exptl Clin Res 1991;17:53–57.
153. Muller-Fassbender H, Bach GL, Haase W, Rovato LC, Setnikar I. Glucosamine sulfate compared to ibuprofen in osteoarthritis of the knee. Osteoarthritis and Cartilage 1994;2:61–69.
154. McAlindon TE, LaValley MP, Gulin JP, Felson DT. Glucosamine and chondroitin for treatment of osteoarthritis: a systematic quality assessment and meta-analysis. JAMA 2000;283(11):1469–1475.
155. Cohen J. Statistical Power Analysis for the Behavioral Sciences, 2nd ed. Erlbaum, Hillsdale, NJ, 1988.
156. Towheed TE, Anastassiades TP, Shea B, Houpt J, Welch V, Hochberg MC. Glucosamine therapy for treating osteoarthritis (Cochrane Review). Cochrane Database Syst Rev 2001;1.
157. Liang MH, Larson MG, Cullen KE, Schwartz JA. Comparative measurement efficiency and sensitivity of five health status instruments for arthritis research. Arthritis Rheum 1985;28(5):542–547.
158. Roos EM, Nilsdotter AK, Toksvig-Larsen S. Patient expectations suggest additional outcomes in total knee replacement. ACR Abstracts, 2002:Abstract 450.
159. Leeb BF, Schweitzer H, Montag K, Smolen JS. A metaanalysis of chondroitin sulfate in the treatment of osteoarthritis. J Rheumatol 2000;27(1):205–211.
160. Reichenbach S, Trelle S, Scherer M, et al. Chondroitin for the treatment of osteoarthritis: meta-analysis. Arthritis Rheum 2006:S1679.
161. Cibere J, Kopec JA, Thorne A, et al. Randomized, double-blind, placebo-controlled glucosamine discontinuation trial in knee osteoarthritis. Arthritis Rheum 2004;51(5):738–745.
162. McAlindon T, Formica M, Kabbara K, LaValley M, Lehmer M. Conducting clinical trials over the internet: feasibility study. BMJ 2003;327(7413):484–487.

163. Hughes R, Carr A. A randomized, double-blind, placebo-controlled trial of glucosamine sulphate as an analgesic in osteoarthritis of the knee. Rheumatology (Oxford) 2002;41(3):279–284.
164. Rindone JP, Hiller D, Collacott E, Nordhaugen N, Arriola G. Randomized, controlled trial of glucosamine for treating osteoarthritis of the knee. West J Med 2000;172(2):91–94.
165. Cibere J, Thorne A, Kopec JA, et al. Glucosamine sulfate and cartilage type II collagen degradation in patients with knee osteoarthritis: randomized discontinuation trial results employing biomarkers. J Rheumatol 2005;32(5):896–902.
166. Towheed T, Maxwell L, Anastassiades T, et al. Glucosamine therapy for treating osteoarthritis. Cochrane Database Syst Rev 2005;2:CD002946.
167. Herrero-Beaumont G, Ivorra JA, Del Carmen Trabado M, et al. Glucosamine sulfate in the treatment of knee osteoarthritis symptoms: a randomized, double-blind, placebo-controlled study using acetaminophen as a side comparator. Arthritis Rheum 2007;56(2):555–567.
168. Clegg DO, Reda DJ, Harris CL, et al. Glucosamine, chondroitin sulfate, and the two in combination for painful knee osteoarthritis. N Engl J Med 2006;354(8):795–808.
169. Reginster JY, Deroisy R, Rovati LC, et al. Long-term effects of glucosamine sulphate on osteoarthritis progression: a randomised, placebo-controlled clinical trial. Lancet 2001;357(9252):251–256.
170. Pavelka K, Gatterova J, Olejarova M, Machacek S, Giacovelli G, Rovati LC. Glucosamine sulfate use and delay of progression of knee osteoarthritis: a 3-year, randomized, placebo-controlled, double-blind study. Arch Intern Med 2002;162(18):2113–2123.
171. Michel BA, Stucki G, Frey D, et al. Chondroitins 4 and 6 sulfate in osteoarthritis of the knee: a randomized, controlled trial. Arthritis Rheum 2005;52(3):779–786.
172. Vignon E. Radiographic issues in imaging the progression of hip and knee osteoarthritis. J Rheumatol Suppl 2004;70:36–44.
173. Reginster JY, Kahan A, Vignon E. A Two-Year Prospective, Randomized, Double-Blind, Controlled Study Assessing the Effect of Chondroitin 4&6 Sulfate (CS) on the Structural Progression of Knee Osteoarthritis: STOPP (STudy on Osteoarthritis Progression Prevention). Ann Rheum Dis 2006;65(4):L42.
174. Spencer CM, Wilde MI. Diacerein. Drugs 1997;53(1):98–106; discussion 7–8.
175. Martel-Pelletier J, Mineau F, Jolicoeur FC, Cloutier JM, Pelletier JP. In vitro effects of diacerhein and rhein on interleukin 1 and tumor necrosis factor-alpha systems in human osteoarthritic synovium and chondrocytes. J Rheumatol 1998;25(4):753–762.
176. Pelletier JP, Mineau F, Fernandes JC, Duval N, Martel-Pelletier J. Diacerhein and rhein reduce the interleukin 1beta stimulated inducible nitric oxide synthesis level and activity while stimulating cyclooxygenase-2 synthesis in human osteoarthritic chondrocytes. J Rheumatol 1998;25(12):2417–2424.
177. Yaron M, Shirazi I, Yaron I. Anti-interleukin-1 effects of diacerein and rhein in human osteoarthritic synovial tissue and cartilage cultures. Osteoarthritis Cartilage 1999;7(3):272–280.
178. Fidelix TS, Soares BG, Trevisani VF. Diacerein for osteoarthritis. Cochrane Database Syst Rev 2006;1:CD005117.
179. Dougados M, Nguyen M, Berdah L, Mazieres B, Vignon E, Lequesne M. Evaluation of the structure-modifying effects of diacerein in hip osteoarthritis: ECHODIAH, a three-year, placebo-controlled trial. Evaluation of the Chondromodulating Effect of Diacerein in OA of the Hip. Arthritis Rheum 2001;44(11):2539–2547.
180. Pham T, Le Henanff A, Ravaud P, Dieppe P, Paolozzi L, Dougados M. Evaluation of the symptomatic and structural efficacy of a new hyaluronic acid compound, NRD101, in comparison with diacerein and placebo in a 1 year randomised controlled study in symptomatic knee osteoarthritis. Ann Rheum Dis 2004;63(12):1611–1617.
181. Mauviel A, Daireaux M, Hartmann DJ, Galera P, Loyau G, Pujol JP. [Effects of unsaponifiable extracts of avocado/soy beans (PIAS) on the production of collagen by cultures of synoviocytes, articular chondrocytes and skin fibroblasts]. Rev Rhum Mal Osteoartic 1989;56(2):207–211.
182. Mauviel A, Loyau G, Pujol JP. [Effect of unsaponifiable extracts of avocado and soybean (Piascledine) on the collagenolytic action of cultures of human rheumatoid synoviocytes and rabbit articular chondrocytes treated with interleukin-1]. Rev Rhum Mal Osteoartic 1991;58(4):241–245.

183. Henrotin YE, Labasse AH, Jaspar JM, et al. Effects of three avocado/soybean unsaponifiable mixtures on metalloproteinases, cytokines and prostaglandin E2 production by human articular chondrocytes. Clin Rheumatol 1998;17(1):31–39.
184. Henrotin YE, Sanchez C, Deberg MA, et al. Avocado/soybean unsaponifiables increase aggrecan synthesis and reduce catabolic and proinflammatory mediator production by human osteoarthritic chondrocytes. J Rheumatol 2003;30(8):1825–1834.
185. Boumediene K, Felisaz N, Bogdanowicz P, Galera P, Guillou GB, Pujol JP. Avocado/soya unsaponifiables enhance the expression of transforming growth factor beta1 and beta2 in cultured articular chondrocytes. Arthritis Rheum 1999;42(1):148–156.
186. Cake MA, Read RA, Guillou B, Ghosh P. Modification of articular cartilage and subchondral bone pathology in an ovine meniscectomy model of osteoarthritis by avocado and soya unsaponifiables (ASU). Osteoarthritis Cartilage 2000;8(6):404–411.
187. Ernst E. Avocado–soybean unsaponifiables (ASU) for osteoarthritis—a systematic review. Clin Rheumatol 2003;22(4–5):285–288.
188. Blotman F, Maheu E, Wulwik A, Caspard H, Lopez A. Efficacy and safety of avocado/soybean unsaponifiables in the treatment of symptomatic osteoarthritis of the knee and hip. A prospective, multicenter, three-month, randomized, double-blind, placebo-controlled trial. Rev Rhum Engl Ed 1997;64(12):825–834.
189. Maheu E, Mazieres B, Valat JP, et al. Symptomatic efficacy of avocado/soybean unsaponifiables in the treatment of osteoarthritis of the knee and hip: a prospective, randomized, double-blind, placebo-controlled, multicenter clinical trial with a six-month treatment period and a two-month followup demonstrating a persistent effect. Arthritis Rheum 1998;41(1):81–91.
190. Appelboom T, Schuermans J, Verbruggen G, Henrotin Y, Reginster JY. Symptoms modifying effect of avocado/soybean unsaponifiables (ASU) in knee osteoarthritis. A double blind, prospective, placebo-controlled study. Scand J Rheumatol 2001;30(4):242–247.
191. Lequesne M, Maheu E, Cadet C, Dreiser RL. Structural effect of avocado/soybean unsaponifiables on joint space loss in osteoarthritis of the hip. Arthritis Rheum 2002;47(1):50–58.
192. Curtis CL, Hughes CE, Flannery CR, Little CB, Harwood JL, Caterson B. n-3 fatty acids specifically modulate catabolic factors involved in articular cartilage degradation. J Biol Chem 2000;275(2):721–724.
193. Curtis CL, Rees SG, Cramp J, et al. Effects of n-3 fatty acids on cartilage metabolism. Proc Nutr Soc 2002;61(3):381–389.
194. Curtis CL, Rees SG, Little CB, et al. Pathologic indicators of degradation and inflammation in human osteoarthritic cartilage are abrogated by exposure to n-3 fatty acids. Arthritis Rheum 2002;46(6):1544–1553.
195. Lippiello L. Lipid and cell metabolic changes associated with essential fatty acid enrichment of articular chondrocytes. Proc Soc Exp Biol Med 1990;195(2):282–287.
196. Lippiello L, Walsh T, Fienhold M. The association of lipid abnormalities with tissue pathology in human osteoarthritic articular cartilage. Metabolism 1991;40(6):571–576.
197. Stammers T, Sibbald B, Freeling P. Efficacy of cod liver oil as an adjunct to non-steroidal anti-inflammatory drug treatment in the management of osteoarthritis in general practice. Ann Rheum Dis 1992;51(1):128–129.
198. Muller-Fassbender H. Double-blind clinical trial of S-adenosylmethionine versus ibuprofen in the treatment of osteoarthritis. Am J Med 1987;83(5A):81–83.
199. Konig B. A long-term (two years) clinical trial with S-adenosylmethionine for the treatment of osteoarthritis. Am J Med 1987;83(5A):89–94.
200. Vetter G. Double-blind comparative clinical trial with S-adenosylmethionine and indomethacin in the treatment of osteoarthritis. Am J Med 1987;83(5A):78–80.
201. Maccagno A, Di Giorgio EE, Caston OL, Sagasta CL. Double-blind controlled clinical trial of oral S-adenosylmethionine versus piroxicam in knee osteoarthritis. Am J Med 1987;83(5A):72–77.
202. Glorioso S, Todesco S, Mazzi A, et al. Double-blind multicentre study of the activity of S-adenosylmethionine in hip and knee osteoarthritis. Int J Clin Pharmacol Res 1985;5(1):39–49.
203. Najm WI, Reinsch S, Hoehler F, Tobis JS, Harvey PW. S-adenosyl methionine (SAMe) versus celecoxib for the treatment of osteoarthritis symptoms: a double-blind cross-over trial. [ISRCTN36233495]. BMC Musculoskelet Disord 2004;5(1):6.

204. Altman RD, Marcussen KC. Effects of a ginger extract on knee pain in patients with osteoarthritis. Arthritis Rheum 2001;44(11):2531–2538.
205. Felson DT. Weight and osteoarthritis. J Rheumatol 1995;22(suppl 43):7–9.
206. Sokoloff L, Mickelsen O. Dietary fat supplements, body weight and osteoarthritis in DBA/2JN mice. J Nutr 1965;85:117–121.
207. Sokoloff L, Mickelsen O, Silverstein E, Jay GE, Jr., Yamamoto RS. Experimental obesity and osteoarthritis. Am J Physiol 1960;198:765–770.
208. Aspden RM, Scheven BA, Hutchison JD. Osteoarthritis as a systemic disorder including stromal cell differentiation and lipid metabolism. Lancet 2001;357(9262):1118–1120.
209. Dumond H, Presle N, Terlain B, et al. Evidence for a key role in leptin in ostoearthritis. Arthritis Rheum 2003;48(9):S282.
210. Messier SP, Loeser RF, Miller GD, et al. Exercise and dietary weight loss in overweight and obese older adults with knee osteoarthritis: the Arthritis, Diet, and Activity Promotion Trial. Arthritis Rheum 2004;50(5):1501–1510.
211. Christensen R, Astrup A, Bliddal H. Weight loss: the treatment of choice for knee osteoarthritis? A randomized trial. Osteoarthritis Cartilage 2005;13(1):20–27.
212. Toda Y, Toda T, Takemura S, Wada T, Morimoto T, Ogawa R. Change in body fat, but not body weight or metabolic correlates of obesity, is related to symptomatic relief of obese patients with knee osteoarthritis after a weight control program. J Rheumatol 1998;25(11):2181–2186.
213. Hooper MM, Stellato TA, Hallowell PT, Seitz BA, Moskowitz RW. Musculoskeletal findings in obese subjects before and after weight loss following bariatric surgery. Int J Obes (Lond) 2007;31(1):114–120.

9 Nutritional Supplementation in Systemic Lupus Erythematosus

Sangeeta D. Sule and Michelle Petri

Summary

- There are interesting data on nutritional supplementation in the treatment of systemic lupus erythematous. However, at this time, there is little convincing human data to support dietary modifications or nutritional supplementation.
- Future research may be helpful to identify potentially beneficial nutritional supplementation therapies in systemic lupus erythematous.

Key Words: Nutritional supplements; systemic lupus erythematous

1. INTRODUCTION

Systemic lupus erythematous (SLE) is an autoimmune disease characterized by inflammation of multiple organs including kidneys, joints, skin, and blood. The course can be quite variable, ranging from intermittent exacerbations to severe, life-threatening disease. Females are affected nine times more frequently than men, and disease prevalence is higher in African Americans, Asians, and Hispanics. The relationship between nutrition and SLE remains obscure, as multiple factors including genetics, environment, and hormones may play a role in pathogenesis. Decreased appetite and weight loss over the previous year are common in newly diagnosed patients with SLE. Weight gain may be problematic in patients taking corticosteroids for SLE therapy. No specific diet for the treatment of SLE exists. However, studies examining the role of dietary modification have shown some promise.

This chapter explores diet in SLE and is arranged into two sections focusing on potentially beneficial nutritional modifications in SLE and potentially harmful nutritional substances in SLE. We review the large animal literature, but only a few clinical trials address the role of nutrition in SLE.

From: *Nutrition and Health: Nutrition and Rheumatic Disease*
Edited by: L. A. Coleman © Humana Press, Totowa, NJ

2. POTENTIALLY BENEFICIAL NUTRITIONAL MODIFICATIONS IN SLE

2.1. Caloric Restriction

The autoimmune-prone NZB/NZW F1 (B/W) mouse is an excellent model for SLE. These mice produce autoantibodies at 2 to 3 months of age. These autoantibodies are deposited in the kidneys by 4 to 5 months of age, leading to nephritis and renal disease by 9 to10 months of age *(1)*. This murine model has been extensively used to study pathogenesis of SLE and to test potential interventions for controlling SLE.

Caloric restriction in this murine model has a profound effect on the onset and progression of nephritis and has been shown to improve survival *(2)*. In B/W mice, the life span is increased from 345 days in controls to 494 days in caloric-restricted mice. The calorie restriction (40% less food) also significantly delays the onset of nephritis. These dietary changes are initiated early (age 2 months). By 14 months of age, 0% of the calorie-restricted mice develop nephritis, compared with 100% of the controls *(3)*.

Calorie restriction diminishes the decline in CD4+ T lymphocytes and stops the decline in CD8+ T lymphocytes that normally occurs with age in NZB/W mice *(4)*. Caloric restriction also inhibits the elevated immunoglobulin (Ig)A and IgG_2 seen in NZB/W mice. Caloric restriction diminishes the rise in Th-1 cytokines, including interferon-γ, interleukin (IL)-10, and IL-12, in older B/W mice *(5)*. Mizutani et al. noted that reducing calories to 32% or less than the control diet in NZB/W mice resulted in decreased antibody production, fewer coronary vascular lesions, and less glomerular involvement *(6)*. However, in order to implement this calorie restriction in humans, 25 to 35% or more of total intake would have to be cut, beginning before adolescence and continuing for life. This makes such strict caloric restriction difficult to impossible to implement in humans with SLE, especially given the long life span.

2.2. Low-Protein Diets

High protein intakes have been associated with acceleration of kidney damage in both humans and experimental animals *(7)*. Low-protein diets are known to improve survival in autoimmune NZB/NZW mice *(8)*. Mice that are fed a protein-restricted diet had delayed development of SLE compared with normal controls. They also had less severe nephritis. In humans, protein restriction has long been a recommended treatment modality in patients with renal failure. In an 18-month study including 64 patients, individuals on a protein-restricted diet had a slower decline in glomerular filtration rate (GFR) compared with controls *(9)*. In another study of moderate renal disease, patients restricted to 0.58 g/kg per day of protein had a slower decline in GFR over long-term, 3-year follow-up compared with normal controls *(10)*.

Restriction of different proteins may have different effects in autoimmune mice. In an effort to study oral tolerance in NZB/W mice, researchers unexpectedly found that casein restriction improved survival in autoimmune mice with 12 of 15 mice fed a casein-free diet alive at 10 months compared with 1 of 10 mice on the control diet. Casein-free mice had less anti-DNA antibody and less nephritis compared with controls *(11)*.

2.3. Dietary Fat Intake

Over the last 20 years, there have been numerous studies of fatty acids and their role in inflammation. Omega-3 (n-3) and omega-6 (n-6) fatty acids are considered essential fatty acids, which means that they are essential to human health but cannot be made in the body and must be obtained from food. Both types of fatty acids play a crucial role in brain function as well as normal growth and development *(12,13)*. The n-3 fatty acids have anti-inflammatory, anti-arrhythmic, and anti-thrombotic properties *(14)*. The n-6 fatty acids are proinflammatory and prothrombotic. The n-3 polyunsaturated fatty acids are found in oily fish and vegetable sources such as the seeds of chia, perilla, flax, and walnuts.

Fatty acids are thought to modulate the immune system. Fish-oil supplementation diminishes the age-related increase in Th-2 (IL-10, IL-5) cytokine production in the NZB/NZW mice *(5)*. n-3 is thought to be important in lowering anti-double-stranded DNA (anti-dsDNA) and circulating immune complexes. In the idiotype induced mouse model of SLE, linseed oil, with 70% n-3 fatty acids, leads to decreased anti-dsDNA antibodies, decreased anti-cardiolipin antibodies and less severe glomerulonephritis compared with other diets, including fish-oil supplementation *(15)*. In the NZB/NZW B/W (F_1) mouse, n-3 fatty acids lower anti-dsDNA and circulating immune complexes *(16)*. Fish-oil supplementation also improves survival in female mice and decreases proteinuria. The anti-inflammatory effects of fish oil seem to depend on the synergistic effects of at least two n-3 fatty acids. NZB/NZW (F_1) mice given diets containing three to one mixtures of eicosapentaenoic acid (EPA-E) and docahexaenoic acid (DHA-E) had less severe glomerulonephritis than mice fed either fatty acid alone *(17)*.

NZB/NZW (F_1) B/W female mice fed fish oil, but not corn oil, had increased survival, reduced proteinuria, and decreased anti-dsDNA antibodies. Fish oil reduces renal transforming growth factor (TGF)-β1 mRNA, renal fibronectin-1, and intracellular adhesion molecule-1 *(18)*. Fish oil also decreases proinflammatory cytokines (IL-1β, IL-6, and tumor necrosis factor-α) and increases antioxidant enzyme gene expression *(19)*. TGF-β1 mRNA decreases in kidneys, but is increased in splenic tissue *(20)*. With increased TGF-β1 in the spleen, programmed cell death (apoptosis) is enhanced. The apoptotic process is thought to be important in SLE disease initiation and propagation and fish-oil supplementation may lead to deletion of self-reactive lymphocytes in lymphoid organs *(21)*.

Clinical trials of fatty acid supplementation in humans with SLE have been reported. Twelve patients with SLE with nephritis were given a 5-week trial of 6 g of fish oil followed by a 5-week washout period, and then 18 g of fish oil. The platelet EPA levels rose. However, platelet arachidonic acid incorporation, platelet aggregation, whole blood viscosity, and neutrophil leukotriene B4 release were reduced. The 18 g of fish-oil supplement reduced triglycerides by 38%, very low-density lipoprotein cholesterol by 39% and increased high-density lipoprotein cholesterol by 28%. There was no effect on immune titers, anti-dsDNA or albuminuria *(22)*. Twenty-six patients with lupus nephritis were given fish oil in a double-blind cross-over trial. No significant effect was seen on proteinuria, GFR, disease activity, or lowering of corticosteroid dose. However, lipid levels did improve *(16)*. In another study of 27 active patients with SLE given 20 g of maxEPA or 20 g of olive oil, 14 patients in the maxEPA group had improvement in "useful or ideal status" *(23)*. Given these mixed results, a future well-designed clinical trial of fatty acid supplementation in SLE would be desirable.

2.4. Vitamin E

Vitamin E, a fat-soluble vitamin, is an antioxidant vitamin involved in the metabolism of all cells. It protects essential fatty acids from oxidation and prevents breakdown of body tissues. In another murine model of lupus, the MRL/*lpr* mice, a single lymphoproliferation (*lpr*) gene is mutated, leading to a lupus-like syndrome and lymphoproliferation. Treating MRL/*lpr* mice with vitamin E delayed the onset of autoimmunity and extended mean survival time *(24)*.

However, treating patients with SLE with vitamin E is controversial. Large doses of vitamin E have been reported beneficial in a few cases. Four discoid lupus patients, treated with 900 to 1,600 IU of vitamin E daily, showed partial or complete clearing of the discoid rash, compared with two patients receiving 300 IU daily *(25)*. However, recurrences of SLE were not abrogated by vitamin E. Additionally, vitamin E may act as an anticoagulant at high doses (above the Reference Daily Intake [RDI] of 30 IU) and may interact with immunosuppressive medication in SLE. A meta-analysis of 135,967 participants in 19 clinical trials identified a dose-dependent relationship between vitamin E and all-cause mortality. There was also a trend toward increasing cardiovascular disease (CVD) in patients supplemented with vitamin E *(26)*. This has important implications in patients with SLE, in whom CVD is more prevalent compared with age-matched controls *(27)*.

2.5. Vitamin A

Vitamin A, a fat-soluble vitamin also called retinol, plays an essential role in vision, growth, and development. The U.S. Recommended Daily Allowance for vitamin A is 900 retinol activity equivalents (RAE) for men and 700 RAE for females (RDI of 5,000 IU). In vitamin A-deficient NZB mice, more severe lupus symptoms were noted including hypergammaglobulinemia and earlier onset of autoantibodies.

In humans, case reports have suggested a beneficial effect of vitamin A in SLE. Three patients with SLE were given 50 mg of β-carotene three times daily and experienced a clearing of skin involvement within 1 week of starting treatment. Others have noted that high levels of vitamin A (100,000 U daily for 2 weeks) in patients with SLE resulted in improved antibody-dependent cell-mediated cytotoxicity and natural killer cell activity. However, high levels of vitamin A are associated with toxicity including anemia, headache, hair loss, dry skin, decreased appetite, and, in extreme cases, death.

In the Physicians Health Study of 18,314 men, there was an increased relative risk of death from any cause in patients taking combination of 30 mg of β-carotene per day and 25,000 IU of retinol (vitamin A) compared with placebo (relative risk [RR] 1.17; 95% confidence interval [CI], 1.03–1.33). Death from lung cancer was also increased in the supplement group compared with controls (RR 1.46;,95% CI, 1.07–2.00); and death from CVD was increased (RR 1.26; 95% CI, 0.99–1.61 *(28)*). Based on these findings, supplementation of vitamin A in patients with SLE is not advised.

2.6. Selenium

Selenium is a natural antioxidant associated with anti-inflammatory properties. Supplementing diets of NZB/W mice with selenium increases their survival. Although the mechanism of action is unclear, higher levels of natural killer cell activity are noted in selenium-supplemented mice. Levels of blood glutathione-peroxidase increase after selenium and vitamin E supplementation. Low levels of glutathione-peroxidase have been noted in some patients with SLE. Some researchers have suggested that selenium and vitamin E supplementation in patients with SLE with skin involvement may be helpful, because decreased levels of glutathione-peroxidase have been noted in the skin of patients with SLE *(29)*. However, there are few studies to support any recommendation of selenium supplementation in SLE. Signs of selenium toxicity include diarrhea, vomiting, hair and nail loss, and lesions of the central nervous system.

2.7. Zinc

Zinc is an essential mineral found in almost every cell. It acts as a catalytic regulatory ion for enzymes, proteins, and transcription factors. Zinc is involved in T-cell development and thymic atrophy *(30)*. NZB/NZW mice fed a zinc-restricted diet had increased survival and less severe glomerulonephritis compared with nonrestricted mice. As opposed to other dietary manipulations, zinc restriction was found to be beneficial both early (after weaning) and later in life (at 6 months of age). In the MRL/*lpr* mouse model, zinc deficiency introduced early in life (4 weeks of age) resulted in decreased titers of antibodies to dsDNA, less severe glomerulonephrirts, and prolonged survival compared with controls. However, if the zinc deficiency was introduced later in life (at 10 weeks of age), it had little beneficial effect on disease progression *(31)*. These data suggest that there is a critical period in which manipulation of dietary zinc can alter the course of autoimmune disease.

2.8. Flaxseed

One animal and one human study suggest that flaxseed may be beneficial in SLE. A 15% flaxseed diet fed to MRL/*lpr* mice results in less proteinuria, spleen lymphocyte proliferation, and mortality compared to control mice. Flaxseed-fed mice also have higher GFR compared to controls. In a double-blind, crossover study, 23 patients with SLE were randomized to receive 30 g of ground flaxseed daily or control (no placebo) for 1 year, followed by a 12-week washout period and the reverse treatment for 1 year. In those who were compliant, serum creatinine during flaxseed administration declined from a mean of 0.97±0.31 mg/dL to a mean of 0.94±0.30 mg/dL and rose in the control phase to a mean of 1.03± 0.28 mg/dL ($p < 0.08$ *(32)*).

2.9. Plant Herb

Tripterygium wilfordii hook F (TWH) is a plant herb that has been used in herbal medicine in China for the treatment of SLE and rheumatoid arthritis (RA *(33)*). *In vitro* tests show that TWH inhibits lymphoproliferation, production of cytokines from monocytes and lymphocytes, and prostaglandin E_2 production *(34)*. The toxicity of TWH would prevent its widespread use for SLE. Reported complications include diarrhea, infertility, and one reported case of death resulting from cardiac shock *(35)*.

2.10. Dehydroepiandrosterone

Autoimmune diseases are more prevalent in women and immune responses may be influenced by sex hormones. Androgens naturally suppress the immune system and dehydroepiandrosterone (DHEA), a weak androgen and intermediate compound in testosterone synthesis, has been evaluated in the treatment of SLE.

Animal studies with NZB/W mice show that DHEA produces similar results to caloric restriction, with decreased antibody production and prolonged survival rates *(36,37)*. In a double-blind, placebo-controlled study of 28 women with SLE who were given DHEA (200 mg per day) for 3 months, there were fewer flares, decreased SLE Disease Activity Index scores, decreased disease activity, and less prednisone use in the DHEA-treated patients. The main side effect was mild acne *(38)*.

In a study exploring whether prednisone doses could be reduced to 7.5 mg or less per day for 2 months or longer while women with SLE were receiving 100 or 200 mg of DHEA, Petri et al. noted that 51% of patients responded in the 200-mg group compared with 29% in the placebo group ($p = 0.031$ *(39)*). In another study to determine whether DHEA impacts SLE disease activity, women with active SLE were randomized to 200 mg DHEA plus standard SLE treatment or placebo plus standard SLE treatment for up to 12 months. Of the 147 women in the DHEA group, 86 (58.5%) showed improvement or stabilization in activity indices compared with 65 of 146 in the placebo group (44.5%; $p = 0.017$ *(40)*). However, the Food and Drug Administration (FDA) has not approved DHEA for the treatment of SLE.

3. POTENTIALLY HARMFUL NUTRITIONAL SUBSTANCES IN SLE

3.1. Iron

Iron is necessary for production of red blood cells. Daily requirements are usually met through routine diets. One animal study suggested that high levels of iron intake (seven times the daily requirement) in MRL/*lpr* mice resulted in increased proteinuria. Renal histopathology was more severe in iron-supplemented mice than in pair-fed control mice. Immunostaining with anti-IgG and anti-C3 in severely iron-deficient mice (fed 3 mg iron/kg, normal: 35 mg/kg) was more intense. Additionally, the concentration of circulating immune complexes in serum was significantly higher in severely iron-deficient mice, compared with controls *(41)*. This suggests that alterations in serum iron concentration can worsen disease in lupus-prone mice.

3.2. Alfalfa

Alfalfa is a perennial herb that grows in a variety of climates. It has been used by the Chinese since the 6th century to treat kidney stones and edema. When studying its effects on cholesterol, investigators noted SLE-like symptoms in laboratory animals. Three of five cynomologous macaques fed alfalfa seeds developed a positive antinuclear antibody, Coombs-positive hemolytic anemia, hypocomplementemia, and positive anti-dsDNA. One animal also developed immune-complex glomerulonephritis *(42,43)*. Autoimmune mice fed L-canavanine had increased autoantibody production and higher renal histology scores compared to normal controls. In vitro experiments suggest that L-canavanine, an amino acid in alfalfa sprouts, suppressed T-cell regulation of antibody synthesis and lymphocyte proliferation *(44)*.

In an analysis of the Baltimore Lupus Environment Study, ingestion of alfalfa sprouts was significantly associated with the development of lupus *(45)*. Two patients with SLE were reported to have worsening of symptoms including malaise, lethargy, and depression after ingesting 8 to 15 alfalfa tablets a day *(46)*.

3.3. Echinacea

Echinacea is a derivative of the coneflower. It is often used for treatments of colds and upper respiratory symptoms. Conflicting data exist regarding efficacy in shortening the duration of cold symptoms *(47–50)*. Echinacea is known to have immunostimulatory effects on natural killer cells, neutrophils, and monocytes *(51–53)*. These cells have been shown to be increased in both the bone marrow and spleen as soon as 1 week after starting therapy. In the Johns Hopkins Lupus Cohort, flares of SLE have been noted in patients taking echinacea, including diffuse proliferative glomerulonephritis requiring subsequent cyclophosphamide therapy *(54)*.

3.4. Noni Juice (Morinda citrifolia)

Noni juice is prepared from the fruit of Morinda citrifolia, a Polynesian plant. Various preparations of noni juice are now sold as wellness drinks. Reported manufacturer health claims include improvement in arthralgias, fibromyalgia, and cancer; however, there is very little scientific data regarding noni juice. One study examining the effect of noni juice on C57BL/6 mice noted that intra-peritoneal injections of noni juice given every day or every other day for a total of four to five injections resulted in increased survival time compared to controls (15 mg per mouse of noni juice 34.7±3.3 days survival compared to 15.9±0.8 days in controls *(55)*). However, two cases of toxic hepatitis have been reported in humans taking noni juice supplements *(56)*. There have been no studies of noni juice in SLE.

4. CONCLUSION

In conclusion, nutritional supplementation is a potentially tantalizing therapeutic option in SLE. However, at this time, there is little convincing human data to support dietary modifications or nutritional supplementation. Future studies are warranted to assess any potential benefit of dietary supplements in SLE.

We recommend that patients with SLE maintain a healthy, balanced diet. As with any healthy diet, fruits and vegetables are the recommended mainstay. Low-fat proteins, such as fish and chicken, are also healthy choices. If appropriate, exercise is also important in the overall health and well-being of patients with SLE.

REFERENCES

1. Holmes MC, Gorie J, Burnett FM. Transmission by splenic cells of an autoimmune disease occurring spontaneously in mice. Lancet 1961;2:638–639.
2. Friend PS, Fernandes G, Good RA, Michael AF, Yunis EJ. Dietary restrictions early and late: effects on the nephropathy of the NZB X NZW mouse. Lab Invest 1978;38(6):629–632.
3. Urao M, Ueda G, Abe M, Kanno K, Hirose S, Shirai T. Food restriction inhibits an autoimmune disease resembling systemic lupus erythematosus in (NZB x NZW) F1 mice. J Nutr 1995;125(9):2316–2324.
4. Muthukumar AR, Jolly CA, Zaman K, Fernandes G. Calorie restriction decreases proinflammatory cytokines and polymeric Ig receptor expression in the submandibular glands of autoimmune prone (NZB x NZW)F1 mice. J Clin Immunol 2000;20(5):354–361.

5. Jolly CA, Fernandes G. Diet modulates Th-1 and Th-2 cytokine production in the peripheral blood of lupus-prone mice. J Clin Immunol 1999;19(3):172–1678.
6. Mizutani H, Engelman RW, Kinjoh K, et al. Calorie restriction prevents the occlusive coronary vascular disease of autoimmune (NZW x BXSB)F1 mice. Proc Natl Acad Sci U S A 1994;91(10): 4402–4406.
7. Ihle BU, Becker GJ, Whitworth JA, Charlwood RA, Kincaid-Smith PS. The effect of protein restriction on the progression of renal insufficiency. N Engl J Med 1989;321(26):1773–1777.
8. Johnson BC, Gajjar A, Kubo C, Good RA. Calories versus protein in onset of renal disease in NZB x NZW mice. Proc Natl Acad Sci U S A 1986;83(15):5659–5662.
9. Ihle BU, Becker GJ, Whitworth JA, Charlwood RA, Kincaid-Smith PS. The effect of protein restriction on the progression of renal insufficiency. N Engl J Med 1989;321(26):1773–1777.
10. Peterson JC, Adler S, Burkart JM, et al. Blood pressure control, proteinuria, and the progression of renal disease. The Modification of Diet in Renal Disease Study. Ann Intern Med 1995;123(10): 754–762.
11. Carr R, Forsyth S, Sadi D. Abnormal responses to ingested substances in murine systemic lupus erythematosus: apparent effect of a casein-free diet on the development of systemic lupus erythematosus in NZB/W mice. J Rheumatol Suppl 1987;14(suppl 13):158–165.
12. Kromann N, Green A. Epidemiological studies in the Upernavik district, Greenland. Incidence of some chronic diseases 1950–1974. Acta Med Scand 1980;208(5):401–406.
13. Black KL, Culp B, Madison D, Randall OS, Lands WE. The protective effects of dietary fish oil on focal cerebral infarction. Prostaglandins Med 1979;3(5):257–268.
14. Kelley VE, Ferretti A, Izui S, Strom TB. A fish oil diet rich in eicosapentaenoic acid reduces cyclooxygenase metabolites, and suppresses lupus in MRL-lpr mice. J Immunol 1985;134(3): 1914–1919.
15. Reifen R, Blank M, Afek A, et al. Dietary polyunsaturated fatty acids decrease anti-dsDNA and anti-cardiolipin antibodies production in idiotype induced mouse model of systemic lupus erythematosus. Lupus 1998;7(3):192–197.
16. Clark WF, Parbtani A. Omega-3 fatty acid supplementation in clinical and experimental lupus nephritis. Am J Kidney Dis 1994;23(5):644–647.
17. Robinson DR, Xu LL, Tateno S, Guo M, Colvin RB. Suppression of autoimmune disease by dietary n-3 fatty acids. J Lipid Res 1993;34(8):1435–1444.
18. Chandrasekar B, Troyer DA, Venkatraman JT, Fernandes G. Dietary omega-3 lipids delay the onset and progression of autoimmune lupus nephritis by inhibiting transforming growth factor beta mRNA and protein expression. J Autoimmun 1995;8(3):381–393.
19. Chandrasekar B, Fernandes G. Decreased pro-inflammatory cytokines and increased antioxidant enzyme gene expression by omega-3 lipids in murine lupus nephritis. Biochem Biophys Res Commun 1994;200(2):893–898.
20. Fernandes G, Bysani C, Venkatraman JT, Tomar V, Zhao W. Increased TGF-beta and decreased oncogene expression by omega-3 fatty acids in the spleen delays onset of autoimmune disease in B/W mice. J Immunol 1994;152(12):5979–5987.
21. Fernandes G, Chandrasekar B, Luan X, Troyer DA. Modulation of antioxidant enzymes and programmed cell death by n-3 fatty acids. Lipids 1996;31(suppl):S91–S96.
22. Clark WF, Parbtani A, Huff MW, Reid B, Holub BJ, Falardeau P. Omega-3 fatty acid dietary supplementation in systemic lupus erythematosus. Kidney Int 1989;36(4):653–660.
23. Walton AJ, Snaith ML, Locniskar M, Cumberland AG, Morrow WJ, Isenberg DA. Dietary fish oil and the severity of symptoms in patients with systemic lupus erythematosus. Ann Rheum Dis 1991;50(7):463–466.
24. Weimann BJ, Hermann D. Inhibition of autoimmune deterioration in MRL/lpr mice by vitamin E. Int J Vitam Nutr Res 1999;69:255–261.
25. Ayres S,Jr, Mihan R. Is vitamin E involved in the autoimmune mechanism? Cutis 1978;21(3):321–325.
26. Miller ER, 3rd, Pastor-Barriuso R, Dalal D, Riemersma RA, Appel LJ, Guallar E. Meta-analysis: high-dosage vitamin E supplementation may increase all-cause mortality. Ann Intern Med 2005;142(1): 37–46.

27. Manzi S, Meilahn EN, Rairie JE, et al. Age-specific incidence rates of myocardial infarction and angina in women with systemic lupus erythematosus: comparison with the Framingham Study. Am J Epidemiol 1997;145(5):408–415.
28. Omenn GS, Goodman GE, Thornquist MD, et al. Effects of a combination of beta carotene and vitamin A on lung cancer and cardiovascular disease. N Engl J Med 1996;334(18):1150–1155.
29. Juhlin L, Edqvist LE, Ekman LG, Ljunghall K, Olsson M. Blood glutathione-peroxidase levels in skin diseases: effect of selenium and vitamin E treatment. Acta Derm Venereol 1982;62(3):211–214.
30. Mocchegiani E, Santarelli L, Muzzioli M, Fabris N. Reversibility of the thymic involution and age-related peripheral immune dysfunction by zinc supplementation in old mice. Int J Immunopharmacol 1995;17:703.
31. Beach RS, Gershwin ME, Hurley LS. Nutritional factors and autoimmunity. III. Zinc deprivation versus restricted food intake in MRL/1 mice—the distinction between interacting dietary influences. J Immunol 1982;129(6):2686–2692.
32. Clark WF, Kortas C, Heidenheim AP, Garland J, Spanner E, Parbtani A. Flaxseed in lupus nephritis: a two-year nonplacebo-controlled crossover study. J Am Coll Nutr 2001;20(2 suppl):143–148.
33. Tao X, Lipsky PE. The Chinese anti-inflammatory and immunosuppressive herbal remedy Tripterygium wilfordii Hook F. Rheum Dis Clin North Am 2000;26(1):29,50, viii.
34. Ho LJ, Chang DM, Chang ML, Kuo SY, Lai JH. Mechanism of immunosuppression of the antirheumatic herb TWHf in human T cells. J Rheumatol 1999;26(1):14–24.
35. Chou WC, Wu CC, Yang PC, Lee YT. Hypovolemic shock and mortality after ingestion of Tripterygium wilfordii hook F.: a case report. Int J Cardiol 1995;49(2):173–177.
36. Yang BC, Liu CW, Chen YC, Yu CK. Exogenous dehydroepiandrosterone modified the expression of T helper-related cytokines in NZB/NZW F1 mice. Immunol Invest 1998;27(4–5):291–302.
37. Matsunaga A, Miller BC, Cottam GL. Dehydroisoandrosterone prevention of autoimmune disease in NZB/W F1 mice: lack of an effect on associated immunological abnormalities. Biochim Biophys Acta 1989;992(3):265–271.
38. van Vollenhoven RF, Engleman EG, McGuire JL. Dehydroepiandrosterone in systemic lupus erythematosus. Results of a double-blind, placebo-controlled, randomized clinical trial. Arthritis Rheum 1995;38(12):1826–1831.
39. Petri MA, Lahita RG, Van Vollenhoven RF, et al. Effects of prasterone on corticosteroid requirements of women with systemic lupus erythematosus: a double-blind, randomized, placebo-controlled trial. Arthritis Rheum 2002;46(7):1820–1829.
40. Petri MA, Mease PJ, Merrill JT, et al. Effects of prasterone on disease activity and symptoms in women with active systemic lupus erythematosus. Arthritis Rheum 2004;50(9):2858–2868.
41. Leiter LM, Reuhl KR, Racis SP,Jr, Sherman AR. Iron status alters murine systemic lupus erythematosus. J Nutr 1995;125(3):474–484.
42. Bardana EJ,Jr, Malinow MR, Houghton DC, et al. Diet-induced systemic lupus erythematosus (SLE) in primates. Am J Kidney Dis 1982;1(6):3453–52.
43. Malinow MR, Bardana EJ,Jr, Pirofsky B, Craig S, McLaughlin P. Systemic lupus erythematosus-like syndrome in monkeys fed alfalfa sprouts: role of a nonprotein amino acid. Science 1982;216(4544):415–417.
44. Morimoto I, Shiozawa S, Tanaka Y, Fujita T. L-canavanine acts on suppressor-inducer T cells to regulate antibody synthesis: lymphocytes of systemic lupus erythematosus patients are specifically unresponsive to L-canavanine. Clin Immunol Immunopathol 1990;55(1):97–108.
45. Petri M, Thompson E, Abusuwwa R, Huang J, Garrett E. BALES: the Baltimore Lupus Environmental Study. Arthritis Rheum 2001; 44(9,suppl):S331.
46. Roberts JL, Hayashi JA. Exacerbation of SLE associated with alfalfa ingestion. N Engl J Med 1983;308(22):1361.
47. Lindenmuth GF, Lindenmuth EB. The efficacy of echinacea compound herbal tea preparation on the severity and duration of upper respiratory and flu symptoms: a randomized, double-blind placebo-controlled study. J Altern Complement Med 2000;6(4):327–334.
48. Schulten B, Bulitta M, Ballering-Bruhl B, Koster U, Schafer M. Efficacy of Echinacea purpurea in patients with a common cold. A placebo-controlled, randomised, double-blind clinical trial. Arzneimittelforschung 2001;51(7):563–568.

49. Turner RB, Riker DK, Gangemi JD. Ineffectiveness of echinacea for prevention of experimental rhinovirus colds. Antimicrob Agents Chemother 2000;44(6):1708–1709.
50. Giles JT, Palat CT, 3rd, Chien SH, Chang ZG, Kennedy DT. Evaluation of echinacea for treatment of the common cold. Pharmacotherapy 2000;20(6):690–697.
51. Currier NL, Miller SC. Natural killer cells from aging mice treated with extracts from Echinacea purpurea are quantitatively and functionally rejuvenated. Exp Gerontol 2000;35(5):627–639.
52. Rininger JA, Kickner S, Chigurupati P, McLean A, Franck Z. Immunopharmacological activity of Echinacea preparations following simulated digestion on murine macrophages and human peripheral blood mononuclear cells. J Leukoc Biol 2000;68(4):503–510.
53. Sun LZ, Currier NL, Miller SC. The American coneflower: a prophylactic role involving nonspecific immunity. J Altern Complement Med 1999;5(5):437–446.
54. Petri M. Diet and systemic lupus erythematosus: from mouse and monkey to woman? Lupus 2001;10(11):775–777.
55. Hirazumi A, Furusawa E. An immunomodulatory polysaccharide-rich substance from the fruit juice of Morinda citrifolia (noni) with antitumour activity. Phytother Res 1999;13(5):380–387.
56. Stadlbauer V, Fickert P, Lackner C, et al. Hepatotoxicity of NONI juice: report of two cases. World J Gastroenterol 2005;11(30):4758–4760.

10 Hyperuricemia, Gout, and Diet

Naomi Schlesinger

Summary

- Dietary trends, increasing obesity and metabolic syndrome prevalence, are contributing to the increasing worldwide prevalence of hyperuricemia and gout.
- There is a strong association of metabolic syndrome with hyperuricemia.
- Dietary intervention is strongly recommended in patients with metabolic syndrome and hyperuricemia. Consumption of meat, seafood, and alcoholic beverages in moderation is useful.
- Controlled weight management has the potential to lower serum urate levels.
- Dairy products may have clinically meaningful antihyperuricaemic effects.
- Further education and studies are needed to improve our understanding of dietary factors and hyperuricemia.

Key Words: Alcohol; diet, gout; resistance; obesity; purines; uric acid; seafood; vegetarian

1. INTRODUCTION

The connection between gout or hyperuricemia and gluttony, overindulgence in food and alcohol, or obesity can be traced back to ancient times. Studies from different parts of the world suggest that the incidence and severity of hyperuricemia and gout may be increasing.

Uric acid (urate) is the end product of purine degradation. Although most uric acid is derived from the metabolism of endogenous purine, eating foods rich in purines contributes to the total pool of uric acid.

Sustained hyperuricemia is a risk factor for acute gouty arthritis, chronic tophaceous gout, renal stones, and possibly cardiovascular events and mortality. Before starting life-long urate-lowering drug therapy, it is important to identify and treat underlying disorders that may be contributing to hyperuricemia. It is relevant to recognize the strong association of the metabolic syndrome (MetS; abdominal obesity, dyslipidemia, hypertension, raised serum insulin levels, and glucose intolerance) with hyperuricemia.

2. CLINICAL FEATURES: HYPERURICEMIA

Uric acid is the end product of purine degradation (referred to as uric acid in urine and urate in serum). Humans have higher levels of serum urate (SU), in part, because they lack the hepatic enzyme, uricase, which converts uric acid to allantoin and a lower fractional excretion of uric acid. Approximately two-thirds of total body urate is produced endogenously, whereas the remaining one-third is accounted for by dietary purines. Approximately 70% of the urate produced daily is excreted by the kidneys, while the rest is eliminated by the intestines. In men, uric acid production is increased after puberty and in women, after menopause. The predominant cause of hyperuricemia in most patients is under-excretion of urate by the kidneys. A lower clearance of urate is seen in patients with gout compared with normal controls (1). Hyperuricemia is defined as an SU concentration in excess of urate solubility. An SU level of more than 7.0 mg/dL (413 µmol/L) in men and more than 6.0 mg/dL (354 µmol/L) in women is considered elevated.

If SU concentration is increased for a sustained period of time, monosodium urate will come out of the solution to form crystals. Micro-tophi will subsequently form, particularly in the cooler parts of the body such as distal extremities, olecranon bursa, and ears. Sustained hyperuricemia is a risk factor for acute gouty arthritis, chronic tophaceous gout, renal stones, and possibly cardiovascular events and mortality. Most patients with hyperuricemia will never have an attack of gout and no treatment is required although it is prudent to determine the cause of hyperuricemia and correct it, if possible.

The correlation between hyperuricemia and cardiovascular events and mortality is currently controversial and under intense investigation. It is suggested that the increased cardiovascular risk linked to hyperuricemia could be related to the association with other vascular risk factors (2).

3. NUTRITIONAL STATUS

3.1. Metabolic Syndrome and Hyperuricemia

The connection of gout and hyperuricemia to gluttony, overindulgence in food and alcohol, and obesity dates from ancient times. In the fifth century BC, Hippocrates attributed gout to excessive intake of food and wine (3). This link has become more obvious in recent times.

It is relevant to recognize the strong association of the MetS with hyperuricemia. Insulin resistance and its metabolic sequel, compensatory hyperinsulinemia and glucose intolerance, represent a unifying link common to type 2 diabetes, coronary artery disease, hypertension, abdominal obesity, and dyslipidemia (increased plasma triglycerides, decreased high-density lipoproteins and smaller, denser low-density lipoproteins [LDL]) (4–6). This cluster of factors is frequently referred to as the metabolic syndrome or Syndrome X (5).

MetS is strongly associated with hyperuricemia (4). Within a normouricemic population, there are significant correlations between resistance to insulin-mediated glucose uptake, the magnitude of the plasma insulin response to an oral glucose challenge, and the SU concentration. The increase in SU concentration is the result of a decrease in urinary uric acid clearance (7). Hyperuricemia may serve as a surrogate marker of insulin-resistance syndrome (8). SU may be involved in the obesity–MetS link (9). Dietary alterations in plasma very LDL levels also modify renal excretion of urate in hyperuricemic–hypertriglyceridemic patients (10).

Insulin resistance, independent of body weight and blood pressure, may play an important role in uric acid metabolism. If there is a significant impairment of glucose tolerance, management will include the use of drugs to increase insulin sensitivity, such as the thiazolidinediones (e.g., rosiglitazone *(11)*). The amelioration of insulin resistance by either a low-energy diet or troglitazone decreased the SU level in overweight hypertensive patients *(12)*.

The effect of diet on SU levels is relevant to the changing worldwide epidemiology of hyperuricemia and gout. Studies from different parts of the world suggest that the incidence and severity of hyperuricemia and gout may be increasing. The association of hyperuricemia and gout with dietary habits and the resulting insulin resistance is a likely cause *(13)*.

3.2. Obesity

Obesity, defined as a body mass index (BMI) of more than 30 kg/m^2, is a major public health problem. Data from the National Health and Nutrition Examination Survey have shown a rise in the age-adjusted prevalence of obesity from 22.9% during 1988–1994 to 30.5% during 1999–2000 *(14)*. Current dietary trends, with higher consumption of meat, seafood, and fat, in combination with inactivity, have contributed to this rising prevalence of obesity.

Epidemiological studies have demonstrated a strong correlation between obesity and hyperuricemia *(15,16)*. Obesity is associated with both increased production and decreased renal excretion of urate *(17)*; 3.4% of subjects with a relative weight below the 20th percentile are hyperuricemic, compared with 11.4% of those above the 80th percentile *(18)*. Weight loss alone has reduced SU levels *(19)*.

The Boston Veterans Administration Normative Aging Study *(20)* prospectively followed 2,280 healthy men, aged 21 to 81 at entry in 1963, and evaluated the incidence of gout and its associated risk factors. Although serum urate level was the most important predictive factor, a proportional hazards regression analysis showed that BMI also was a significant independent predictor for the development of gout. Similarly, data from the Johns Hopkins Precursors Study *(21)* on 1,216 men and 121 women with 40,000 person-years of follow-up noted a strong dose–response effect of BMI on the development of gout. The cumulative prevalence rose from 3.2 per 100 with a BMI of less than 22 kg/m^2 to 14.8 per 100 among men with a BMI of more than 25 kg/m^2. In addition to the absolute BMI, the relative increase in BMI over time was also associated with an increased risk for gout, with the cumulative prevalence rising to 14.5 per 100 for men who gained more than 1.88 BMI units.

The prevalence of gout in relation to BMI was assessed using the data from the Health Professionals Follow-up Study *(22)*. A clear dose–response relationship was noted between BMI and the risk for gout, with the age-adjusted relative risk (RR) increasing from 1.4 to 3.26 for BMIs of 21 to 23 and 30 to 35 kg/m^2, respectively. Compared with those with stable weight over time, men who gained more than 30 lb since age 21 had a RR of 2.47 for gout after adjusting for age and weight at age 21 years. In contrast, a loss of more than 10 lb since the study entry was associated with a 30% reduction in the risk of gout (RR 0.61). Similarly, the Nurses Health Study *(23)* of 92,224 women with no history of baseline gout found a similar dose–response relationship between BMI and the risk of gout, with RRs of 6.13 and 10.59 for BMIs of 30 to 35 and more than 35 kg/m^2, respectively. These observations have led to further support of weight loss to prevent recurrent gout attacks.

Fat and total calorie intake, in combination with decreased physical activity, lead to overall obesity with centripetal deposition of fat *(24)*. In a study from Taiwan, waist-to-height ratio, which indicates central obesity, was found to have a significant linear effect on gout occurrence, independent of BMI *(25)*. Centripetal obesity, in turn, is a powerful stimulus to increased insulin plasma levels and therefore, to hyperuricemia *(26)*.

3.3. Dehydration/Starvation

Dehydration can cause hyperuricemia *(26)*. The SU levels return to normal following the administration of normal saline over a period of 3 to 4 days. Hydration is often recommended as part of a conservative treatment for gout. Hydration is well known to assist in the prevention of hyperuricemia in the setting of malignancy, chemotherapy treatment, and nephrolithiasis.

Diuretics are associated with hyperuricemia. Diuretics have an inhibitory effect on renal excretion of uric acid. Some foods have a diuretic property that can potentially increase SU levels. Such foods include caffeine (coffee, tea—especially green tea—and colas), cranberry juice, asparagus, celery, eggplant, lemon, garlic, cucumbers, and licorice.

Fasting is also associated with a rise in SU. This is presumably owing to the inhibitory effect of ketones on uric acid excretion by the renal tubules *(27)*. Acetoacetic and β-hydroxybutyric acidemia associated with fasting results in inhibition of renal urate excretion and a rise in SU level. This study *(27)* suggests that the combination of fasting and alcohol appears to be mutually potentiating with regard to their effect on uric acid metabolism.

4. HYPERURICEMIA AND DIET

The introduction of the Western lifestyle to non-Western people has been associated with increases in SU levels, the incidence of gout, or both hyperuricemia and gout. Such is the case of the Maori of New Zealand. In the 19th century, the lean and physically active Maori ate mainly sweet potato, taro, fern root, birds, and fish. Hyperuricemia and gout were unknown. After the introduction of a diet low in dairy products and high in fatty meats and carbohydrates in the early 1900s, an epidemic of obesity, hyperuricemia, and gout developed *(28)*. Immigration of Filipino and Japanese people to North America, in parallel with a shift to a diet containing greater amounts of meat and saturated fat *(29)*, has caused an increase in SU levels as well as a rise in the incidence of gout.

Hyperuricemia and gout were rare among blacks in Africa, especially in rural areas where traditional agricultural and dairy-based diets were common. However, the frequency of hyperuricemia and gout is now increasing, particularly in urban communities, in parallel with hypertension and cardiovascular disease *(30)*.

4.1. Purine-Rich Foods

A diet low in meat and high in dairy products was proposed as a means to prevent gout by the philosopher John Locke (1632–1704), who encouraged milk drinking and "eating very little flesh but abundance of herbs"; similar diets were proposed by George Cheyne in the 1700s and by Alexander Haig in the late 1800s.

The suspicion that there is a link between purine-rich diets (high in meats and seafood) and gout has been based on metabolic experiments in animals and humans that examined the effect of the artificial short-term loading of purified purine on the SU level. The administration of an oral purine load to humans can increase the SU level by 1.0 to 2.0 mg/dL (59–118 µmol/L) within 24 hours *(31–34)*.

The Dutch Nutritional Surveillance Study suggested that, in women, higher consumption of meat and fish was associated with an increased SU level *(35)*. Purine-rich foods (beef liver and haddock) increased SU at 2 to 4 hours post meals *(36)*. A purine-rich diet will produce a transient elevation in SU levels by 1.0 to 2.0 mg/dl (59–118 µmol/L) and conversely, a purine-free diet, containing the same amount of calories, taken for 7 to 10 days, decreases SU level by the same amount *(17)*. Such small changes in SU levels may suggest that purine content is not the main contributing factor in the occurrence of acute gout.

The relationship between the consumption of purine-rich foods and the risk of developing gout was evaluated in the Health Professionals Study *(37)*. During the 12-year follow-up, validated semi-quantitative food-frequency questionnaires were used to obtain dietary information every 2 years. Men with the highest quintiles of meat and seafood intake were noted to have an increased risk of gout compared with those in the lowest quintile, with odds ratio (OR) of 1.41 (95% confidence interval [CI], 1.07–1.86) and 1.51 (95% CI, 1.17–1.95), respectively.

Little is known about the precise identity and quantity of individual purines in most foods, especially when they are cooked or processed *(38)*. Additionally, the bioavailability of purines contained in different foods varies substantially. For example, dietary experiments have shown that the bioavailability is greater for RNA than for an equivalent amount of DNA *(34,39)* and greater for adenine than for guanine *(31)*. The variation in hyperuricemia and gout with different purine-rich foods may be explained by the variation in the amounts and types of purine content and their bioavailability for purine-to-uric-acid metabolism *(31–34)*.

Research on cooking and purine content is very limited. Animal studies in this area have shown changes in purine content following the boiling and broiling of beef, beef liver, haddock, and mushrooms. However, although these cooking processes affect purine content, the nature of the changes is not clear. On the one hand, boiling high-purine foods in water can cause a break down of the purine-containing components (called nucleic acids) and eventual freeing up of the purines for absorption. For example, in some animal studies, where rats were fed cooked versus noncooked foods, the animals eating the cooked version experienced greater absorption and excretion of purine-related compounds. From this evidence, it might be tempting to conclude that cooking of high-purine foods actually increases the risk of purine overload. On the other hand, when foods were boiled, some of the purines were released into the cooking water and never ingested in the food. From this evidence, the exact opposite conclusion would make sense: Cooking of high-purines reduces the purine risk *(39)*. An observational study found that a strict purine-free diet will reduce the SU by 15 to 20% *(19)*. However, a rigid purine-free diet can rarely be sustained for a long period of time. Moderation in dietary purines rather than a strict purine-free diet may be helpful *(13)*.

4.2. Dairy Products

The ingestion of milk proteins (casein and lactalbumin) has been shown to reduce SU levels in healthy subjects because of their uricosuric effect *(40)*. There may be an inverse association between the level of consumption of dairy products and the SU level *(40,41)*. In women, lower consumption of bread and milk products was associated with increased SU level *(41)*.

In a 12-year cohort study using biannual questionnaires, it was concluded that having more than two glasses of milk per day was associated with a 50% risk reduction in gout *(37)*. Dairy intake was inversely correlated with the risk of gout, with an OR of 0.56. This protective effect was only evident with low-fat dairy products, such as skim milk and low-fat yogurt. Hyperuricemia was not addressed because SU levels were not measured *(37)*. Conversely, a significant increase in SU level was induced by a dairy-free diet in a 4-week randomized clinical trial (RCT *(42)*). Because dairy products are low in purine content, dairy protein may exert its urate-lowering effect without providing the concomitant purine load contained in other protein sources such as meat and seafood.

A prospective study of 92,224 women in the Nurses Health Study *(43)* noted a similar protective effect of dairy product consumption—especially low-fat dairy products—on the incidence of gout (OR 0.82).

This apparent protective effect of dairy products against hyperuricemia may be multifactorial. In addition to the postulated uricosuric effect of milk proteins, the vitamin D content in milk may also play a key role. One study suggests that patients with gout may have significantly lower levels of 1,25-dihydroxyvitamin (OH)-2-vitamin D_3 *(44)*. The year-long administration of urate-lowering drugs in this study caused a decrease in the SU concentration, which was associated with a significant elevation in the levels of 1,25-(OH)2-vitamin D_3. Serum 25-(OH)-vitamin D_3 and parathyroid hormone levels were not altered by the administration of urate-lowering agents. This may suggest that urate interferes with the hydroxylation of 25-(OH)-vitamin D_3 by inhibiting the activity of 1-hydroxylase. Whether the supplementation of vitamin D can prevent hyperuricemia has not yet been studied.

4.3. Fruits and Vegetables

The ability of dietary changes to modulate the SU levels in species that lack uricase may explain why the SU levels in the great apes (1.5–3.0 mg/dL; 89–177 µmol/L) are lower than those in the general human population of the United States (mean: 4.0 mg/dL [236 µmol/L] among women and 5.5 mg/dL [325 µmol/L] among men). The diet of the great apes consists of fruits and vegetation, with only small amounts of animal protein. It is likely that some hunting-and-gathering societies that subsist on traditional diets, primarily derived from fruits and vegetables with sporadic additions of fish and game, have SU levels approaching those of the great apes *(45)*.

4.3.1. FRUITS

According to a 1950 study of 12 people with gout, eating one-half pound of cherries or drinking an equivalent amount of cherry juice prevented attacks of gout. Black, sweet yellow, and red sour cherries were all effective *(46)*. Clinical case reports of three patients with gout showed that consumption of 227 g of cherry products daily for 3 days to 3 months reduced plasma urate to normal levels and alleviated attacks of gouty arthritis *(46)*. It is not known what compounds in cherries are responsible for these alleged actions. In an RCT *(47)*, cherries provoked a significant decrease in plasma urate over 5 hours post-dose, whereas the other fruits (grapes, strawberries, and kiwifruit) produced no change. These findings support the claim that consumption of cherry products may benefit individuals who suffer from high levels of SU and gout.

4.3.2. VEGETABLES

Tofu (soybean curd) is rich in protein, but most of the purines are lost during processing, and ingestion of tofu produces only a small rise of SU in both healthy individuals and gout sufferers *(48)*.

Lyu et al. *(25)* suggested that purines are not an important risk factor for hyperuricemia and gout because, in their study of Taiwanese vegetarians who eat mainly plant food and soybean products (a diet high in purines), the risk of developing hyperuricemia and gout was reduced. They concluded that food sources rich in dietary fiber, folate, and vitamin C, such as fruit and vegetables, protect against hyperuricemia and gout. An increased waist-to-hip ratio, which indicates central obesity, has a significant linear effect on gout occurrence, independent of BMI *(25)*. Neither total protein intake nor consumption of purine-rich vegetables was associated with an increased risk of gout. Men with the highest quintile of vegetable protein had a lower risk of gout compared with those with the lowest quintile (OR 0.73 *(37)*).

Another study compared the insulin-sensitivity indices between Chinese vegetarians and omnivores. The omnivores had higher SU levels than vegetarians. The vegetarians were more insulin sensitive than their omnivore counterparts. The degree of insulin sensitivity appeared to correlate with years on a vegetarian diet *(49)*.

The metabolic effects of diets high in vegetable protein were assessed by an RCT of wheat gluten on serum lipids and SU concentrations. The study found that high intakes of vegetable protein from gluten reduced oxidized LDLs, serum triglycerides, and SU levels *(50)*.

With respect to fatty acids, red blood cell omega-6 (n-6) polyunsaturated fatty acids (PUFAs) were independently associated with SU. n-6 PUFAs are mostly found in vegetables, while their content is fairly limited in meat products, which are the main sources of purines and saturated fatty acids *(51)*. Thus, it is plausible that subjects whose diet is mainly rich in vegetables will have lower SU and triglyceride levels and higher 6-PUFA levels than those who are preferential meat consumers.

One murine model study suggested that diets fortified with γ-linolenic acid (GLA) and eicosapentaenoic acid (EPA) decreased the inflammatory response induced by monosodium urate crystals. GLA is found in plant seed oils, such as flaxseed oil, and EPA is found in fish oils, such as salmon. It has not been studied whether humans who consume relatively high amounts of these oils have lower levels of SU or a lower incidence of gouty arthritis *(52)*.

4.4. High-Protein Diets

High-protein diets are associated with increased urinary uric acid excretion and may reduce the blood uric acid level *(53–55)*. It is suggested that a high-protein diet lowers triglycerides *(56)*, is satiating *(57,58)*, and promotes weight loss *(59)*. Increasing evidence supports the notion that it also may improve insulin sensitivity *(60)*.

One observational study followed gouty patients on a diet moderately decreased in calories and increased in protein *(61)*. Dietary changes included calorie restriction (to 1,600 calories per day), macronutrient modification (40% calories from carbohydrate, 30% from protein, and 30% from fat), replacement of refined carbohydrates (e.g., white flour, white rice) with complex ones (e.g., whole wheat flour, brown rice) and replacement of saturated fats (e.g., dairy fats, meat fat) with mono- and polyunsaturated ones (e.g., macadamia nuts, almonds, peanuts and peanut butter, olive oil, canola oil, and avocados). The mean SU decreased by 18% in gouty patients after 4 months of dietary intervention. This was accompanied by a 67% reduction in monthly gouty attack frequency. The authors suggested re-evaluation of the current dietary recommendations for patients with gout. They advocated limitation of carbohydrate intake, an increased proportional intake of protein, and the use of unsaturated fat, because these modifications all enhance insulin sensitivity and therefore, may promote a reduction in SU. They suggested that lowered insulin resistance could increase uric acid clearance from the renal tubule as a result of stimulation by insulin of tubular ion exchange *(61)*.

Forms of the latest popular diet programs include high-protein/high-fat/low-carbohydrate diets, such as Atkins™, South Beach™, and Zone™. In contrast to the American Heart Association's (AHA) recommendation that a diet should be composed of 50 to 60% carbohydrates, less than 30% fat and 12 to 18% protein (based on total daily caloric intake), the unmodified Atkins diet is composed of 5% carbohydrates, 60% fat, and 35% protein *(62)*. These diets encourage patients to take in foods that are rich in purine, such as meat and seafood, which have been associated with a higher risk of gout. Moreover, these diets are high in fat and can induce ketosis and subsequent hyperuricemia. The official Atkins Website *(63)* cautions patients about the potential flares of gout with the diet.

Unfortunately, to date, there are no controlled studies on the impact of these ketogenic diets on serum urate levels and frequency of gout flares. A major question is whether reduction in BMI by such diets outweighs the theoretical risk of induced ketosis in worsening hyperuricemia.

5. DIETARY SUPPLEMENTS

5.1. Herbs

Garlic (*Allium sativum*) has been widely used for gout and rheumatism. According to *Alternative Medicine: The Definitive Guide (64)*, there are general benefits from almost any type of garlic, be it raw or dried garlic, garlic oil, or a prepared commercial product. However, odorless or odor-controlled garlic preparations have a high degree of activity and may be more appropriate.

Autumn crocus (*Colchicum autumnale*) is the herb from which the drug colchicine was originally isolated. Colchicine, strong anti-inflammatory compound, is used as a conventional treatment for gout. Both the herb and the drug have significant toxicity.

5.2. Vitamin/Mineral Supplements

Large amounts of supplemental folic acid (up to 80 mgper day) have reduced SU levels in preliminary research *(65)*. However, other studies have failed to confirm the effectiveness of folic acid in treating gout *(66)*.

The effect of vitamin C on serum uric acid level was evaluated in a double-blind placebo-controlled study *(67)* of 184 participants who received either placebo or 500 mg per day of vitamin C for 2 months. Both groups had similar intakes of protein, purine-rich foods, and dairy products at baseline. The SU level, however, was lowered only in the vitamin C group. Among those who had hyperuricemia at baseline (SU >7 mg/dL), vitamin C supplementation resulted in a mean SU reduction of 1.5 mg/dL ($p = 0.0008$, adjusted for age, gender, and baseline SU and ascorbic acid level). It has been postulated that vitamin C may decrease SU by both increasing renal secretion and decreasing renal reabsorption of uric acid through competitive binding activities.

In one small study, people who took 4 g of vitamin C (but not lower amounts) had an increase in urinary excretion of uric acid within a few hours and those who took 8 g of vitamin C per day for several days had a reduction in SU levels *(68)*. Thus, supplemental vitamin C could, in theory, reduce the risk of gout attacks. However, the authors of this study warned that taking large amounts of vitamin C could also trigger an acute attack of gout by abruptly changing SU levels. Despite this concern, some doctors recommend vitamin C supplementation (sometimes starting with 1 g per day) as a method for reducing elevated SU levels.

6. ALCOHOL

"Gout attacks such old men indulging freely in high living, wine and other generous drinks, at length, from inactivity, the usual attendant of advanced life, have left off altogether the bodily exercises of their youth" (Thomas Sydenham).

The Dutch Nutritional Surveillance Study suggested that in men, higher consumption of alcohol was associated with increased SU levels *(35)*. The exact incidence of alcohol-induced gouty arthritis is not known, but it is estimated that half the gout sufferers drink excessively *(69)*. Hyperuricemia was found to be a significant correlate of alcohol abuse in an unselected group of men admitted to a general hospital *(70)*.

Consumption of alcohol, but not of purines, was found to be a significant dietary risk factor for gout *(25)*. In a 12-year cohort study using biannual questionnaires, the Health Professionals Follow-up Study found that even moderate regular consumption of beer was associated with a high risk of development of gout (multivariate relative risk of 1.49 per 12-oz beer serving per day *(71)*). Consumption of spirits was associated with a multivariate relative risk of incident gout of 1.15 per shot *(70)*. In contrast, moderate wine consumption of one to two glasses per day was not associated with significant change in the risk of incident gout *(71)*. Beer has a high purine content, predominantly as readily absorbable guanosine, and beer intake heightens urate production, compounding the stimulatory effects of alcohol metabolites on renal urate reabsorption. There have been no adequate direct comparisons of the effects of beer and wine on urate production and SU levels in this study *(71)*.

Beer ingestion causes an increase in the plasma concentrations and urinary excretion of hypoxanthine, xanthine, and uric acid *(72)*. Beer, unlike most other forms of alcohol, has a high content from malt of the readily absorbable purine guanosine, which can further increase uric acid production. These findings indicated that purines in the beer increased the production of uric acid, which resulted in increases in the plasma concentration and urinary excretion of uric acid. This problem is not avoided by the use of reduced-carbohydrate "light beer."

Another small study *(73)* noted differing effects of different types of alcohol on serum urate. Four gout patients were given regular beer, liquor (vodka with orange juice), nonalcoholic beer ,or orange juice on separate occasions. Patients were monitored for both serum and urine urate levels. The serum urate rose significantly only after the ingestion of regular beer. Additionally, both regular and nonalcoholic beer reduced the urinary excretion of urate.

A number of mechanisms have been implicated in the pathogenesis of alcohol-induced hyperuricemia. Acute alcohol excess may cause temporary lactic acidemia, reduced renal urate excretion, and hyperuricemia, whereas chronic alcohol intake stimulates purine production by accelerating the degradation of adenosine triphosphate to adenosine monophosphate via the conversion of acetate to acetyl-coenzyme A in the metabolism of alcohol *(69)*. Ethanol increases urate synthesis by enhancing the turnover of adenine nucleotides *(74)*. Additionally, people who binge tend to forget to take their urate-lowering drugs *(69)*.

IN SUMMARY

Dietary trends, increasing obesity and MetS prevalence are contributing to the increasing worldwide prevalence of hyperuricemia and gout. Before starting life-long urate-lowering drug therapy, it is important to identify and treat underlying disorders that may be contributing to hyperuricemia. It is also relevant to recognize the strong association of MetS (abdominal obesity, hypertension, dyslipidemia, raised serum insulin levels, and glucose intolerance) with hyperuricemia. An elevated SU level may serve as a surrogate marker of MetS.

Given the prognostic ramifications of MetS in terms of cardiovascular morbidity, dietary intervention is strongly recommended in these patients. Consumption of meat, seafood, and alcoholic beverages in moderation is useful. Restriction of alcoholic beverages plays a key role in the management of gout; a high intake of alcohol can result in refractoriness to urate-lowering effects of both allopurinol and uricosurics *(75)*. Moderation in the consumption of not only beer but also other forms of alcohol is essential. Moderate beer consumption is acceptable in most patients.

Patients with hyperuricemia need to pay attention to weight management, including moderation in the intake of meat and seafood rich in cholesterol and saturated fatty acids and restraint in consumption of foods and drinks with noncomplex carbohydrates. In the obese, controlled weight management and reduction in alcohol consumption have the potential to lower SU in a quantitatively similar way to relatively unpalatable "low-purine" diets. There is growing evidence that a low-energy, calorie-restricted, low-carbohydrate (40% of energy), high-protein (120 g per day or 30% of energy) diet, with unsaturated fat (30% of energy) and high dietary fiber, are more beneficial in terms of lowering SU, than the conventional low-purine diet, with its unlimited intake of carbohydrates and saturated fat *(8,75)*. Non-fat milk and low-fat yogurt also have a variety of health benefits. Dairy products may have clinically meaningful antihyperuricaemic effects. Unfortunately, only 20% of patients seeking medical care are ready to change unhealthy behavior, including hazardous alcohol use and unhealthy eating habits *(76)*. Further education and studies are needed to improve our understanding of dietary factors and hyperuricemia.

REFERENCES

1. Perez-Ruiz F, Calabozo M, Erauskin GG, Ruibal A, Herrero-Beites AM. Renal underexcretion of uric acid is present in patients with apparent high urinary uric acid output. Arthritis Rheum 2002;47: 610–613.
2. Tinahones FJ, Vazquez F, Soriguer FJ, Collantes E. Lipoproteins in patients with isolated hyperuricemia. Adv Exper Med Biol 1998;431:61–67.
3. Kersley GD. A short history of gout. In: Gutman AB, Fessel WJ, Hall AP, et al, eds. Gout: A Clinical Comprehensive. Medcom, New York, 1971, pp. 8–13.
4. Reaven GM. Role of insulin resistance in human disease. Diabetes 1988;37:1495–1607.
5. Reaven GM. Syndrome X: 6 years later. J. Internal Med 1994;236, 13–22.
6. DeFronzo RA, Ferrannini E. Insulin resistance. A multifaceted syndrome responsible for NIDDM, obesity, hypertension, dyslipidemia, and atherosclerotic cardiovascular disease. Diabetes Care 1991;14:173–194.
7. Reaven GM, Chen Y-DI, Jeppesen J, Maheux P, Krauss RM. Insulin resistance and hyperinsulinemia in individuals with small, dense, low density lipoprotein particles. J Clin Invest 1993;92:141–146.
8. Vuorinen-Markkola H, Yki-Jarvinen H. Hyperuricemia and insulin resistance. J Clin Endocrinol Metab 1994;78:25–29.
9. Lee J, Sparrow D, Vokonas PS, Landsberg L, Weiss ST. Uric acid and coronary heart disease risk: evidence for a role of uric acid in the obesity-insulin resistance syndrome. The Normative Aging Study. Am J Epidemiol 1995;142:288–294.
10. Tinahones JF. Perez-Lindon G. C-Soriguer FJ. Pareja A. Sanchez-Guijo P. Collantes E. Dietary alterations in plasma very low density lipoprotein levels modify renal excretion of urates in hyperuricemic-hypertriglyceridemic patients. J Clin Endocrinol Metab 1997;82:1188–1191.
11. Sunayama S, Watanabe Y, Daida H, Yamaguchi H. Thiazolidinediones, dyslipidaemia and insulin resistance syndrome. Curr Opin Lipidol 2000;11:397–402.
12. Tsunoda S, Kamide K, Minami J, Kawano Y. Decreases in serum uric acid by amelioration of insulin resistance in overweight hypertensive patients: effect of a low-energy diet and an insulin-sensitizing agent. Am J Hypertens 2002;15:697–701.
13. Fam AG. Gout, diet, and the insulin resistance syndrome. J Rheumatol 2002;29:1350–1355.
14. Flegal KM, Carroll MD, Ogden CL, Johnson CL. Prevalence and trends in obesity among US adults, 1999–2000. JAMA 2002;288:1723–1727.
15. Myers AR, Epstein FH, Dodge HJ, Mikkelsen WM. The relationship of serum uric acid to risk factors in coronary heart disease. Am J Med 1968;45:520–528.
16. Roubenoff R, Klag MJ, Mead LA, Liang KY, Seidler AJ, Hochberg MC. Incidence and risk factors for gout in white men. JAMA 1991;266:3004–3007.
17. Emmerson BT. The management of gout. N Engl J Med 1996;334:445–451.
18. Myers AR, Epstein FH, Dodge HJ, Mikkelsen WM. The relationship of serum uric acid to risk factors in coronary heart disease. Am J Med 1968;45:520–528.
19. Nicholls A, Scott JT. Effect of weight-loss on plasma and urinary levels of uric acid. Lancet 1972;2:1223–1224.
20. Campion EW, Glynn RJ, DeLabry LO. Asymptomatic hyperuricemia: risks and consequences in the Normative Aging Study. Am J Med 1987;82:421–426.
21. Roubenoff R. Gout and hyperuricemia. Rheum Dis Clin North Am 1990;16:539–550.

22. Choi HK, Atkinson K, Karlson EW, Curhan G. Obesity, weight change, hypertension, diuretic use, and risk of gout in men. Arch Intern Med 2005;165:742–748.
23. Choi H, Curhan G. Adiposity, hypertension, diuretic use and risk of incident gout in women: The Nurses Health Study. Arthritis Rheum 2005;52(suppl 9):S733.
24. Carey DGP. Abdominal obesity. Curr Opin Lipidol 1998;9:35–40.
25. Lyu LC, Hsu CY, Yeh CY, Lee MY, Huang SH, Chen CL. A case–control study of the association of diet and obesity with gout in Taiwan. Am J Clin Nutr 2003;78:690–701.
26. Feinstein El, Quion-Verde H, Kaptein EM, Massry SG. Severe hyperuricemia in patients with volume depletion. Am J Nephrol 1984;4:77–80.
27. Maclachlan MJ, Rodnan GP. Effects of food, fast and alcohol on serum uric acid and acute attacks of gout. Am J Med 1967;42:38–57.
28. Lennane GAQ, Rose BS, Isdale IC. Gout in the Maori. Ann Rheum Dis 1960;19:120–125.
29. Kagan A, Harris BR, Winkelstein W Jr, et al. Epidemiologic studies on coronary heart disease and stroke in Japanese men living in Japan, Hawaii and California: demographic, physical, dietary and biochemical characteristics. J Chronic Dis 1974;27:345–364.
30. Cassim B, Mody GM, Deenadayalu VK, Hammond MG. Gout in black South Africans: a clinical and genetic study. Ann Rheum Dis 1994;53:759–762.
31. Clifford AJ, Riumallo JA, Young VR, Scrimshaw NS. Effect of oral purines on serum and urinary uric acid of normal, hyperuricemic and gouty humans. J Nutr 1976;106:428–434.
32. Clifford AJ, Story DL. Levels of purines in foods and their metabolic effects in rats. J Nutr 1976;106:435–442.
33. Zollner N. Influence of various purines on uric acid metabolism. Bibl Nutr Dieta 1973;19:34–43.
34. Zollner N, Griebsch A. Diet and gout. Adv Exp Med Biol 1974;41:435–442.
35. Brule, D, Sarwar G, Savoie L. Changes in serum and urinary uric acid levels in normal human subjects fed purine-rich foods containing different amounts of adenine and hypoxanthine. J Am Coll Nutr 1992;11:353–358.
36. Gibson T, Rodgers AV, Simmonds HA, Court-Brown F, Todd E, Meilton V. A controlled study of diet in patients with gout. Ann Rheum Dis 1983;42:123–127.
37. Choi HK, Atkinson K, Karlson EW, Willett W, Curhan G. Purine-rich foods, dairy and protein intake, and the risk of gout in men. N Engl J Med 2004;350:1093–1103.
38. Griebsch A, Zollner N. Effect of ribomononucleotides given orally on uric acid production in man. Adv Exp Med Biol 1974;41:443–449.
39. Sarwar G, Brule D. Assessment of the uricogenic potential of processed foods based on the nature and quantity of dietary purines. Prog Food Nutr Sci. 1991;15:159–181.
40. Garrel DR, Verdy M, PetitClerc C, Martin C, Brule D, Hamet P. Milk- and soy-protein ingestion: acute effect on serum uric acid concentration. Am J Clin Nutr 1991;53:665–669.
41. Loenen HM, Eshuis H, Lowik MR, Schouten EG, Hulshof KF, Odink J, Kok FJ. Serum uric acid correlates in elderly men and women with special reference to body composition and dietary intake (Dutch Nutrition Surveillance System). J Clin Epidemiol 1990;43:1297–1303.
42. Choi H, Curhan G. Dairy consumption and risk of incident gout in women: the Nurses Health Study. Arthritis Rheum 2005;52(suppl 9):S101.
43. Ghadirian P, Shatenstein B, Verdy M, Hamet P. The influence of dairy products on plasma uric acid in women. Eur J Epidemiol 1995;11:275–281.
44. Takahashi S, Yamamoto T, Moriwaki Y, Tsutsumi Z, Yamakita J, Higashino K. Decreased serum concentrations of 1,25(OH)2-vitamin D_3 in patients with gout. Metabolism 1998;47:336–338.
45. Blau LW. Cherry diet control for gout and arthritis. Tex Rep Biol Med 1950;8:309–311.
46. Johnson RJ, Rideout BA. Uric acid and diet-insights into the epidemic of cardiovascular disease. N Eng J Med 2004;350:1071–1073.
47. Jacob RA, Spinozzi GM, Simon VA, et al. Consumption of cherries lowers plasma urate in healthy women. J Nutr 2003;133:1826–1829.
48. Yamakita J, Yamamoto T, Moriwaki Y, Takahashi S, Tsutsumi Z, Higashino K. Effect of tofu (bean curd) ingestion and on uric acid metabolism in healthy and gouty subjects. Adv Exp Med Biol 1998;431:839–842.

49. Kuo CS, Lai NS, Ho LT, Lin CL. Insulin sensitivity in Chinese ovo-lactovegetarians compared with omnivores. Eur J Clin Nutr 2004;58:312–316.
50. Jenkins DJ, Kendall CW, Vidgen E, et al. High-protein diets in hyperlipidemia: effect of wheat gluten on serum lipids, uric acid, and renal function. AM J Clin Nutr 2001;74:57–63.
51. Ulbricht TLV, Southgate DAT. Coronary heat disease: seven dietary factors. Lancet 1991;338: 985–892.
52. Tate GA, Mandell BF, Karmali RA, et al. Suppression of monosodium urate crystal-induced acute inflammation by diets enriched with gamma-linolenic acid and eicosapentaenoic acid. Arthritis Rheum 1988;31:1543–1551.
53. Waslien CI, Calloway DH, Margen S. Uric acid production of men fed graded amounts of egg protein and yeast nucleic acid. Am J Clin Nutr 1968;21:892–897.
54. Lewis HB, Doisy EA. Studies in uric acid metabolism. I. The influence of high protein diets on the endogenous uric acid elimination. J Biol Chem 1918;36:1–7.
55. Raiziss GW, Dubin H, Ringer AI. Studies in endogenous uric acid metabolism. J Biol Chem 1914;19:473–485.
56. Wolfe BM, Piche LA. Replacement of carbohydrate by protein in a conventional-fat diet reduces cholesterol and triglyceride concentrations in healthy normolipidemic subjects. Clin Invest Med 1999;22:140–148.
57. Porrini M, Santangelo A, Crovetti R, Riso P, Testolin G, Blundell JE. Weight, protein, fat, and timing of preloads affect food intake. Physiol Behav 1997;62:563–70.
58. Crovetti R, Porrini M, Santangelo A, Testolin G. The influence of thermic effect of food on satiety. Eur J Clin Nutr 1998;52:482–488.
59. Skov AR, Toubro S, Ronn B, Holm L, Astrup, A. Randomized trial on protein vs carbohydrate in ad libitum fat reduced diet for the treatment of obesity. Int J Obes Relat Metab Disord 1999;23: 528–536.
60. Reaven GM. Do high carbohydrate diets prevent the development or attenuate the manifestations (or both) of syndrome X? A viewpoint strongly against. Curr Opin Lipidol 1997;8:23–27.
61. Dessein PH, Shipton EA, Stanwix AE, Joffe BI, Ramokgadi J. Beneficial effects of weight loss associated with moderate calorie/carbohydrate restriction, and increased proportional intake of protein and unsaturated fat on serum urate and lipoprotein levels in gout: a pilot study. Ann Rheum Dis 2000;59:539–543.
62. Blackburn GL, Phillips JCC, Morreale S. Physician's guide to popular low-carbohydrate weight-loss diets. Cleve Clin J Med 2001;68:761, 765–766, 768–769, 773–774.
63. www.atkins.com
64. Burton Goldberg Group. Alternative Medicine: The Definitive Guide. Future Medicine Publishing Co., Puyallup, WA, 1994.
65. Oster KA. Xanthine oxidase and folic acid. Ann Intern Med 1977;87:252–253.
66. Huang HY, Appel LJ, Choi MJ, et al. The effects of vitamin C supplementation on serum concentrations of uric acid. Arthritis Rheum 2005;52:1843–1847.
67. Boss GR, Ragsdale RA, Zettner A, Seegmiller JE. Failure of folic acid (pteroylglutamic acid) to affect hyperuricemia. J Lab Clin Med 1980;96:783–789.
68. Stein HB, Hasan A, Fox IH. Ascorbic acid-induced uricosuria: a consequence of megavitamin therapy. Ann Intern Med 1976;84:385–388.
69. Sharpe CR. A case–control study of alcohol consumption and drinking behavior in patients with acute gout. Can Med Assoc J 1984;131:563–567.
70. Drum DE, Goldman PA, Jankowski CB. Elevation of serum uric acid as a clue to alcohol abuse. Arch Intern Med 1981;141:477–479.
71. Choi HK, Atkinson K, Karlson EW, Willett W, Curhan G. Alcohol intake and risk of incident gout in men: a prospective study. Lancet. 2004;363:1277–1281.
72. Eastmond CJ, Garton M, Robins S, Riddoch S. The effects of alcoholic beverages on urate metabolism in gout sufferers. Br J Rheumatol 1995;34:756–759.
73. Yamamoto T, Moriwaki Y, Ka T, et al. Effect of sauna bathing and beer ingestion on plasma concentrations of purine bases. Metabolism: Clin Exper 2004;53:772–776.

74. Faller J, Fox IH. Ethanol-induced hyperuricemia: evidence for increased urate production by activation of adenine nucleotide turnover. N Engl J Med 1982;307:1598–1602.
75. Ralston SH, Capell HA, Sturrock RD. Alcohol and response to treatment of gout. BMJ 1988;296: 1641–1642.
76. Levinson W, Cohen MS, Brady D, Duffy FD. To change or not to change: "Sounds like you have a dilemma." Ann Intern Med 2001;135:386–391.

11 Fibromyalgia and Diet

Osmo Hänninen and Anna-Lissa Rauma

Summary

- The pathophysiology of fibromyalgia is not known. Its prevalence is approx 3 to 5%. Females are affected more often than males.
- The most pathogenomic features are multiple bilateral tender points. The other symptoms include chronic pain, sleep disturbances, and fatigue, which may lead to psychological distress.
- Fibromyalgia symptoms and time course are individually variable.
- Gastrointestinal symptoms may also occur, and circulatory disturbances in the brain have been described.
- There is no special therapeutic diet for this disease. All patients with rheumatoid diseases may have nutritional deficiencies. Vegan diets may be helpful for pain relief and modification in fibromyalgia. Physical activity helps maintain proper food intake and rest.

Key Words: Brain metabolism; dietary supplements; gut microflora; vegan diets; vitamins

1. INTRODUCTION

The pathophysiology of rheumatoid diseases is still only partially known [1]; in fibromyalgia, it is even more so. Some 3 to 5% of the population has fibromyalgia. Most of the patients are females who develop the illness between 40 and 60 years of age [2]. The incidence increases with advancing age. Actually, fibromyalgia is more common than rheumatoid arthritis (RA [1]). The symptoms of fibromyalgia include chronic burning or gnawing pain, multiple tender points, sleep disturbances, and fatigue. The tender points are located in the muscle insertions at both sides of the body [3]. No clear structural abnormalities have been found in their biopsies and no inflammation can be detected [4]. Gastrointestinal (GI) symptoms may also occur, and circulatory disturbances in the brain have been described [1]. Pain and fatigue often lead to psychological disturbances and depression is a common problem. Fibromyalgia symptoms are individually variable. During pregnancy, the symptoms may, however, be alleviated. There seems to be a familiar component in fibromyalgia. Approximately every second patient attributes the onset of symptoms to an injury, infection, or other stress [4,5].

Unfortunately there is no "gold standard" in the diagnosis of fibromyalgia. The individual course of symptoms is variable, which also makes the diagnosis difficult.

From: *Nutrition and Health: Nutrition and Rheumatic Disease*
Edited by: L. A. Coleman © Humana Press, Totowa, NJ

Nine (previously 7) bilateral and now 18 tender points found in characteristic locations are the key findings in the diagnosis *(3,6)*. If the tenderness in palpation of at least 11 of these is found in a patient whose diffuse musculoskeletal pains have lasted at least 3 months, then the fibromyalgia diagnosis can be made. Fibromyalgia as a diagnostic entity is, unfortunately, poorly known by many practicing physicians *(4)*, and as a result, it may take a long time before the diagnosis is made. Simply identifying the diagnosis helps significantly in alleviating the patient's suffering by assuring the patient that this disease is not dangerous, despite the suffering and the limited ability to work that it causes. Patients should be encouraged to continue working because it has been shown that when they stop working, their symptoms seem to worsen *(4)*.

As a nutritional approach for the treatment of rheumatoid diseases in general is poorly understood, it is easy to understand that the dietary treatment of fibromyalgia in particular is also not known. In all chronic diseases, nutritional status tends, however, to be altered and physical activity tends to be depressed. The rheumatoid diseases are no exception *(7)*. The first course of action should always be the correction of nutritional deficits, and only then should drug treatment be considered. Often, patients have tried a variety of drug treatments themselves, albeit with limited success. The regulation of food intake is a multifaceted problem. Many drugs may interfere with the normal regulation of food intake, which exacerbates the effect of the disease, per se, on nutritional status *(8)*.

There is no special therapeutic diet for fibromyalgia. Instead, patients are advised to eliminate or supplement their diet depending on their symptoms. Typically, patients with fibromyalgia have looked for alleviation of their symptoms by using different kinds of vegetarian diets or having specific "remedy" foods or supplements such as herbs, wheatgrass juice, or purified antioxidants.

Theories on the pathophysiology of fibromyalgia have included alterations in neurotransmitter regulation (especially serotonin); hormonal control problems (especially of the hypothalamic–pituitary–adrenal and growth hormone axes); immune system dysfunction; problems in sleep physiology; abnormal perception of bodily sensations; stress; viral pathologies; local hypoxia; and disturbances in muscle microcirculation, adenosine monophosphate, and creatinine concentrations. Current evidence most strongly supports a neurochemical or neurohormonal hypothesis *(1,9)*.

The following sections focus on the brain functions, followed by nutritional interventions for patients with fibromyalgia, especially vegan and vegetarian approaches. We also discuss the possible roles of antioxidants and gut flora.

2. PATHOPHYSIOLOGY OF FIBROMYALGIA

Despite of the symptoms, the findings in the tender points and muscles have been minor in fibromyalgia *(1,4)*. Therefore, at present more attention is being directed to the central nervous system (CNS) and its role in pain perception. Metabolism and blood circulation in the CNS are both high. The CNS contributes to the regulation of most body functions, making it easy to understand that adequacy of vitamins and minerals (i.e., the cofactors) is essential. Furthermore, the CNS is high in lipid content; approx 50% of the fatty acids are unsaturated (n-3 series) that are found in fish oil *(10)*. If an adequate intake is not achieved, various symptoms including fatigue and depression as well as abnormal pain sensation can be expected.

Patients with fibromyalgia have lowered blood circulation in the pain-sensitive areas of their brains, which may be the origin of several symptoms reported, including pain and fatigue *(11)*. Pain signals reach the consciousness only when the signals are handled in the brain. Therefore, the pain affects many functions of the CNS. Patients with fibromyalgia have exaggerated pain responses to various stimuli and show allodynia (i.e., signals that normally do not cause pain, cause it now *(4)*). Substance P is one of the chemicals related to pain sensation. Patients with fibromyalgia have higher Substance P levels. Massage may be helpful in lowering its levels *(12)*. The autonomic nervous system shows higher activity of the sympathetic component, and blocking of these fibers alleviates the pain sensation in patients. As one can expect, pain causes poor sleep quality *(12)*, which is one of the most common problems reported in fibromyalgia.

Serotonin, norepinephrine, and corticotrophin-releasing hormone are examples of hormones that have a role in fatigue, pain, sleep, and also in mood. Serotonin levels are low in the CNS in fibromyalgia. All of the hormones mentioned are amino acid derivatives. Serotonin itself is synthesized from tryptophan. Schwarz et al. *(13)* have provided evidence for altered tryptophan metabolism in fibromyalgia. Excessive serotonin levels are not desirable either, however, because serotonin causes vasoconstriction, as in migraine headaches *(14)*.

Blood platelets share some properties of neurons and therefore, they can be used as a model for studying fibromyalgia. A significant increase in benzodiazepine receptors occurs in platelet membranes of patients affected by primary fibromyalgia, and this seems to be related to the severity of fibromyalgic symptoms *(15)*.

Patients with fibromyalgia also have lower growth hormone (GH) levels than healthy controls *(16)*, and its administration may alleviate the symptoms. GH is released from the hypothalamus; the hypothalamus regulates the release of GH in the hypophysis and the hormones, in turn, regulate the functions of many glands (i.e., the adrenal gland). Patients with fibromyalgia have some similarities with subjects whose glucocorticoid administration has been withdrawn in that both cause fatigue, sleep disturbances, and pain.

Persistent pain and poor sleep quantity and quality make it easy to understand the feeling of fatigue. A vicious cycle is created whereby fatigue leads to reduced physical activity and poor appetite, which then further exacerbate feelings of fatigue and lethargy. It has been shown that fibromyalgia symptoms are alleviated by exercise and physical therapy *(4)*. Nutrition therapy can be helpful by promoting physical activity, which creates a positive feedback loop and reduces symptoms.

At present, no effective drug therapy is available for fibromyalgia. Therefore, patients with fibromyalgia tend to search for help from alternative and complementary methods, including herbal remedies. Alcohol and caffeine are not effective remedies in fibromyalgia.

Chronic fatigue syndrome is a related, and common, problem *(4)*. In chronic fatigue syndrome, subjects complain of muscle and joint pain, headache, tender lymph nodes, poor sleep, and several other symptoms similar to those that occur in fibromyalgia. Actually, both conditions can exist simultaneously. The discussion here may thus be helpful in chronic fatigue syndrome, too.

3. NUTRITION AND FIBROMYALGIA

In all chronic diseases, nutrition seems to be affected. This can be expected in fibromyalgia, too. The aim of nutrition therapy in rheumatoid diseases is to maintain optimal nutritional status. This can be achieved by following recommendations on healthy eating. Supplements may also be needed to speed up the correction.

There is no special therapeutic diet for fibromyalgia. Instead, patients are advised to eliminate or supplement the diet depending on their symptoms. Commonly, it is advised that patients avoid gas-forming foodstuffs such as onions, cabbage, pulses, or carbonated drinks, and increase the consumption of fiber-rich foods such as roots and vegetables, whole-grain products, bran, linseeds, plums, and fruits because of obstipation. It is also recommended to consume adequate liquids and to participate in exercises *(17,18)*. Balanced nutrition promotes the intake of all necessary nutrients and no supplementation is needed. However, if some basic items such as fish are not preferred, patients can be encouraged to consume fish oil as preparations.

Because in many cases medication is not effective enough to relieve the symptoms, one can try to relieve them either by using the elimination diet or supplementing the diet. Elimination diets are used in order to avoid substances that possibly increase the inflammation, whereas the beneficial effect of certain food supplements are thought to result from their ability to decrease inflammation. Consequently, it is typical that patients with rheumatoid diseases try various forms of alternative therapy or dietary manipulation in order to relieve their pain.

3.1. Vegetarian Diets

Vegetarianism includes a wide variety of eating patterns, and today there is widespread dissemination of information demonstrating that appropriately planned plant-rich omnivorous diets and plant-based lactovegetarian and semi-vegetarian diets are equally successful in promoting health. Plant-only diets, without nutrient fortification, do not necessarily promote health, because they often do not supply adequate amounts of energy and essential nutrients, such as vitamin B_{12}, vitamin D, calcium, and iron. The positive physiological health consequences of vegetarian diets include the high body antioxidant capacity owing to dietary antioxidants such as vitamins C and E, and β-carotene, avoidance of overweight, low blood pressure, and low serum glucose and cholesterol levels, and positively changed microflora in the colon *(19)*, which are discussed later in this chapter.

The health-promoting effects of plant foods are thought to be to the result of various compounds found in them, only some of which are nutrients in the classic sense. The mechanisms of action include several physiological processes such as their antioxidant effect, modulation of biotransformation enzymes, changes in colon microflora, and alteration of hormone metabolism, to name a few.

Consumption of a vegetarian diet is a typical alternative therapy among patients with rheumatoid diseases, including patients with fibromyalgia. Fasting has also been used because it may decrease inflammation owing to energy deprivation. There are two studies where the effects of vegan and lactovegetarian diets on rheumatoid disease have been studied *(20,21)*, and two raw-food dietary interventions conducted on patients with fibromyalgia *(22,23)*. In all of these studies, there have been patients who have both subjectively and objectively benefited from a vegetarian regimen.

Administration of dietary supplements including eicosapentaenic acid (EPA *(24–28)*, *Chlorella pyrenoidosa (29)*, and γ-linolenic acid *(30)* has also resulted in positive responses in some patients with rheumatoid diseases. The possible mechanisms behind these treatments have been suggested to be of neurological, immunological, and/or hormonal of origin *(9,17,18,29)*. Some supplements have been shown to nonspecifically inhibit inflammation *(29)*, so benefits are not limited to patients with fibromyalgia.

3.1.1. Raw-Food Diets and Dietary Supplements in Fibromyalgia

We have been studying in detail an extreme type of vegan diet called the living food diet (LFD). Our studies are based on a series of clinical trials conducted among healthy subjects *(31–33)*, patients with RA *(34)* and patients with fibromyalgia *(22)*. Some studies have been conducted on long-term users of the LFD *(35–37)*. Additionally, we have also conducted analyses of several LFD items. The research interest has varied from the nutrient content to the possible therapeutic effects of the diet. Some of the interest in the LFD regimen has been owing to its antioxidant properties and its effects on the colon microflora.

The LFD consists of germinated seeds, cereals, sprouts, vegetables, fruits, and berries *(33)*; Table 1). Some items are fermented, and therefore the LFD is high in lactobacilli content. The diet contains dietary fiber in amounts up to 80 g per day. The diet is very low in sodium content and contains no cholesterol. Food items such as berries and wheat grass juice are rich in antioxidants including carotenoids and flavonoids *(38)*. For example, cranberry, bog whortleberry, lingonberry, black currant, and crowberry have total contents of flavonols quercetin, kaempherol, and myricetin of 100 to 263 mg/kg, which is higher than that of the common fruits and vegetables, except onions and broccoli *(39)*.

The first intervention conducted on patients with rheumatoid diseases *(7,21)* as well as the other one on patients with fibromyalgia *(22)* revealed that Finnish rheumatoid patients' energy and some nutrient intakes were below the recommended levels of intake. Patients with rheumatoid disease ($n = 43$) consumed less than recommended amounts of iron, zinc, and niacin *(7)* and patients with fibromyalgia ($n = 29$) consumed less carbohydrate (E-%), fiber, vitamin D, iron, potassium, calcium, and copper *(40)*. The amount and quality of fat also did not meet the recommendations.

Dietary modification among patients with fibromyalgia led to an increased intake of vegetables, fruits, and berries such that twice the amount consumed on a mixed diet was achieved *(40)*. On an LFD, patients received less saturated and more unsaturated fat. There was no change in the total intake of energy, but the proportion of energy from carbohydrates was higher and that from protein lower during the intervention. The LFD also provided significantly more fiber, β-carotene, vitamins C, B_1, B_6, iron, and copper, and significantly less cholesterol, vitamins D and B_{12}, iodine, selenium, and sodium chloride *(40)*.

Consequently, from the nutritional point of view, patients benefited from the LFD. The LFD had positive effects on serum lipids, which may also be helpful to some patients with fibromyalgia *(31,41)*. Furthermore, patients achieved a remarkable weight reduction. There was significant reduction in body mass index in both studies.

Table 1
Food Intake (Grams per Day) by the Female Vegans and Their Matched Controls, mean±SD (mean-max)

	Vegans (n = 20)	Controls (n = 20)
Cereal products	263±189 (22–1029)	167±53 (73–254)
Whole-meal bread	2±5*** (0–17)	60±36 (0–118)
Wheat bread	0***	16±18 (0–60)
Other cereal products[a]	261±290* (23–1029)	91±53 (17–241)
Vegetables and roots	676±207*** (398–1099)	258±112 (43–512)
Potato	7±15*** (0–57)	60±41 (0–156)
Root crops	207±132*** (6–549)	57±65 (0–300)
Vegetables	224±103** (77–487)	122± 75(8–286)
Pulses and nuts	169±68*** (60–330)	11±17 (0–74)
Mushrooms	8±13 (0–44)	3±5 (0–21)
Vegetable products[b]	61±47*** (0–162)	6±6 (0–19)
Fruits and Berries	579±290** (276–1588)	259±242 (0–1069)
Fruits	479±246*** (214–1314)	205±143 (0–544)
Berries	99±76** (0–274)	33±109 (0–544)
Jam and juices	1±3** (0–12)	21±54 (0–247)
Fats and oils	4±7*** (0–25)	37±17 (20–71)
Butter	0.2±0.6*** (0–2)	8±6 (0–20)
Margarine	0.7±2*** (0–8)	16±13 (2–53)
Vegetable oils	2±4* (0–14)	5±4 (0–14)
Other fats	0.8±13** (0–10)	7±9 (0–34)

Wilcoxon test for matched pairs (*** $p < 0.001$, ** $p < 0.01$, * $p < 0.05$)
[a]Including sprouted wheat, rice, and macaroni
[b]Including (e.g., soy sauce and vegetable foodstuffs)
From reference (33).

Vitamin B_{12} intake was compromised (36), and the iodine status was variable in some long-term users of the LFD (35), so attention must be given to these nutrients. In addition, Ågren et al. (37) reported significantly lower proportions of EPA and docohexaenoic acid (DHA) in the erythrocytes, platelets, and serum lipids of living-food eaters.

In both studies, subjects in the intervention groups ate living food for 3 months, wheras the control patients continued on their omnivorous diet. The fibromyalgia intervention was an open, nonrandomized controlled study that presumably helped patients to follow the diet more strictly and longer compared with the rheumatoid study where patients were randomized. The therapeutic effect of the LFD was recorded in both studies. The patients with RA eating the LFD reported amelioration of their pain ($p = 0.03$), swelling of joints ($p = 0.003$), and morning stiffness ($p = 0.0008$), which all worsened after finishing the LFD. The composite indices of objective measures also showed improvement of the patients with RA during the intervention (34). In fibromyalgia-intervention patients, joint stiffness ($p = 0.001$), pain (visual analog scale; $p = 0.003$), the quality of sleep ($p = 0.0001$), the Health Assessment questionnaire (HAQ; $p = 0.03$), and general health Questionnaire (GHQ; $p = 0.021$) all improved (22).

Donaldson and co-workers have also *(23)* studied the effects of a raw-food diet on patients with fibromyalgia. In their intervention study, 30 subjects were eating mostly raw salads, carrot juice, tubers, grain products, nuts, seeds, and dehydrated barley grass juice products for 2 to 4 months. The fibromyalgia impact questionnaire score was reduced by 46%, from 51 to 28 ($n = 20$). The quality-of-life survey score rose highly significantly ($n = 20$). Significant improvements were seen in shoulder pain at rest and after motion, abduction range of motion of shoulder, flexibility, and in the 6-minute walk. Of the whole group, 19 subjects were responders who showed significant improvement on all measured outcomes, whereas rest did not benefit from the diet. The authors concluded that many patients with fibromyalgia can be helped by a mostly raw vegetarian diet. If these two studies are compared, one probably significant difference has been the content of lactobacilli in the intervention diet. Lactobacilli seem to have a significant role according to our studies *(42)*.

The results of a small pilot study in 18 patients with fibromyalgia *(29)* suggested that the addition of *Chlorella pyrenoidosa* to their diet produced a significant reduction in pain after only 2 months. Almost 50% of the patients expressed that some of their other symptoms had improved. The principal health components in *Chlorella pyrenoidosa* are thought to be chlorophyll, β-carotene and chlorella growth factor (CGF). Presumably, the healing takes place because of its capacity to nonspecifically enhance immunological reactions *(29)*. *C. pyrenoidosa* is an algae and can be found as purified in chlorella tablets.

In another small case study ($N = 4$) the elimination of monosodium glutamate (MSG) and other excitotoxins, such as aspartame, from the diets of patients with fibromyalgia resulted in a dramatic recovery. Based on their study, Smith et al. *(9)* suggest that there might be a subgroup of patients with fibromyalgia who are sensitive to MSG and these patients need to be identified by physicians and other health care providers in order to initiate appropriate dietary adjustments that may lead to significant improvements of symptoms. However, identification of similar patients and much more research must be performed before definitive conclusions concerning causation can be made.

3.1.2. Antioxidants

Human metabolism is based on the consumption of oxygen and the aerobic production of energy-rich compounds like adenosine triphosphate (ATP), which drives metabolic reactions by hydrolysis. The oxygen consumption produces intermediates which are reactive (i.e., reactive oxygen species [ROS]). They are also released by neutrophils and macrophages when they fight against bacteria and other agents causing inflammation. Although in RA, inflammation is a significant source of symptoms, in fibromyalgia it is not.

Plants are an important source of antioxidants. They receive high amounts of exposure to ultraviolet light that generates radicals in tissues. Furthermore, during photosynthesis, oxygen *in statu nascendi* is generated in their chloroplasts. When the plants are oxidizing nutrients, their mitochondria are releasing oxygen-derived radicals, as do animal cells. This means that the plants must be very well prepared to meet the challenges of the radical-induced stress. The plants contain, therefore, a broad variety of antioxidant chemicals in addition to the enzymes catalysing their interaction. The plants must also defend themselves against the attacks of microorganisms and animals, and in order to do so, they use radicals. Oxygen-derived radicals are part of life in all aerobic organisms, humans included.

Measurements of antioxidant levels in vegetarians show that a vegetarian diet maintains higher antioxidant vitamin status (vitamins C and E and β-carotene) but variable antioxidant trace element status as compared with an omnivorous diet *(43)*. In our study, the calculated dietary antioxidant intakes by the long-term users of the LFD ($N = 21$), expressed as percentages of the U.S. Recommended Dietary Allowances, were as follows: 305% vitamin C, 247% vitamin A, 313% vitamin E, 92% zinc, 120% copper, but only 49% selenium. Consequently, compared with the matched omnivores, the living-food eaters had significantly higher blood concentrations of β-carotene and vitamins C and E, as well as higher erythrocyte superoxide dismutase activity *(38)*. Intervention on patients with fibromyalgia also showed that an LFD provided significantly more β-carotene, vitamin C, and copper *(40)*.

On an LFD, antioxidants come from cereals, fruits, berries, and vegetables. A good individual source is also a wheatgrass juice, which contains a lot of lycopene and β-carotene. In our study *(38)* we found that some long-term vegans had serum β-carotene concentrations exceeding those achieved by supplementation with 20 to 30 mg pure β-carotene. The mean dietary intake of β-carotene was 11.9 mg (1.3–29) per day. In Donaldson's et al. *(23)* study, patients with fibromyalgia consumed even more β-carotene per day (52 mg) from the carrot juice, which they consumed daily (480–960 mL). LFD patients show uniquely high-serum patterns of lutein and xanthines *(39)*.

3.1.3. INTESTINAL MICROFLORA

Fibromyalgia is not an infectious disease. The GI problems in fibromyalgia are not caused by microbial infection *(4)*. The GI tract carries out digestion, which is necessary for the absorption of nutrients. Additionally, it houses a rich microflora environment that carries out valuable tasks (e.g., breaking down dietary fiber *(44)*, but it also produces toxic components such as phenol and cresols. The intestinal microflora changes depending on the diet *(32)*. In our study on patients with rheumatoid disease, we found a correlation between the change in colon microflora and the therapeutic effect of the diet. A greater change in the colon microflora was associated with a greater reduction in symptoms *(42)*.

Plant fibers serve as substrates for the synthesis of lignans and other polyphenols in gut bacteria. A number of these compounds have weak estrogenic activity *(45)*. It is known that some patients with fibromyalgia experience an alleviation of their symptoms during pregnancy *(4)*. Pregnancy causes extensive systemic exposure to steroid hormones. The alleviation and altered nature of the pain during an LFD intervention providing plant estrogenic-acting compounds, and the response, may perhaps be partially explained in this way.

4. DISCUSSION

There are only few dietary studies conducted on patients with fibromyalgia *(9,22,23, 29)*. There is obviously a need for more such studies. Based on our data *(7,40)* we see that patients with fibromyalgia, similarly to the other patients with rheumatoid disease, have nutritional deficiencies that can be overcome by increasing the consumption of foods of vegetarian origin such as whole-grain products, vegetables, fruits, and berries. Refereed studies also show that rheumatic symptoms can be relieved by consuming supplements containing EPA *(24–28)*. Based on our study *(22)* and that of Donaldson et al. *(23)* we see that raw vegan diets can be helpful in the treatment of fibromyalgia at least in some patients with fibromyalgia.

We cannot, however, identify the food item or nutrient behind this response. Some typical common features in these vegan diets can be, however, described. For example, the low energy intake, the high intake of antioxidants, especially β-carotene, and the high intake of chlorophyll-containing wheat grass juice are common features. Additionally, in our study we found a correlation between the change in the colon microflora and the therapeutic effect of the diet *(42)*. Consumption of an LFD contains several benefits, however, its consumption over the long term may also have some negative consequences in terms of nutritional status. The supply of vitamin B_{12} is insufficient and because the diet does not contain animal products, the intake of EPA and DHA is reduced; both of these nutrients are known to be important for brain health. Furthermore, even if the vegan diets may be helpful in intervention studies, their practical use is unclear as no, or limited, commercial support systems are available at present.

Based on the literature and our own studies, we have summarized our dietary recommendations for fibromyalgia..

5. DIETARY RECOMMENDATIONS IN FIBROMYALGIA

Practitioners should check the nutritional status of all patients with fibromyalgia and recommend the following advice to their patients:

1. Follow a balanced diet.
2. If you cannot consume adequate amounts of ordinary food, use nutritive preparations in order to maintain good nutritional status.
3. Increase the consumption of foods of plant origin such as cereals, vegetables, roots, fruits, and berries.
4. If following a vegetarian diet, ensure that the intake of all nutrients and energy is adequate.
5. Use dietary supplementation only if it is necessary because of inadequate nutrient status.
6. Consume fish regularly.
7. An LFD cannot be recommended without the additional use of dietary supplementation (vitamins B_{12} and D, calcium, and in some circumstances also with iron). Also fish-oil supplementation is recommended.
8. Food allergies are not uncommon, and they must be kept in mind.

In dietary supplementation remember:

1. Before starting supplementing make sure that you need the nutrient.
2. If supplementation is warranted, use the supplement regularly.
3. Do not supplement the same nutrient from two different preparations.
4. Follow the instructions.

5. Tell your physicians about the supplement.
6. Take care that while consuming the supplement you still follow a healthy diet. Supplements do not replace a balanced diet.

REFERENCES

1. McCance KL, Mourad LA. Alterations of musculoskeletal function. In: Huether SE, McCance KL, eds. Understanding Pathophysiology 2nd ed. Mosby, St. Louis, MO, 2000, pp. 1031–1074.
2. Wolfe F. The clinical syndrome fibrositis. Am J Med 1986:81(suppl 3A);7–14.
3. Smythe H. Tender points: evolution of concepts of the fibrositis/fibtromyalgia syndrome. Am J Med 1986:81(suppl 3A):2–6.
4. Goldenberg DL. Fibromyalgia, a Comprehensive Guide Based on Over 20 Years of Clinical Research. A Leading Expert's Guide to Understanding and Getting Relief from the Pain Thanks Won't Go Away. The Berkley Publishing Group, Penguin Putnam Inc., New York, 2002, pp. 1–244.
5. Goldenberg DL Fibromylagia syndrome. An emerging but controversial condition. JAMA 1987:257:2782–2787.
6. Wolfe F, Smythe HA, Yunus MB, et al. The American College of Rheumatology 1990 Criteria for the Classification of Fibromyalgia. Report of the Multicenter Criteria Committee. Arthritis Rheum 1990;33(2):160–172.
7. Rauma AL, Nenonen M, Helve T, Hänninen O. Effect of a strict vegan diet on energy and nutrient intakes by Finnish rheumatoid patients. Eur J Clin Nutr 1993:47,747–749.
8. Halford JC, Cooper GD, Dovey TM. The pharmacology of human appetite expression. Curr Drug Targets 2004;5(3):221–240. Review.
9. Smith JD, Terpening CM, Schmidt SOF, Gums J. Relief of fibromyalgia symptoms following discontinuation of dietary excitoxins. Ann Pharmacol 2001;35:702–706.
10. Salvati S, Attorri L, Di Benedetto R, Di Biase A, Leonardi F. Polyunsaturated fatty acids and neurological diseases. Mini Rev Med Chem 2006;6(11):1201–1211. Review.
11. Kwiatek R, Barnden L, Tedman R, et al. Regional cerebral blood flow in fibromyalgia: single-photon-emission computed tomography evidence of reduction in the pontine tegmentum and thalami. Arthritis Rheum 2000;43(12):2823–2833.
12. Field T, Diego M, Cullen C, Hernandez-Reif M, Sunshine W, Douglas S. Fibromyalgia pain and substance P decrease and sleep improves after massage therapy. J Clin Rheumatol 2002;8(2):72–76.
13. Schwarz MJ, Offenbaecher M, Neumeister A, et al. Evidence for an altered tryptophan metabolism in fibromyalgia. Neurobiol Dis 2002;11(3):434–442.
14. Singhal AB, Caviness VS, Begleiter AF, Mark EJ, Rordorf G, Koroshetz WJ. Cerebral vasoconstriction and stroke after use of serotonergic drugs. Neurology 2002;58(1):130–133.
15. Bazzichi L, Giannaccini G, Betti L, et al. Peripheral benzodiazepine receptors on platelets of fibromyalgic patients. Clin Biochem 2006 Jul 13 [Epub ahead of print].
16. Jones KD, Deodhar P, Lorentzen A, Bennett RM, Deodhar AA. Growth hormone perturbations in fibromyalgia: a review. Semin Arthritis Rheum 2007 Jan 12 [Epub ahead of print].
17. Buchanan, HM, Preston SJ, Brooks PM, Buchanan WW. Is diet important in rheumatoid arthritis? Br J Rhematol 1991;30:125–134.
18. Darlington LG, Ramsey WR. Review of dietary therapy for rheumatoid arthritis. Br J Rheumatol 1993;32;507–514.
19. Rauma A-L. Vegetarianism and vegan diet. vegetarianism and vegan diet, in (physiology and maintenance). In: Hänninen O, ed. Encyclopedia of Life Support Systems (EOLSS). Developed under the Auspices of the UNESCO, 2003. URL https://www.eolss.net.
20. Kjeldsen-Kragh J, Haugen M, Borchgrevink CF, et al. Controlled trial of fasting and one-year vegetarian diet in rheumatoid arthritis. Lancet 1991;338:899–902.
21. Nenonen MT, Helve TA, Rauma A-L, Hänninen O. Uncooked, lactobacilli-rich, vegan food and rheumatoid arthritis. Br JRheumatol1998;37:274–281.

22. Kaartinen K, Lammi K, Hypen M, Nenonen M, Hänninen O, Rauma A-L. Vegan diet alleviates fibromyalgia symptoms. Scand J Rheumatol 2000;29:308–313.
23. Donaldson MS, Speight N, Loomis S. Fibromyalgia syndrome improved using a mostly raw vegetarian diet: an observational study. BMC Complement Altern Med 2001;1:7.
24. Kremer JM, Jubiz W, Michalek A, et al. Fish-oil ftty acid supplementation in active rheumatoid arthritis. A double-blinded, controlled, crossover study. Ann Inter Med 1987;106:497–503.
25. Kremer JM. Clinical studies of omega 3 fatty acid supplementation in patients who have rheumatoid arthritis. Rheum Dis Clin North Am 1990;17(2):391–401.
26. Fahrer H, Hoeflin F, Lauterburg BH, Pehaim E, Levy A, Vischer TL. Diet and fatty acids: can fish substitute for fish oil? Clin Exp Rheumatol 1991;9:403–406.
27. Lau CS, Morley KD, Belch JJF. Effects of fish oil supplementation on non-steroidal anti-infallamtory drug requirement in patients with mild rheumatoid arthritis–a double blind placebo controlled study. Br J Rheumatol 1993;32:982–989.
28. Fortin PR, Lew RA, Liang MH et al. Validation of Meta-analysis: The Effects of Fish Oil in Rheumatoid Arthritis. Jornal of Clinical Epidemiology 1995; 48;1376–1390.
29. Merchant RE, Carmack CA, Wise CM. Nutritional supplementation with *Chlorella pyrenoidosa* for patients with fibromyalgia syndrome: a pilot study. Phytotherapy Research 2000;14:167–173.
30. Zurier RB, Rossetti RG, Jacobson EW, et al. Gamma linolenic acid treatment of rheumatoid arthritis. A randomized, placebo controlled trial. Arthritis Rheum 1996;39(11:1808–1817.
31. Hänninen O, Nenonen M, Ling W-H,, Li D-S,, Sihvonen L. Effects of eating an uncooked vegetable diet for 1 week. Appetite 1992;19:243–254.
32. Peltonen R, Ling W-H, Hänninen O, Eerola E. An uncooked vegan diet on human fecal microflora: computerized analysis of direct stool sample gas-liquid chromatography on bacterial cellular fatty acids. Appl Environ Microbiol 1992;58:3660–3666.
33. Rauma A-L. Nutrition and biotransformation in strict vegans (eaters of "living food"). PhD dissertation. Kuopio University Publications D. Med Sci 1996;102:114..
34. Nenonen MT. Vegan diet rich in lactobacilli ("living food"): metabolic and subjective responses in healthy subjects and in patients with rheumatoid arthritis. PhD dissertation. Kuopio University Publications D. Med Sci 1995;76:155.
35. Rauma A-L, Törmälä M-L, Nenonen M, Hänninen O. Iodine status in vegans consuming a living food diet. Nutr Res 1994;14:1789–1795.
36. Rauma A-L, Törrönen R, Hänninen O, Mykkänen H. Vitamin B-12 status of long-term adherents of a strict uncooked vegan diet ("Living food diet") is compromised. J Nutr 1995;125:2511–2515.
37. Ågren JJ, Törmälä M-L, Nenonen MT, Hänninen OO. Fatty acid composition of erythrocyte, platelet, and serum lipids in strict vegans. Lipids 1995;30:365–369.
38. Rauma A-L, Törrönen R, Hänninen O,Verhagen H, Mykkänen H. Antioxidant status in long-term adherents to a strict uncooked vegan diet. Am J Clin Nutr 1995:62;221–227.'
39. Hänninen O, Kaartinen K, Rauma A-L, et al. Antioxidants in vegan diet and rheumatic disorders. Toxicology 2000;155:45–53.
40. Rauma A-L, Lammi K, Kaartinen Kati, Nenonen M, Hänninen O. Food and nutrient intake of fibromyalgic females on a vegetarian regimen. Eur Cong Nutr, Lillehammer 1999;6:17–20.
41. Ling W-H, Laitinen M, Hänninen O. Shifting from conventional diet to an uncooked vegan diet reversibly alters serum lipid and apolipoprotein levels. Nutrition Res. 1992;12:1431–1440.
42. Peltonen R, Nenonen M, Helve T, Hänninen O, Toivanen P, Eerola E. Faecal microbial flora and disease activity in rheumatoid arthritis during a vegan diet. Brit J Rheumatol 1997:36:64–68.
43. Rauma A-L, Mykkänen HM. Antioxidant Status in Vegetarians Versus Omnivores. Nutrition 2000;16:111–119.
44. Hänninen O, Nenonen M, Rauma A-L, etal. Health effects of uncooked vegan diet, rich in Lactobacilli. In: Mälkki Y, Cummings JH, eds. Dietary Fibre and Fermentation in the Colon, Proceedings of COST Action 92 Workshop, Espoo, Finland. European Commission, Directorate-General XII, Science, Research and Development, B-1049, Brussels, 1996, pp. 254–262.
45. Slavin J, Jacobs D, Marquart L. Whole-grain consumption and chronic disease: protective mechanisms. Nutr Cancer 1997;27(1):14–21. Review

12 Nutrition and Polymyositis and Dermatomyositis

Ingela Loell and Ingrid Lundberg

Summary

- Chronic muscle inflammation in polymyositis or dermatomyositis causes muscle weakness and fatigue.
- The chronic inflammation could lead to a catabolic state and additional loss of muscle mass.
- The chronic muscle inflammation could induce a metabolic myopathy.
- Body weight may not be reliable to measure muscle loss, rather measurement of body composition is recommended.
- For patients with polymyositis or dermatomyositis it is important to provide the body with the right amount of macronutrients and trace elements for maintenance and improvement of body functions.
- One recommendation is supplementation with calcium and vitamin D.
- Another recommendation is regular physical exercise that during limited periods can be combined with supplements such as creatine, if done under the care of a physician.

Key Words: Creatine supplement; dermatomyositis; exercise; glutamine; inflammatory myopathies; polymyositis; vitamin D

1. INTRODUCTION

Polymyositis and dermatomyositis are chronic, rheumatic muscle disorders that are characterized by slowly progressive, symmetrical muscle weakness and fatigue in the arms, legs and neck, and by inflammation in muscle tissue. Other organs are frequently involved, such as the skin in dermatomyositis. In both polymyositis and dermatomyositis the inflammation may also affect the lungs, the heart, and joints. The gastrointestinal (GI) tract is frequently involved and may cause problems that affect nutritional status. Chronic inflammation may also lead to general symptoms such as weight loss, fatigue, and fever, all of which could potentially affect nutritional status. In most cases, these chronic conditions require life-long immunosuppressive treatment and side effects are common.

1.1. Epidemiology

Polymyositis and dermatomyositis are relatively rare diseases with a yearly onset of approximately 1 case per 100.000 people per year. Women are two to three times more often affected than men. The peak of incidence is in the 60s although polymyositis or dermatomyositis may start at any age, even in children. These forms of myositis are worldwide disorders, but there is a latitude gradient of polymyositis and dermatomyositis. The latter form occurs more frequently closer to the equator and polymyositis is more frequent in northern countries *(1,2)*.

1.2. Etiology

Both polymyositis and dermatomyositis are autoimmune diseases, where the immune system that normally protects us from foreign agents is directed against our own tissues, causing inflammation and damage. Further support for polymyositis and dermatomyositis being autoimmune diseases is the presence of autoantibodies in serum, which can be seen in two-thirds of the patients. Some of these autoantibodies are specific for myositis and are not present in other diseases. One of these myositis-specific autoantibodies is anti-Jo-1 autoantibody, directed against histidyl-tRNA-synthetase. This autoantibody is present in approx 20% of patients with myositis and is often associated with the presence of arthritis in finger joints, lung disease, Raynaud's phenomenon, and skin problems of the hands (mechanic's hands) *(3)*.

The mechanisms that cause autoimmune reactions are not known, but both genetic and environmental factors are likely to be involved. The role of genes as a risk factor for polymyositis or dermatomyositis is supported by familial association with other rheumatic or autoimmune diseases. Moreover, genetic traits have been found to be associated with polymyositis and dermatomyositis but the traits vary between populations *(4,5)*. Furthermore, the same genetic traits are also associated with other autoimmune diseases, such as Sjögren's syndrome (SS) and systemic lupus erythematosus (SLE), suggesting that other genetic as well as environmental factors are important for the development of myositis.

One such environmental factor is exposure to ultraviolet (UV) light. This is based on the observation of the aforementioned regional differences in the ratio between polymyositis and dermatomyositis, which is correlated to latitude. The higher frequency of dermatomyositis is directly correlated with high UV light irradiation *(2)*. This observation suggests that UV light may be an environmental risk factor for the development of dermatomyositis.

Another environmental risk factor that has been suggested is viral infections. One viral infection associated with polymyositis is HIV *(6,7)*. Myositis could also develop together with some parasite infections such as trypanosome cruzi. In most patients with polymyositis or dermatomyositis no infections have been detected.

2. HISTORICAL PERSPECTIVES

Dermatomyositis and polymyositis were first described as disease entities in the 19th century, characterized by symmetrical edema, stiffness, pain, and limited motion of muscles. Lung and skin involvement were described in the first reports. No specific treatment was available until the introduction of adrenocorticotropic hormone and glucocorticoids as therapeutic possibilities in the early 1950s. Before this, different therapies were used, such as amino acids, vitamin E, and anabolic steroids, without any consistent beneficial effect. During this time, the mortality rate in these disorders was high. The major cause of death was pulmonary infection resulting from involvement of respiratory muscles and inflammation of the lungs.

Treatment with glucocorticoids made a remarkable difference in the survival of patients with myositis. Although treatment with glucocorticoids improved the survival rate, the frequent and profound side effects soon became evident. Features reminiscent of Cushing's syndrome became apparent; glucose intolerance requiring dietary control or a small dose of insulin was also quite common. To prevent toxicity of glucocorticoids, supplements such as potassium and antacids were given frequently. Later on, anabolic steroids were used in addition to glucocorticoid treatment in an attempt to preserve body protein but the value of this therapy was never determined.

From 1950 to 1965, supportive therapy for patients with myositis included dietary management. Patients experiencing difficulties with swallowing, for instance, were fed with a high-calorie liquid diet. Some patients experienced constipation owing to weakness of abdominal musculature or lack of physical activity; this was treated with a gentle enema. The improved muscle function with glucocorticoid treatment was not seen in all patients; some only had a limited beneficial effect and others did not improve at all.

During the 1980s, therapies started to include additional immunosuppressants, such as azathioprine and methotrexate, to achieve both a steroid-sparing effect and additional benefits when glucocorticoid treatment was not sufficient. Treatment was based on high doses of glucocorticoids with the supplementation of antacids and potassium. During the last two decades, several new immunosuppressive agents have been tested in patients with myositis with inconsistent results, as is discussed further, and improved therapy is still required *(8–12)*.

3. CLINICAL AND LABORATORY FEATURES

3.1. Clinical Features

The predominant clinical features of myositis are muscle weakness, muscle fatigue, and sometimes muscle pain, mainly affecting thigh, shoulder, arm, and neck muscles. The onset of symptoms is often slow over weeks to months. Although muscle symptoms predominate, other organ systems are frequently affected. As the name implies, the skin is involved in dermatomyositis. The type of skin rash varies and could affect all parts of the body, although the most characteristic rash is localized to the eyelids, characterized by a red or purple rash with edema, called heliotropic exanthema. Another typical skin rash for dermatomyositis is seen on the dorsal side of the finger joints or hand and is characterized by small red to purple slightly elevated papules (Gottron´s papules).

Other organ systems that are frequently involved are lungs, joints, heart and the GI tract. Lung involvement could be caused by different mechanisms. Chronic noninfectious inflammation causing symptoms like cough or breathlessness is common and could vary from mild to severe. Involvement of the respiratory muscles of the chest may also cause breathlessness and impairment of physical activities. The muscle inflammation may also affect muscles in the GI tract, most frequently in the throat and esophagus resulting in problems with swallowing and regurgitation, and ultimately leading to nutritional problems. The arthritis may affect one or several joints. It is often mild and does not cause deformities. Although the heart is a muscle, clinical manifestations of heart involvement are less common, but may occur and give rise to symptoms such as arrhythmia or congestive heart failure.

3.2. Muscle Tissue Features

A typical finding in polymyositis and dermatomyositis is inflammation in muscles and muscle fiber damage. The inflammation is characterized by the presence of inflammatory cells such as lymphocytes and macrophages. This can be seen in muscle biopsies, which are helpful both for diagnosis and to exclude other muscle disorders. In the muscle tissue of patients with myositis, several inflammatory and immune-mediating molecules are produced. These are likely to be important for the clinical symptoms and for the muscle fiber damage and loss of muscle strength. These molecules are of interest as targets for new therapies that are more specific than glucocorticoids and other immunosuppressants that are used today. Such new therapies can be developed by modern molecular biology technology, as has successfully been the case, for example, in rheumatoid arthritis (RA) and Chrohn´s disease. A better understanding of the key molecules that cause the disease could lead to the development of new and better therapies for patients with polymyositis or dermatomyositis.

3.3. Molecules Present in Muscle Tissue in Inflammatory Conditions

Cytokines are important signaling molecules in inflammatory responses and immune regulation. These molecules have also become successful targets of therapy in several other autoimmune diseases such as RA, pelvospondylitis, psoriasis, and Crohn´s disease. The most frequently observed cytokines in the muscle tissue of patients with inflammatory myopathies are cytokines with proinflammatory properties, namely, interleukin (IL)-1α, IL-1β, high-mobility group box1, and tumor necrosis factor (TNF)-α *(13–18)*. These cytokines are secreted by cells in the immune system and by endothelial cells in the lining of blood vessels. Endothelial cells control the passage of compounds and white blood cells into and out of the bloodstream *(19)*.

Cytokines stimulate several inflammatory responses, such as the production of other families of molecules: chemokines, which regulate adhesion of white blood cells to muscle tissue, and adhesion molecules that allow trafficking of circulatory inflammatory cells to endothelial cells, thus letting inflammation pass from the blood into the tissue. One possible mechanism leading to an increased local expression of proinflammatory cytokines might be found in an enhanced activation of the signal substance regulator of DNA transcription, nuclear factor (NF)-κB. This transcription factor regulates the expression of proinflammatory cytokines, for example, TNF-α and IL-1β *(20)*. NF-κB occurs in chronic muscle diseases and is believed to be involved in the reduced maturation and regeneration of skeletal muscle by activating cytokine production *(20)*.

IL-1β and TNF-α also induce the production of prostaglandin E_2 (PGE_2), a molecule that mediates pain, fever and inflammation. PGE_2 is the most common PG and is produced in various cells, such as fibroblasts and macrophages *(21–23)*. There are several enzymes involved in the PG-production pathway converting different fatty acids to biologically active metabolites, including PGs and thromboxanes. In muscle tissue, PGE_2 in concert with these other mediators, controls blood flow in the microvessels, and thereby the nutrient supply, to the muscle tissue. PGE_2 also has a role in muscle regeneration upon injury and in the early inflammatory response in order to remove damaged tissue and to induce tissue formation *(24,25)*.

Similar inflammatory responses with IL-1 and TNF expression in muscle tissue could also be induced by hypoxia and, interestingly, hypoxia could be a consequence of chronic inflammation in affected tissues *(26)*. This is well established in the membrane of joints in chronic arthritis *(27)*. Hypoxia could also be a consequence of loss of microvessels, capillaries, in muscle tissue that is a typical finding in dermatomyositis. Interestingly, a loss of capillaries seems to be an early event in dermatomyositis. More recently, we have also observed a reduced number of capillaries in muscle tissue in patients with polymyositis (unpublished data). As oxygen supply is crucial for aerobic muscle metabolism, hypoxia can have several negative consequences that affect the working capacity of muscles and could also affect the nutritional status of patients with chronic muscle inflammation.

3.4. Pharmacological Treatment

As presented earlier, glucocorticoids have become the cornerstone of treatment since 1950 when they were first introduced. Although treatment with glucocorticoids made a dramatic improvement in patient survival, it soon became apparent that some patients with myositis do not respond at all and very few patients recover their former muscle performance. Furthermore, as also discussed previously, a disadvantage of high-dose glucocorticoid treatment is the substantial risk of side effects. For these reasons, combination therapies with other immunosuppressive agents have been developed. Today, glucocorticoids are still recommended as baseline treatment (starting doses of 0.75–1 mg/kg body weight per day), although most authors recommend combination with another immunosuppressant from the start as a glucocorticoid-saving drug and to improve the efficacy of treatment. The most often used immunosuppressants are azathioprine and methotrexate. Other therapies that are used in severe cases are cyclophosphamide, cyclosporine A, mycophenylate mofetile, tacrolimus or infusions with high doses of intravenous immunoglobulin. Only a few of these drugs have been tested in controlled trials of adequate size and duration to show beneficial effects. They are mostly used based on observed beneficial effects in occasional individuals or reported case series. Glucocorticoids can have profound negative effects on metabolism, making the immunosuppressive treatment of myositis an important issue with regard to nutritional status in patients with polymyositis and dermatomyositis. These topics are discussed further.

3.5. Prognosis

Currently, there is only limited information available on the survival rate of patients with polymyositis and dermatomyositis. The few studies are mainly based on cohorts from one hospital; they are not population based and they include only a small number of patients. With this limitation in mind, the 5-year survival was estimated to be 95% and 10-year survival to be 85 or 89% in two recent papers *(28,29)*.

4. NUTRITIONAL STATUS

As with other chronic inflammatory diseases, many patients with polymyositis and dermatomyositis experience general symptoms such as muscle fatigue and weight loss. This may be a catabolic effect caused by the systemic chronic inflammation, or it may be a side effect of long-term glucocorticoid treatment, which is a well-known muscle catabolic agent.

In patients with myositis, muscle wasting may also be caused by muscle atrophy and damage as a consequence of muscle inflammation, or to nutritional deficits depending on difficulties with swallowing. Inactivity, lack of physical activity, and at worst, bed rest, together with inappropriate nutrition, may further play a part in the metabolic alterations as seen in critically ill patients. Because of the inflammatory process and to glucocorticoid treatment, muscle mass may be replaced by fat and muscle wasting may not always be signaled by weight loss. A more appropriate way to follow nutritional status is by assessment of body composition. This can be done by a dual energy X-ray absorptiometry scan, typically used for bone densitometry.

Little detailed information on nutritional status is available in the literature that is specific for polymyositis and dermatomyositis. Here, we summarize available information that we find relevant for patients with myositis after a literature survey.

4.1. Muscle Metabolism

The use of muscles for all kinds of movement requires energy. The major source of energy for muscles is adenosine triphosphate (ATP) and creatine phosphate (CP). Every muscle contraction demands an enormous amount of ATP that cannot be stored in the body and therefore needs to be generated continuously. The body only contains small amounts of energy stores, ATP, and CP, and these stores only last for about 1 minute during muscle work. After the first minute of work, the skeletal muscle is dependent on oxygen-generated ATP. The oxygen is provided to muscle by blood vessels including the small capillaries. By using the macronutrients— carbohydrates (glycogen), proteins (amino acids) and fat (fatty acids and glycerol)—energy is produced in the mitochondria in muscle cells, and the muscle will be able to contract *(30)*.

4.2. Glucocorticoids

A special problem in patients with myositis that may affect nutritional status is their need for long-term (often over months to years), high-dose, glucocorticoids. Glucocorticoids are used to suppress muscle inflammation by acting on most cell types.

The effects on T lymphocytes and macrophages are both direct and indirect, by influencing the mediators released by these cells *(31,32)*. The anti-inflammatory and immunosuppressive effects of glucocorticoids in myositis are mediated by inhibiting the expression of IL-1β, TNF-α, IL-6 and interferon-γ. One way to achieve this inhibition is to interfere with the inflammatory pathway directed by NF-κB through promoting the production of the specific NF-κB inhibitory factor, or by binding directly to NF-κB itself, to restrain the inflammatory action *(33)*. Via this mechanism, blocked gene expression of proinflammatory cytokines will occur and therefore the amount of these inflammatory molecules will decrease.

Glucocorticoids can also inhibit inflammatory cells to migrate over the endothelium, from the bloodstream into the muscle tissue and further into sites of inflammation. Glucocorticoids also suppress cyclooxygenase (COX)-2, one of the enzymes involved in the regulation of PGE_2 synthesis, as well as other lipid mediators synthesized from the same fatty acid precursor *(34)*. As mentioned previously, it was noticed early that treatment with glucocorticoids had negative effects on muscles and may induce muscle atrophy and also a catabolic state. Glucocorticoids act in several ways to retard growth and promote muscle protein breakdown *(35)*. Some strategies that could possibly be undertaken to counteract these negative effects of glucocorticoids are discussed later.

4.3. Role of Exercise

The catabolic effect of glucocorticoids on muscle tissue is likely to contribute to muscle wasting in patients with myositis who are also affected by catabolism from the muscle inflammation and from physical inactivity as well. In patients who have undergone renal transplant, the negative effect of low or moderate doses (10–12 mg per day) of glucocorticoids on muscles was reversed by physical exercise. Whether this is true for patients with myositis is not known *(36,37)*.

Physical exercise was, until recently, believed to be harmful for patients with chronic inflammation in muscles, but during the 1990s, it was determined that instead of being harmful, it could even be beneficial for patients with myositis to exercise with improved performance and health-related quality of life *(38,39)*. There are numerous benefits of exercise in terms of nutritional status in healthy individuals. Although many of these effects have not been evaluated specifically in patients with myositis, they could be assumed to be attributable to these patients.

Beneficial effects of exercise in healthy individuals include the following:

- improvement of insulin sensitivity and glucose uptake *(40–42)*;
- increased angiogenesis (blood vessel growth) *(43–45)*, which improves blood flow, oxygen and nutrient supply to the muscle;
- improved endothelial function *(46)*;
- altered stress, immune, and inflammatory mediators and cytokine production *(47)*;
- counteracts muscle protein wasting *(48,49)*; and
- improved function *(50,51)*.

In healthy individuals, the muscle protein metabolism after exercise is negative and food intake is needed in order to gain muscle mass. Because patients with myositis already experience a catabolic state owing to glucocorticoid treatment, the post-exercise meal could be even more important to prevent further muscle protein breakdown. This is best achieved by digesting a combination of carbohydrates and protein after the exercise bout *(52)*. For most rapid availability, a liquid, dietary shake can be used but also dietary carbohydrates with a high glycemic index, like rice cakes, with some protein-rich cottage cheese, suits the purpose fine. It seems as if early post-exercise ingestion of a nutrient supplement, as opposed to ingestion 2 hours after training, enhances the anabolic effect of whole-body protein *(53,54)*. The fact that patients with myositis are in a catabolic state caused by inflammation and steroid use, this approach, otherwise mostly used by athletes, might be of use in these patients.

4.4. Dietary Management

A diet achieving energy balance with a content of approx 30% fat, 50 to 60% carbohydrates and 10 to 20% protein of total energy is recommended for healthy individuals in Nordic European countries and is likely to be appropriate for patients with myositis as well *(52,55)*. Dietary supplements have become popular and some of these have been tested in clinical trials in patients with various chronic inflammatory diseases. There are a few reports on effects of supplements in patients with polymyositis or dermatomyositis.

4.4.1. GLUTEN

Celiac disease or gluten-sensitivity is a chronic intestinal disorder where the upper small intestine is damaged, leading to impaired nutrient uptake in these patients. The predominant antigen triggering an autoimmune response in celiac disease has been identified as the enzyme transglutaminase 2 (TG2). Several studies have established a close association between celiac disease and other autoimmune disorders, such as SS and SLE.

An elevated expression of TG2 has been found in muscle tissue from patients with myositis compared to normal muscle, and TG2 is suggested to be a marker of idiopathic inflammatory myopathies *(56–58)*. There have been reports of an increased frequency of gluten-sensitivity among patients with myositis but screening for autoantibodies against TG2 in serum has so far been negative and needs to be further investigated.

Anti-gliadin, another antibody associated with celiac disease, has been found with increased frequency in patients with myositis. Thus, celiac disease should be considered in patients with myositis who experience intestinal problems such as diarrhea or weight loss that cannot be explained otherwise. Celiac disease is diagnosed by presence of anti-TG2 autoantibodies or anti-gliadin autoantiboides and a small bowel biopsy. Implementation of a gluten-free diet is important in these cases to avoid malnutrition *(59)*.

4.5. Supplements

In healthy individuals, it is crucial to support the body with adequate nutrients in order to optimize physical exercise and increase muscle mass or muscle endurance. Body builders, fitness competitors, and marathon runners have, for decades, been using dietary and nutritional supplements to sculpt massive muscles or to be able to undertake strenuous endurance exercise. Supplements have become an enormously profitable industry and the effect of most supplements on the market can be questioned. Through basic research, the safety of several different supplements for use in healthy people has been established *(60)*. There is limited information available that is specific to patients with polymyositis and dermatomyositis; information that is available is presented further on in this chapter.

4.5.1. CREATINE

A commonly used supplement among athletes is creatine. A large number of studies have been published on the subject, describing the ergogenic outcome on muscle strength and size when using creatine in combination with resistance training [61–64].

As mentioned earlier, energy is stored as CP in muscle cells. The effect of creatine supplements in exercise is the result of increased muscle creatine levels that make it possible to perform more repetitions during weight training by increasing the resynthesis of ATP. This provides the ability to work out at an enhanced level and results in a greater gain in muscle mass *(65)*.

Some patients with myositis have a metabolic disturbance that gives them significantly lower levels of stored creatine in muscles and a defect in the production of ATP, impairing their muscle energy supply *(66,67)*. Creatine supplements have recently been evaluated in a placebo-controlled trial in patients with myositis, in combination with stable immunosuppressive treatment and/or steroids *(68)*. The creatine and the placebo groups performed the same home exercise program. The creatine-supplemented group had a significant improvement, compared with the placebo group, in the primary outcome that reflected the ability to undertake high-intensity exercise.

Side effects of creatine supplements, for example, muscle cramps and heat intolerance, have been described. These side effects may be related to an increase in water retention during the initial days of supplementation. Water retention and an increase in muscle mass may cause weight gain while supplementing with creatine *(69)*. The use of creatine supplements with exercise among patients with myositis was without significant side effects and was considered effective and inexpensive *(68,70)*.

In animal models with arthritis, it was suggested that creatine supplementation might have an anti-inflammatory action; similar suggestions have been made based on research using cell cultures in which creatine supplementation also had an anti-inflammatory action on endothelial cells. These effects may arise from the ability of creatine-supplemented cells to inhibit endothelial permeability and expression of adhesion molecules, decreasing the traffic of proinflammatory cells and mediators from the bloodstream into the tissue *(71)*.

The optimal duration of creatine supplementation during exercise is not known. In the controlled trial, a beneficial effect of creatine, in combination with exercise, was observed after 3 months, and no significant side effects were reported over 5 months.

Regarding creatine supplementation in general, the literature is based on adults, so there is a lack of data regarding safety of creatine use in growing adolescents. Therefore, no conclusions can be drawn for patients with juvenile dermatomyositis and creatine supplementation *(72)*. In a placebo-controlled study including 50 boys between ages 4 and 10 years diagnosed with Duchenne muscular dystrophy (DMD), creatine supplementation was well tolerated *(73)*. Although creatine is a common supplement, commercially marketed creatine products might not meet the same quality control standards as pharmaceuticals, and because of possible impurities or differences in dosage, caution is urged. Patients should always discuss use of any dietary supplement with their physician.

4.5.2. ANABOLIC STEROIDS

Anabolic steroids increase muscle mass and strength, and have been used by athletes for decades. The use of anabolic steroids in sports was banned by the International Olympic Committee in 1974. Use of these hormones may generate several side effects, such as severe acne, increased body hair, and aggressive behavior that may occasionally trigger violent behavior *(74)*.

Until the 1990s, anabolic steroids were manufactured solely by pharmaceutical companies, but the variety of prohibited anabolic steroids in sports has expanded because of steroid production by nonpharmaceutical companies *(75)*. Without a prescription from a doctor, anabolic steroids are an illegal drug, and the use of hormones without a physician's surveillance could involve major risks.

In recent years, anabolic steroids have been investigated in terms of possible benefits for patients with disease-related muscle wasting. Testosterone administration has had positive results in different patient populations, but because it is a natural androgen hormone, it possesses virilizing effects, which limits the population that can be treated. An alternative is oxandrolone, a synthetic testosterone analog, that also can be used in treating women and children with chronic muscle-wasting conditions *(76)*.

One placebo-controlled study performed mainly on male subjects with inclusion body myositis (IBM), another subset of chronic muscle inflammation, showed some effect in improving whole-body and upper extremity strength *(77)*. Under the controlled conditions of the trial, the adverse effects were minimal and the drug was considered safe and classified as a treatment of possible benefit *(77)*.

No controlled studies have been performed in patients with polymyositis or dermatomyositis, so whether oxandrolone has any effect in these disorders is not known. Results similar to those in the IBM trial were documented in boys with DMD with the conclusion that oxandrolone may have some beneficial effect in slowing the progress of weakness *(78)*. Patients with chronic obstructive pulmonary disease (COPD) also experience muscle wasting, which is further enhanced by glucocorticoid therapy. A study using another anabolic steroid, nandrolone decanoate, for supplementary treatment in patients with COPD, resulted in a significant increase in fat-free mass and an overall positive effect on body composition relative to placebo *(79)*.

4.5.3. GLUTAMINE

Glutamine is a conditionally essential amino acid, meaning that it is essential during conditions of trauma, sepsis, or cancer. The majority of free glutamine is synthesized and stored in skeletal muscle. Glutamine provides the body with new precursors for energy substrates, antioxidants (mostly glutathione), and acute-phase proteins found in the blood shortly after onset of an infection *(80)*. This mobilization leads to an intramuscular glutamine depletion, resulting in a decrease in lean muscle mass *(81)*.

Patients in intensive care may develop severe myopathies and muscle biopsies from these patients show low levels of muscle glutamine *(82)*. The previously mentioned proinflammatory cytokines IL-1 and TNF that are upregulated in myositis, mediate a decrease in protein synthesis and an increase in protein degradation in skeletal muscles. Muscle infusions of glutamine in an animal model of sepsis attenuated the expression of proinflammatory cytokines by suppressing the signaling pathway of NF-κB, and might therefore have therapeutic potential for various inflammatory diseases *(83)*.

Patients with myositis are treated primarily with glucocorticoids, which induce the release of glutamine into the blood at the expense of muscle protein degradation. Branched chain amino acids (BCAA; valine, leucine, and isoleucine) serve as precursors of glutamine *(84)*, and contribute to approx 20% of the amino acids released during muscle protein breakdown, the major part of which is used for glutamine synthesis.

The systemic availability of dietary glutamine is reduced by uptake in the gut and liver; thus, the whole-body glutamine availability largely depends on the rate of glutamine synthesis in skeletal muscle. Supplementation of either glutamine or BCAA might counteract the muscle degradation caused by inflammation, steroid treatment, and physical inactivity, but the field has to be further investigated. No studies have been performed in patients with myositis, but glutamine, as well as amino acid supplementation, over 10 days inhibited whole-body protein degradation in patients with DMD *(85)*.

4.5.4. FATTY ACIDS

Fat is the most calorically dense food component and is known as the most efficient way for the body to store excess energy. Fat is more than just energy storage, however, because every cell within the body has a membrane around the surface and surrounding the nucleus. These membranes are built of fatty acids, called phospholipids, which can be released from the membrane by different enzymes and used for multiple tasks, depending on the fatty acid type. Arachidonic acid (AA), the precursor of the proinflammatory PGE_2, is an omega-6 (n-6) polyunsaturated fatty acid (PUFA) and is metabolized from linoleic acid, found in nuts, seeds, and vegetable oils, such as corn oil *(86)*.

Fish oil and flaxseed oil are rich sources of anti-inflammatory omega-3 (n-3) PUFA, eicosapentaenoic acid (EPA) and docosahexaenoic acid (DHA/DHCA), both metabolized from α-linolenic acid. Both linoleic and α-linolenic acid are essential fatty acids, which means that the body cannot synthesize them.

In a modern Western diet the ratio between n-6 and n-3 fatty acids is about 20 to 1, and this may have an effect on eicosanoid synthesis. A diet containing a higher intake of n-3s may shift AA-derived proinflammatory mediators to the more anti-inflammatory properties of EPA and DHA metabolites. A number of animal trials have been performed showing that diets containing a higher intake of n-3, or fish-oil supplements, reduces AA content in cell membranes and inhibits the synthesis of proinflammatory prostaglandins. Prior to consuming any dietary supplements, patients should consult with their physician and with their nation's dietary guidelines *(86,89–91)*.

4.5.5. VITAMIN D

Osteoporosis and fractures are common consequences of glucocorticoid therapy and of physical inactivity. Thus, patients with polymyositis and dermatomyositis are at high risk for developing this complication. Prevention of bone loss should be considered as part of the therapy for these patients.

Prevention of steroid-induced bone loss is based on calcium and vitamin D supplementation, adequate protein intake, and regular physical exercise *(92)*. The classic function of vitamin D is to regulate bone formation and resorption through regulating calcium homeostasis. For children and adolescents, glucocorticoid treatment may cause failure to reach a normal peak bone mass with an increased risk for hip and spine fractures later in life, which makes supplementation of calcium and vitamin D even more important in this population *(93,94)*.

Vitamin D is also an important immune system regulator. The vitamin D receptor is present on various immune cells, producing and releasing the active hormone. Vitamin D status has been linked to autoimmune diseases in humans where low vitamin D intake is associated with increased susceptibility to develop autoimmune diseases such as multiple sclerosis and RA *(93,95)*. Moreover, vitamin D insufficiency can lead to disturbed muscle metabolism *(96)*. In different animal models of autoimmune disease, it has been shown that supplementation with vitamin D or treatment with D-hormone analogs acts in an immunosuppressive way, decreasing the disease symptoms *(93,95,97,98)*.

Major dietary sources of vitamin D are fortified dairy products, fatty fish, and fish liver oils. The main supply of D hormone is obtained through sun exposure of the skin where the UV light converts a pro-vitamin to the active D vitamin. The sunlight exposure is significantly less in northern climates and especially low during winter months *(93,99)*. The serum level of vitamin D is the best indicator for defining any deficiency, insufficiency, or toxicity. Concentrations below 40 to 50 nmol/L reflect vitamin D insufficiency and intoxication levels are clearly above 200 nmol/L. There have been no reports of intoxication from sunlight exposure; all of the observed cases are owing to excessive oral intake *(96)*.

Most dietary guidelines for vitamin D are based on maintaining bone health, and differ throughout a lifetime. Important variables are season, latitude, and the food fortification of the country *per se (100)*. To our knowledge, no reports of vitamin D effects on the immune system in patients with polymyositis or dermatomyositis have been published, but as patients with dermatomyositis may be sensitive to UV light exposure, they are at risk of vitamin D deficiency and as a consequence at high risk to develop osteoporosis. This is another strong indication for vitamin D supplementation in patients with dermatomyositis.

4.5.6. Vitamin E

Aggressive distribution of vitamin E was used for treatment of polymyositis and dermatomyositis during the early 20th century for several decades. An explanation for this could probably be that one of the primary manifestations of vitamin E deficiency is myopathy *(101,102)*.

Reversible human myopathy caused by vitamin E deficiency has been described in a couple of cases *(103,104)*. Vitamin E is a soluble lipid that acts primarily as an antioxidant and as a scavenger of products from lipid peroxidation preventing cell damage, but in recent years, non-antioxidant functions such as signaling and gene regulation have been discovered *(105)*.

Vitamin E covers eight structurally related isomers, the most active of which is α-tocopherol. Rich sources of vitamin E are vegetable oils, such as sunflower oil. Nuts are also a good source of vitamin E, whereas fruits, vegetables, and meat contain lesser amounts.

Vitamin E deficiency is rare in humans and does not occur as a result of a dietary deficiency, but rather, from genetic abnormalities, or secondary to fat malabsorption syndromes such as chronic cholestasis, cystic fibrosis, and celiac disease. Another aspect to consider in determining the need for vitamin E supplementation is the antioxidant needs during exercise. Reactive oxygen species are generated in contracting muscles and mediate muscle damage and inflammatory responses after a demanding exercise bout. Dietary supplementation with vitamin E in order to negate this contraction-induced muscle damage has been controversial because of dissimilar test parameters including age and fitness of the subjects, dose and duration of the antioxidant, and type of exercise performed *(106–108)*. As myositis therapy, vitamin E is no longer used because it is not considered effective *(109)*.

4.5.7. HERBAL SUPPLEMENTS

Herbal supplements are widely used and among the most popular products are supplements with immune-stimulatory properties. The field of research evaluating alternative medicine and autoimmunity is limited but there have been some cases reported.

4.5.7.1. Polyphenols. Polyphenols are a group of micronutrients with similar molecular structure, found in plants where they act as a defense against pathogens and UV radiation. Dietary polyphenols can be divided into four subgroups: flavonoids, stillbenes, lignas, and phenolic acids *(110)*.

It has been determined both epidemiologically and experimentally that polyphenols have anti-inflammatory activity. The suggested mechanism of this activity is the inhibition of NF-kB signaling and COX activity, thus reducing PG production *(111)*. One group of polyphenols is the flavonoids that can be found in fruits, vegetables, wine, tea, and dark chocolate. Their presumed beneficial effects are mainly antioxidative in disorders such as stroke, cancer, and inflammatory diseases *(111)*.

Another polyphenol found in green tea extract is epigallocatechin gallate (EGCG). EGCG has not yet been tested in humans, but in an animal model of DMD, supplementation of green tea extract for 5 weeks decreased degenerating muscle fibers and infiltrating immune cells in muscle tissue *(112)*. The researchers also noted that the muscles were more fatigue resistant and concluded that this feature was owing to an improved structure of muscle tissue.

In yet another study, EGCG induced expression of mPGES-1 leading to induction of PGE_2 in pulmonary cells *(113)*. We found no reports on EGCG in inflammatory myopathies, but based on these observations, we believe that some caution should be taken if used for myositis as this EGCG could work in both a proinflammatory as well as an anti-inflammatory manner.

4.5.7.2. Immunostimulatory Preparations. There are herbal supplements with immunostimulatory activity. Potent immune-activating properties have been shown in algae (*Spirulina platensis* and *Aphanizomenon flos-aquae*), both in human (chemoprotective effects) and animal studies (increased macrophage activity *(114,115)*).

Support for an immunostimulatory property is based on reports that patients suffering from autoimmune skin disorders have experienced flares and discomfort such as blisters after taking supplements containing *Spirulina* or echinacea (purple cornflower), another popular immune-boosting herbal supplement *(115)*. In one case report, a woman taking algae in a combined dietary supplement developed heliotrope rash and was later diagnosed with dermatomyositis. Although this could be a coincidence, the well-known immune-enhancing properties of these algae supplements, in combination with the clinical history of this woman, could indicate that these substances could induce an autoimmune disease *(115)*.

5. CONCLUDING REMARKS AND RECOMMENDATIONS

As a general recommendation, it is of great importance to consume an adequate amount of macronutrients and trace elements for maintenance and improvement of body functions. This is particularly true for patients with polymyositis or dermatomyositis. A well-balanced diet, with moderate intake of all of the food groups, is generally recommended. There are some additional actions that the patient with myositis can undertake in an attempt to influence the clinical symptoms and treatment-related side effects of this disease. One such recommendation is to supplement with calcium and vitamin D, to reduce the risk of developing steroid-induced osteoporosis. Another suggested supplement is folic acid, in order to counteract deficiencies caused by methotrexate treatment.

Another supplement, although less well studied, is creatine. Creatine has been shown to have a beneficial effect, without negative side effects, on patients with myositis when used as a supplemental treatment in combination with conventional pharmacological treatment and physical exercise.

As a general recommendation, we also emphasize that it is important that people suffering from inflammatory myopathies do not experiment with supplements, trace elements, or excess ingestion of certain foodstuffs without consulting their personal physician first, as there are potential risks of some supplements that may cause adverse events.

Some of the substances mentioned should only be supplemented if there is an existing state of deficiency that can be determined by a blood sample. Some nutrients and trace elements share the same receptors and/or transport molecules in a competitive manner, and an excess intake of one can lead to a deficiency of another, with serious consequences. One compound may affect multiple mechanisms.

Certain foods can also interact with drug metabolism in unfavorable ways, in which case it is absolutely necessary for health care providers to inquire about the intake of any health foods or supplements. The authors do not encourage patients with inflammatory myopathies to undertake unsupervised experiments with any of the above mentioned nutrients. In some instances (i.e., anabolic steroids), possession and distribution is considered a crime. The information presented in this chapter is solely a review of the field of research, based on studies performed primarily on patients suffering from disorders other than myositis, and healthy persons. Thus, the authors cannot be held responsible for any events caused by disuse of this knowledge.

REFERENCES

1. Hengstman G, van Venrooij W, Vencovsky J. The relative prevalence of dermatomyositis and polymyositis in Europe exhibits a latitudinal gradient. Ann Rheum Dis, 2000;59(2):141–142.
2. Okada S, et al. Global surface ultraviolet radiation intensity may modulate the clinical and immunologic expression of autoimmune muscle disease. Arthritis Rheum 2003;48(8):2285–2293.
3. Love LA, et al. A new approach to the classification of idiopathic inflammatory myopathy: myositis-specific autoantibodies define useful homogeneous patient groups. Medicine (Baltimore), 1991;70(6):360–374.
4. Arnett FC, Targoff IN, Mimori T. Interrelationship of major histocompatibility complex class II alleles and autoantibodies in four ethnic groups with various forms of myositis. Arthritis Rheum 1996;39(9):1507–1518.
5. Miller FW. Humoral immunity and immunogenetics in the idiopathic inflammatory myopathies. Curr Opin Rheumatol 1991;3(6):902–910.
6. Authier FJ, Chariot P, Gherardi RK. Skeletal muscle involvement in human immunodeficiency virus (HIV)-infected patients in the era of highly active antiretroviral therapy (HAART). Muscle Nerve 2005;32(3):247–260.

7. Reveille JD, Williams FM. Infection and musculoskeletal conditions: Rheumatologic complications of HIV infection. Best Pract Res Clin Rheumatol 2006;20(6):1159–1179.
8. Sheard C. Jr. Dermatomyositis. AMA Arch Intern Med 1951;88(5):640–658.
9. Logan RG, et al. Polymyositis: a clinical study. Ann Intern Med 1966;65(5):996–1007.
10. Pearson CM. Patterns of Polymyositis and Their Responses to Treatment. Ann Intern Med 1963;59:827–838.
11. Rose AL, Walton JN. Polymyositis: a survey of 89 cases with particular reference to treatment and prognosis. Brain 1966;89(4):747–768.
12. Pearson CM, Bohan A. The spectrum of polymyositis and dermatomyositis. Med Clin North Am 1977;61(2):439–457.
13. Lundberg I, Brengman JM, Engel AG. Analysis of cytokine expression in muscle in inflammatory myopathies, Duchenne dystrophy, and non-weak controls. J Neuroimmunol 1995;63(1):9–16.
14. Lundberg I, et al. Cytokine production in muscle tissue of patients with idiopathic inflammatory myopathies. Arthritis Rheum 1997;40(5):865–874.
15. De Bleecker JL, Meire VI, Declercq W. Immunolocalization of tumor necrosis factor-alpha and its receptors in inflammatory myopathies. Neuromuscul Disord 1999;9(4):239–246.
16. Nyberg P, et al. Increased expression of interleukin 1alpha and MHC class I in muscle tissue of patients with chronic, inactive polymyositis and dermatomyositis. J Rheumatol 2000;27(4):940–948.
17. Englund P, et al. Interleukin-1alpha expression in capillaries and major histocompatibility complex class I expression in type II muscle fibers from polymyositis and dermatomyositis patients: important pathogenic features independent of inflammatory cell clusters in muscle tissue. Arthritis Rheum 2002;46(4):1044–1055.
18. Ulfgren A, et al. Down-regulation of the aberrant expression of the inflammation mediator high mobility group box chromosomal protein 1 in muscle tissue of patients with polymyositis and dermatomyositis treated with corticosteroids. Arthritis Rheum 2004;50(5):1586–1594.
19. Figarella-Branger D, et al. Cytokines, chemokines, and cell adhesion molecules in inflammatory myopathies. Muscle Nerve 2003;28(6):659–682.
20. Spate U, Schulze PC. Proinflammatory cytokines and skeletal muscle. Curr Opin Clin Nutr Metab Care 2004;7(3):265–269.
21. Murakami M, Kudo I. Recent advances in molecular biology and physiology of the prostaglandin E2-biosynthetic pathway. Prog Lipid Res 2004;43(1):3–35.
22. Tilley SL, Coffman TM, Koller BH. Mixed messages: modulation of inflammation and immune responses by prostaglandins and thromboxanes. J Clin Invest 2001;108(1):15–23.
23. Harris SG, et al. Prostaglandins as modulators of immunity. Trends Immunol 2002;23(3):144–150.
24. Karamouzis M, et al. The response of muscle interstitial prostaglandin E(2)(PGE(2)), prostacyclin I(2)(PGI(2)) and thromboxane A(2)(TXA(2)) levels during incremental dynamic exercise in humans determined by in vivo microdialysis. Prostaglandins Leukot Essent Fatty Acids 2001;64(4–5):259–263.
25. Kalliokoski KK, Ryberg LH, Scheede-Bergdahl AK, Doessing C, Kjaer A, Boushel R. Nitric oxide and prostaglandins influence local skeletal muscle blood flow during exercise in humans: coupling between local substrate uptake and blood flow. Am J Physiol Regul Integr Comp Physiol 2006(291):R803–R809.
26. Lundberg IE. The physiology of inflammatory myopathies: an overview. Acta Physiol Scand 2001;171(3):207–213.
27. Taylor PC, Sivakumar B. Hypoxia and angiogenesis in rheumatoid arthritis. Curr Opin Rhematol 2005;17(3):293–298.
28. Sultan SM, et al. Outcome in patients with idiopathic inflammatory myositis: morbidity and mortality. Rheumatology 2002;41(1):22–26.
29. Danko K, et al. Long-term survival of patients with idiopathic inflammatory myopathies according to clinical features: a longitudinal study of 162 cases. Medicine 2004;83(1):35–42.
30. De Feo P, et al. Metabolic response to exercise. J Endocrinol Invest 2003;26(9):851–854.
31. Almawi WY, et al. Regulation of cytokine and cytokine receptor expression by glucocorticoids. J Leukoc Biol 1996;60(5):563–572.

32. Joyce DA, Gimblett G, Steer JH. Targets of glucocorticoid action on TNF-alpha release by macrophages. Inflamm Res 2001;50(7):337–340.
33. Barnes PJ. Corticosteroid effects on cell signalling. Eur Respir J 2006;27(2):413–426.
34. Ristimaki A, Narko K,Hla T. Down-regulation of cytokine-induced cyclo-oxygenase-2 transcript isoforms by dexamethasone: evidence for post-transcriptional regulation. Biochem J 1996;318 (Pt 1):325–331.
35. Hasselgren PO. Glucocorticoids and muscle catabolism. Curr Opin Clin Nutr Metab Care 1999;2(3):201–205.
36. Horber FF, et al. Evidence that prednisone-induced myopathy is reversed by physical training. J Clin Endocrinol Metab 1985;61(1):83–88.
37. Horber FF, et al. Impact of physical training on the ultrastructure of midthigh muscle in normal subjects and in patients treated with glucocorticoids. J Clin Invest 1987;79(4):1181–1190.
38. Alexanderson H. Exercise: an important component of treatment in the idiopathic inflammatory myopathies. Curr Rheumatol Rep 2005;7(2):115–124.
39. Alexanderson H, et al. The safety of a resistive home exercise program in patients with recent onset active polymyositis or dermatomyositis. Scand J Rheumatol 2000;29(5):295–301.
40. Ryder JW, Chibalin AV, Zierath JR. Intracellular mechanisms underlying increases in glucose uptake in response to insulin or exercise in skeletal muscle. Acta Physiol Scand 2001;171(3):249–257.
41. Christ-Roberts CY, Mandarino LJ. Glycogen synthase: key effect of exercise on insulin action. Exerc Sport Sci Rev 2004;32(3):90–94.
42. Wojtaszewski JF, et al. Insulin signalling: effects of prior exercise. Acta Physiologica Scandinavica 2003;178(4):321–8.
43. Gustafsson T, et al. Exercise-induced expression of angiogenesis-related transcription and growth factors in human skeletal muscle.(see comment). Am J Physiol 1999;276(2 Pt 2):H679–H685.
44. Apor P, Radi A. [Vascular effects of physical activity]. Orv Hetil 2005;146(2):63–67.
45. Prior BM, Yang HT, Terjung RL. What makes vessels grow with exercise training? J Appl Physiol 2004;97(3):1119–1128.
46. Mills PJ, et al. Physical fitness attenuates leukocyte–endothelial adhesion in response to acute exercise. J Appl Physiol 2006,101(3):785–788.
47. Petersen AM, Pedersen BK. The anti-inflammatory effect of exercise. J Appl Physiol 2005;98(4):1154–1162.
48. Hargreaves M, Cameron-Smith D. Exercise, diet, and skeletal muscle gene expression. Med Sci Sports Exerc 2002;34(9):1505–1508.
49. Yarasheski KE. Exercise, aging, and muscle protein metabolism. J Gerontol A Biol Sci Med Sci 2003;58(10):M918–M922.
50. Blair SN, et al. How much physical activity is good for health? Annu Rev Public Health 1992;13: 99–126.
51. Alexanderson H, Stenstrom CH, Lundberg I. Safety of a home exercise programme in patients with polymyositis and dermatomyositis: a pilot study. Rheumatology 1999;38(7):608–611.
52. Rennie MJ, Tipton KD. Protein and amino acid metabolism during and after exercise and the effects of nutrition. Annu Rev Nutr 2000;20:457–483.
53. Levenhagen DK, et al. Postexercise nutrient intake timing in humans is critical to recovery of leg glucose and protein homeostasis. Am J Physiol Endocrinol Metab 2001;280(6):E982–E993.
54. Wilborn CD, Willoughby DS. The role of dietary protein intake and resistance training on myosin heavy chain expression. J Int Soc Sports Nutr 2004;1(2):27–34.
55. Becker W, et al. Nordic nutrition recommendations. Ugeskrift for Laeger 2006;168(1):76–77; author reply 77.
56. Gendek EG, Kedziora J, Gendek-KubiakH. Can tissue transglutaminase be a marker of idiopathic inflammatory myopathies? Immunol Lett 2005;97(2):245–249.
57. Facchiano F, Facchiano A, Facchiano AM. The role of transglutaminase-2 and its substrates in human diseases. Front Biosci 2006;11:1758–1773.
58. Kim SY, New target against inflammatory diseases: transglutaminase 2. Arch Immunol Ther Exp (Warsz) 2004;52(5):332–337.

59. Selva-O'callaghan A, et al. Celiac disease and antibodies associated with celiac disease in patients with inflammatory myopathy. Muscle Nerve 2006;11.
60. Lombardo JA, Supplements and athletes. South Med J 2004;97(9):877–879.
61. Demant TW, Rhodes EC. Effects of creatine supplementation on exercise performance. Sports Med 1999;28(1):49–60.
62. Williams MH, Branch JD. Creatine supplementation and exercise performance: an update.(see comment). J Am Coll Nutr 1998;17(3):216–234.
63. Mesa JL, et al. Oral creatine supplementation and skeletal muscle metabolism in physical exercise. Sports Med 2002;32(14):903–944.
64. Kreider RB, Effects of creatine supplementation on performance and training adaptations. Mol Cell Biochem 2003;244(1–2):89–94.
65. Volek JS, Rawson ES. Scientific basis and practical aspects of creatine supplementation for athletes. Nutrition 2004;20(7–8):609–614.
66. Park JH, et al. Use of magnetic resonance imaging and P-31 magnetic resonance spectroscopy to detect and quantify muscle dysfunction in the amyopathic and myopathic variants of dermatomyositis. Arthritis Rheum 1995;38(1):68–77.
67. Park JH, Vital TL, Ryder NM, Hernanz-Schulman M, Partain CL, Price RR, Olsen NJ. Magnetic resonance imaging and P-31 magnetic resonance spectroscopy provide unique quantitative data useful in the longitudinal management of patients with dermatomyositis. Arthritis Rheum 1994;37(5):736–746.
68. Chung YL, Alexanderson H, Pipitone N et al. Creatine supplements in patients with idiopathic inflammatory myopathies who are clinically week after conventional pharmacologic treatment: Six-month, double-blind, randomized, placebo-controlled trial. Arthritis Rheum. 2007 May 15;57(4);694-702.
69. Wyss M, Kaddurah-Daouk R. Creatine and creatinine metabolism. Physiol Rev 2000;80(3): 1107–1213.
70. Chung Y-L,Pipitone AH, MorrisonN, et al. Creatine supplements improve muscle function in idiopathic inflammatory myopathies in a 6-month double blind, randomized placebo-controlled study. Arthritis Care Res 2006.
71. Nomura A, et al. Anti-inflammatory activity of creatine supplementation in endothelial cells in vitro. Br J Pharmacol 2003;139(4):715–720.
72. DesJardins M Supplement use in the adolescent athlete. Curr Sports Med Rep 2002;1(6):369–373.
73. Escolar DM, et al. CINRG randomized controlled trial of creatine and glutamine in Duchenne muscular dystrophy. Ann Neurol 2005;58(1):151–155.
74. Hartgens F,Kuipers H. Effects of androgenic-anabolic steroids in athletes. Sports Med 2004;34(8): 513–554.
75. Van Eenoo P, Delbeke FT. Metabolism and excretion of anabolic steroids in doping control–new steroids and new insights. J Steroid Biochem Mol Biol 2006;101(4–5):161–178.
76. Sheffield-Moore M et al. Short-term oxandrolone administration stimulates net muscle protein synthesis in young men. J Clin Endocrinol Metab 1999;84(8):2705–2711.
77. Rutkove SB, et al. A pilot randomized trial of oxandrolone in inclusion body myositis. Neurology 2002;58(7):1081–1087.
78. Fenichel GM, et al. A randomized efficacy and safety trial of oxandrolone in the treatment of Duchenne dystrophy. Neurology 2001;56(8):1075–1079.
79. Creutzberg EC et al. A role for anabolic steroids in the rehabilitation of patients with COPD? A double-blind, placebo-controlled, randomized trial. Chest 2003;124(5):1733–1742.
80. Newsholme EA, Calder PC. The proposed role of glutamine in some cells of the immune system and speculative consequences for the whole animal. Nutrition 1997;13(7–8):728–730.
81. Biolo G, et al. Muscle glutamine depletion in the intensive care unit. Int J Biochem Cell Biol 2005;37(10):2169–2179.
82. Burnham EL, Moss M, Ziegler TR. Myopathies in critical illness: characterization and nutritional aspects. J Nutr 2005;135(7):1818S–1823S.
83. Singleton KD, Beckey VE, Wischmeyer PE. Glutamine prevents activation of NF-kappaB and stress kinase pathways, attenuates inflammatory cytokine release, and prevents acute respiratory distress syndrome (ARDS) following sepsis.Shock 2005;24(6):583–589.

84. Burnham EL, Moss M, Ziegler TR. Myopathies in critical illness: characterization and nutritional aspects. J Nutr 2005;135(7):1818S–1823S.
85. Mok E, et al. Oral glutamine and amino acid supplementation inhibit whole-body protein degradation in children with Duchenne muscular dystrophy. Am J Clin Nutr 2006;83(4):823–828.
86. DeFilippisAP, Sperling LS. Understanding omega-3's. Am Heart J 2006;151(3):564–570.
87. Doshi M, et al. Effect of dietary enrichment with n-3 polyunsaturated fatty acids (PUFA) or n-9 PUFA on arachidonate metabolism in vivo and experimentally induced inflammation in mice. Biol Pharm Bull 2004;27(3):319–323.
88. Kelley VE, et al. A fish oil diet rich in eicosapentaenoic acid reduces cyclooxygenase metabolites, and suppresses lupus in MRL-lpr mice. J Immunol 1985;134(3):1914–1919.
89. Arterburn LM, Hall EB, Oken H. Distribution, interconversion, and dose response of n-3 fatty acids in humans. Am J Clin Nutr 2006;83(6 suppl):1467S–1476S.
90. Simopoulos AP, Essential fatty acids in health and chronic diseases. Forum Nutr 2003;56:67–70.
91. Calder PC, n-3 polyunsaturated fatty acids, inflammation, and inflammatory diseases. Am J Clin Nutr 2006;83(6 suppl):1505S–1519S.
92. Pennisi P, Trombetti A, Rizzoli R. Glucocorticoid-induced osteoporosis and its treatment. Clin Orthop Relat Res 2006;443:39–47.
93. Cantorna MT, et al. Vitamin D status, 1,25-dihydroxyvitamin D3, and the immune system. Am J Clin Nutr, 2004;80(6 suppl):1717S–20S.
94. Alsufyani KA, et al. Bone mineral density in children and adolescents with systemic lupus erythematosus, juvenile dermatomyositis, and systemic vasculitis: relationship to disease duration, cumulative corticosteroid dose, calcium intake, and exercise. J Rheumatol 2005;32(4):729–733.
95. Cantorna MT, Mahon BD. D-hormone and the immune system. J Rheumatol Suppl 2005;76:11–20.
96. Zittermann A, Vitamin D in preventive medicine: are we ignoring the evidence? Br J Nutr 2003;89(5):552–572.
97. CantornaMT, Mahon BD. Mounting evidence for vitamin D as an environmental factor affecting autoimmune disease prevalence. Exp Biol Med (Maywood) 2004;229(11):1136–1142.
98. Larsson P, et al. A vitamin D analogue (MC 1288) has immunomodulatory properties and suppresses collagen-induced arthritis (CIA) without causing hypercalcaemia. Clin Exp Immunol 1998;114(2):2772–83.
99. Adorini L, Intervention in autoimmunity: the potential of vitamin D receptor agonists. Cell Immunol 2005;233(2):115–124.
100. Grant WB, Holick MF. Benefits and requirements of vitamin D for optimal health: a review. Altern Med Rev 2005;10(2):94–111.
101. Schneider C, Chemistry and biology of vitamin E. Mol Nutr Fod Res 2005;49(1):7–30.
102. Traber MG, Sies H. Vitamin E in humans: demand and delivery. Annu Rev Nutr 1996;16:321–347.
103. Tomasi LG, Reversibility of human myopathy caused by vitamin E deficiency. Neurology 1979;29(8):1182–1186.
104. Osoegawa M, et al. [A patient with vitamin E deficient, myopathy presenting with amyotrophy]. Rinsho Shinkeigaku 2001;41(7):428–431.
105. Schneider C, Chemistry and biology of vitamin E. Mol Nutr Food Res 2005;49(1):7–30.
106. Sacheck JM, Blumberg JB. Role of vitamin E and oxidative stress in exercise. Nutrition 2001;17(10):809–814.
107. Jackson MJ, et al. Vitamin E and the oxidative stress of exercise. Ann N Y Acad Sci 2004;1031:158–168.
108. Beaton LJ, et al. Contraction-induced muscle damage is unaffected by vitamin E supplementation. Med Sci Sports Exerc 2002;34(5):798–805.
109. Haas DC, Vitamin E therapy in polymyositis. South Med J 1977;70(9):1148–1149.
110. Manach C, et al. Polyphenols: food sources and bioavailability. Am J ClinNutr 2004;79(5):727–747.
111. Nam NH, Naturally occurring NF-kappaB inhibitors. Mini Rev Med Chem 2006;6(8):945–951.
112. Dorchies OM, et al. Green tea extract and its major polyphenol (-)-epigallocatechin gallate improve muscle function in a mouse model for Duchenne muscular dystrophy. Am J Physiol Cell Physiol 2006;290(2):C616–C625.

113. Moon Y, Lee M, Yang H. Involvement of early growth response gene 1 in the modulation of microsomal prostaglandin E synthase 1 by epigallocatechin gallate in A549 human pulmonary epithelial cells. Biochem Pharmacol 2007;73(1):125–135.
114. Pugh N, et al. Isolation of three high molecular weight polysaccharide preparations with potent immunostimulatory activity from Spirulina platensis, aphanizomenon flos-aquae and Chlorella pyrenoidosa. Planta Med 2001;67(8):737–742.
115. Lee AN, Werth VP. Activation of autoimmunity following use of immunostimulatory herbal supplements. Arch Dermatol 2004;140(6):723–727.

13 Nutritional Issues in Vasculitis

Paul F. Dellaripa and Donough Howard

Summary
- Gastrointestinal involvement is common in systemic vasculitis.
- Chronic systemic inflammation is common in vasculitis and frequently leads to weight loss and cachexia.
- Immunosuppressive medications can cause gastrointestinal toxicity.
- There is little evidence of any dietary manipulations or supplementations having any impact on the course of vasculitis.

Key Words: Churg-Strauss vasculitis; corticosteroids; giant cell arteritis; microscopic polyangitis; polyarteritis nodosa; vasculitis; Wegener's granulomatosis

1. INTRODUCTION

The vasculitides are a group of disorders characterized by the presence of destructive inflammation in blood vessel walls *(1–4)*. The possibility of a systemic vasculitis should be considered in a patient with systemic complaints and dysfunction of any and often multiple organ systems, frequently in the context of constitutional symptoms such as fever, malaise, and weight loss. Vasculitic syndromes are often classified by the size of vessel involved. Although there may be overlap in the vessel size, diseases may affect predominately large vessels (Takayasu's arteritis [TA] and giant cell arteritis [GCA]), predominately medium arteries (such as polyarteritis nodosa [PAN] and central nervous system [CNS] vasculitis), or predominately small vessels (Wegener's granulomatosis [WG], microscopic polyangiitis [MPA], Churg-Strauss syndrome [CSS], cryoglobulinemia, and drug-induced vasculitis).

Disorders not discussed herein but that may mimic the presentation of vasculitis include embolism caused by endocarditis, cardiac myxoma, hypercoagulable states including the antiphospholipid antibody syndrome, hyperviscosity syndromes, vitamin C deficiency, and cholesterol embolism, among other syndromes *(5,6)*.

2. POLYARTERITIS NODOSA

PAN is a systemic necrotizing arteritis involving predominantly medium-sized vessels, although it may affect smaller vessels. Vasculitic lesions characteristically occur at the bifurcations or branches of vessels and are often segmental. The skin, peripheral nerves, kidneys, gastrointestinal (GI) tract, and joints are the principal organs affected *(7)*.

Patients generally complain of malaise, weight loss, fevers, abdominal or lower extremity pain, myalgias, or arthralgias. Clinical parameters include hypertension and azotemia with proteinuria but rarely glomerulonephritis. Neurological manifestations include peripheral neuropathy, seizures, and altered mental status *(8,9)*. Musculoskeletal symptoms including arthralgias and less frequently arthritis can occur *(7)*. Vasculitis of skeletal muscles may cause severe myalgias and muscle biopsy can be useful diagnostically *(10)*. Abdominal pain may be caused by intestinal angina, mesenteric thrombosis, and localized gallbladder or liver disease. Acute GI bleeding, perforation, and infarction are rare but are associated with a high mortality if the diagnosis is not established promptly *(11)*. Cardiac involvement may be clinically silent but includes congestive heart failure (CHF), pericarditis, myocardial infarction, and conduction abnormalities *(12,13)*. Cutaneous lesions include nonspecific palpable purpura, livedo reticularis, tender nodular lesions, digital infarcts, and ulcers *(14)*.

The pathogenesis of polyarteritis is unknown. Hepatitis B surface antigen (HBsAg) has been found in a minority of patients with PAN. The presence of circulating immune complexes of HBsAg and deposition of surface antigen and immunoglobulin in vessel walls has been noted *(15,16)*. Hepatitis C has rarely been associated with PAN *(17)*. Pathologically, fibrinoid necrosis, pleomorphic cellular infiltration in small and medium vessels, thrombosis, and aneurysms are noted *(18)*.

The diagnosis of PAN focuses on the most frequent areas of involvement, namely, nerve, skin, and GI systems. Laboratory parameters usually present include elevated sedimentation rate, elevated C-reactive protein (CRP), and thrombocytosis. Mesenteric angiography often shows evidence of aneurysms including the renal, hepatic, and mesenteric arteries and areas of arterial stenosis alternating with normal or dilated vessels *(18)*. Sural nerve biopsies are easily accessible sources of nerve tissue when a mononeuritis is present.

Although there is no consensus in the treatment of PAN, administration of corticosteroids at 1 mg per kg per day orally is indicated in nearly all cases. In the presence of GI involvement, intravenous dosing may need to be continued especially in life threatening cases. The use of a second drug is guided by the severity of presentation and if there is failure to respond to steroids alone. A severity of illness scoring system (the Five Factor Score) has been developed based on five different parameters, namely, proteinuria greater than 1 g per day, azotemia, GI involvement, cardiomyopathy, and CNS involvement. The presence of two or more of these factors portends a mortality of nearly 50% *(7)*. A review of long-term follow-up of these patients suggests that those with more severe illness as defined with one of the above factors have a higher survival rate when treated with cyclophosphamide *(19)*. Plasmapheresis (PE) in combination with antiviral therapy is indicated in hepatitis B virus (HBV)-associated PAN, although PE has not shown to improve outcome in non HBV PAN *(20,21)*.

It must also be noted that a variety of drugs, viral infections, connective tissue disease such as rheumatoid arthritis (RA), and underlying malignancies may cause a necrotizing angiitis, which may be indistinguishable from polyarteritis *(22–27)*.

3. MICROSCOPIC POLYANGIITIS

MPA is a necrotizing vasculitis that involves small vessels, including arterioles, capillaries, and venules. Cases of MPA previously classified as part of the PAN classification are distinguished mainly by the presence of segmental necrotizing glomerulonephritis. Clinical presentations may involve concomitant capillaritis with or without alveolar hemorrhage and rapidly progressive glomerulonephritis, the so-called pulmonary renal syndrome. Glomerulonephritis occurs in most cases, and pulmonary involvement ranging from cough and dyspnea to frank hemoptysis occurs in up to 30% of cases. Neuropathy and cutaneous vasculitis occur in up to 50% of cases *(14,26,27)*. Antineutrophilic cytoplasmic antibodies (ANCA) are found in about 75% of cases, mostly specific for myeloperoxidase (MPO), although occasionally ANCA proteinase 3 (PR3) has been described *(27)*.

Diagnosis is typically made with a biopsy of lung, kidney, skin, or nerve in conjunction with a positive ANCA result. Treatment involves corticosteroids at 1 mg/kg per day orally or intravenous methylprednisolone, and cyclophosphamide orally or intravenously with transition to azathioprine or other similar agent after induction of remission *(27)*. PE may have a role in severe renal disease with evidence suggesting a lower rate of dialysis requirement though no evidence of mortality benefit *(28)*. In relapsing disease, intravenous immunoglobulin may be of benefit *(29)*.

4. CHURG-STRAUSS SYNDROME

CSS is characterized by the presence of eosinophilic infiltrates and granulomas in the respiratory tract, and necrotizing vasculitis in the setting of asthma and peripheral eosinophilia. Typically, patients have a preceding history of asthma and allergic rhinitis and then develop constitutional symptoms of fatigue, weight loss, and then systemic symptoms such as mononeuritis, cardiomyopathy, pulmonary infiltrates, or abdominal pain *(14)*. Pulmonary disease includes fleeting or diffuse infiltrates, nodular lesions, and peripheral infiltrates occur in up to 75% of patients *(30,31)*. Peripheral neuropathy is frequent, in up to 75% of patients with CSS, whereas renal involvement is much less common than in MPA and WG. Other sources of morbidity and mortality include GI involvement with bleeding and bowel perforation, cardiac involvement causing arrhythmias, pericarditis, and CHF *(30)*.

The etiology of CSS is unknown. ANCA is positive in approx 38 to 60% of cases, mostly MPO *(31–34)*. As mentioned earlier, the presence of any of the five prognostic factors has been associated with a higher mortality and should guide the choice of treatment, suggesting corticosteroids for limited disease and the addition of cyclophosphamide in the setting of severe disease *(19)*.

5. CRYOGLOBULINEMIC VASCULITIS

Cryoglobulins are immunoglobulins that precipitate below 37°C. There are three types: type I, seen in myeloproliferative disorders; type II, or mixed essential cryoglobulins; and type III, mixed polyclonal. Types II and III are most closely associated with hepatitis C infection. Typical involvement includes cutaneous vasculitis, arthritis, and peripheral neuropathy and less likely renal, GI or pulmonary involvement *(35–38)*.

Abnormal liver enzymes suggest hepatitis C infection; complement levels, especially C4, are decreased *(39,40)*. Therapy in severe cases consists of corticosteroids and cyclophosphamide with careful attention to the potential risk of increased hepatitis C replication and treatment with antiviral therapy if hepatitis C is present. In severe cases involving progressive glomerulonephritis, plasmapheresis or cryofiltration may be of additional benefit *(41,42)*.

6. WEGENER'S GRANULOMATOSIS

WG is a disease of unknown etiology characterized by granulomatous vasculitis of the upper and lower respiratory tract, segmental necrotizing glomerulonephritis, and systemic vasculitis of small blood vessels *(43)*. Although the disease may affect individuals of a wide range of ages, the disease most commonly affects persons in their fourth or fifth decades of life with a slight predominance for men over women *(44,45)*.

The etiology of WG is unknown. Possible infectious etiological associations with *Staphylococcus aureus* have been proposed but are as yet unproven *(46)*. ANCA is present in more than 90% of patients with systemic WG, and in 70 to 80% with active limited disease. Correlation of ANCA titers with clinical remission is controversial, with the most recent data suggesting that in treated patients with negative titers relapse is unlikely, whereas those with rising or recurrently positive titers have a higher risk of relapse, although the timing of relapse is not predictable *(47,48)*. There is also increasing evidence of the pathogenecity of ANCA in the vasculitic component of WG *(49)*.

Most patients (approx 85 to 90%) present with symptoms referable to the upper respiratory tract, including sinusitis, nasal obstruction, rhinitis, otitis, hearing loss, ear pain, gingival inflammation, epistaxis, sore throat, laryngitis, and nasal septal deformity. Fever, in addition to being caused by the underlying disease, may result from suppurative otitis or *S. aureus* sinusitis *(50)*. Granulomatous vasculitis of the upper respiratory tract may lead to damage of nasal cartilage resulting in the "saddle-nose" deformity, sore throat, and oral and nasal mucosal ulcers *(51)*. Chondritis of the nose or ear may develop and laryngeal involvement may result in severe narrowing of the upper respiratory tract *(52–54)*. WG may also be associated with inflammation and subsequent scarring/stenosis of the subglottic region, in about 25% of patients *(55)*. This complication is distinctly more common in younger adult and pediatric populations.

Approximately 10% of patients present with only nonspecific constitutional symptoms such as arthralgias, myalgias, fever, and weight loss. Skin lesions of WG include distinctive punched-out ulcerative skin lesions appearing as pyoderma gangrenosum and painless subcutaneous nodules occurring in approx 2 to 5% *(56)*.

Although only one-third of patients present with symptomatic lung involvement (including cough, sputum production, dyspnea, chest pain, hemoptysis, and even life-threatening pulmonary hemorrhage), lower respiratory tract disease is found in almost all patients after evaluation. Renal manifestations are often asymptomatic although urinalysis reveals renal involvement in approximately 80% of patients at presentation. Functional renal impairment may progress rapidly if appropriate therapy is not instituted promptly *(57)*.

Diagnosis is usually based on the clinical findings of upper and lower respiratory tract noninfectious, inflammation with glomerulonephritis and positive anti-PR3 antibodies

(58). In cases with more limited involvement, or where ANCA titers are negative or show the less typical MPO specificity, tissue diagnosis may be necessary.

Recent advances in the treatment of WG have led to the development of a biphasic approach with an initial remission-induction phase using a combination of cyclophosphamide and corticosteroids for 3 to 6 months followed by a remission-maintenance phase using a less toxic immunosuppressive agent, usually methotrexate or azathioprine, for a further 12 to 24 months *(59)*.

Cyclophosphamide therapy is associated with significant morbidity and patients or their proxy need to be counseled prior to consent for treatment. There is overall a 2.4-fold increase in malignancy with an 11-fold increase in the risk of leukemia or lymphoma *(59,60)* and a significant increased risk of bladder cancer occurring in 1 to 3% of patients with WG who are treated with cyclophosphamide. Hemorrhage cystitis has been reported in 12 to 43% of patients treated for WG. In one study, 57% of women of childbearing age became infertile *(59)*. Opportunistic infection, particularly with pneumocystis carinii, was reported in 6% of patients in initial trials with combination cyclophosphamide and corticosteroids *(61)* and it is now standard of care for patients to be prophylactically treated with double strength trimethoprim/sulfamethoxazole, three times per week or one single-strength tablet daily.

7. DRUG-INDUCED VASCULITIS

Cases of vasculitis associated with the use of certain drugs, vaccines, and toxins have long been recognized. Previously, these have been described as hypersensitivity reactions causing small-vessel vasculitis *(62)*. More recent work in drug-induced vasculitis has broadened the group to include a large variety of small- and medium-vessel syndromes. There are no specific pathological or clinical features that distinguish this group from other forms of vasculitis. Cases ranging from self-limiting cutaneous involvement to severe multiorgan failure have been reported. Diagnosis is simply based on the development of vasculitis where a causal drug/agent can be identified, which in most cases leads to resolution of the vasculitis after drug discontinuation. There is a large variation in the length of drug exposure before symptoms develop, with many reports of years of exposure before the apparent sudden onset of vasculitis.

The most commonly reported medications causing drug-induced vasculitis include hydralazine, propylthiouracil, allopurinol, cefaclor, minocycline, D-penicillamine, phenytoin, isotretinoin, and methotrexate with colony-stimulating factors *(63)*, quinolone antibiotics and leukotriene inhibitors more recently added to the list *(64)*. Other cases have been reported following vaccination, particularly for hepatitis B *(65)* and influenza *(66)*.

8. CENTRAL NERVOUS SYSTEM VASCULITIS

CNS vasculitis is a rare condition that can present as a primary form confined to the CNS, known as primary angiitis of the CNS (PACNS) or as a secondary form associated with a systemic vasculitis or other systemic illness. Connective tissue disease such as systemic lupus erythematosus, RA, and Sjogren's syndrome can all be associated with a variety of CNS manifestations including stroke, seizure, encephalopathy, and aseptic meningitis *(67–69)*. Other secondary causes of CNS vasculitis and syndromes mimicking CNS vasculitis include sarcoidosis, antiphospholipid antibody syndrome, lymphoma, atrial myxoma, artheroemboli, Lyme disease, HIV infection, herpes zoster, tuberculosis and a variety of drugs including cocaine, methamphetamines, ergotamine, pseudoephredrine, and heroin *(70)*.

The clinical presentation associated with PACNS is broad and includes subacute memory loss, acute encephalopathy, and other cognitive and behavioral changes. Seizures, cranial nerve abnormalities, focal deficits involving the cerebrum, cerebellum, and brainstem, spinal cord lesions, meningismus, headache, auditory and vestibular disturbances, intracranial or subarachnoid hemorrhage, and reduced visual acuity or blindness caused by retinal and optic nerve vasculitis have been described *(71,72)*. Frequently, patients have hypertension that aggravates their underlying disease or raises questions about their primary diagnosis. Disease manifestations may develop precipitously but often can present with a long prodrome over months involving subtle mental status changes and cognitive dysfunction *(71,72)*. The disease has a predilection for the small and medium vessels especially of the leptomeninges. Diagnosis is made utilizing a combination of cerebrospinal fluid analysis, magnetic resonance imaging (MRI), angiography, and brain biopsy *(72–76)*.

Treatment of PACNS involves corticosteroids as the initial treatment of choice, ranging from doses of 1 mg/kg per day orally to 1 g intravenously daily for 3 days followed by oral corticosteroids. Cyclophosphamide may be added in severe cases or with progressive disease, although firm recommendations are limited by a lack of prospective trials *(77)*.

9. GIANT CELL ARTERITIS

GCA is a large-vessel vasculitis that principally affects the aorta and the extracranial branches of the carotid arteries and is the most common systemic vasculitis. Individuals are typically over the age of 50 and present with symptoms of headache, jaw claudication, scalp pain or tenderness, and a host of constitutional symptoms including fever, weight loss (50%), and fatigue *(78)*. A significant number of patients will develop proximal pain in the shoulder and hip girdle consistent with polymyalgia rheumatica (PMR) during the course of their illness and it is believed that PMR and GCA represent a spectrum of a similar clinical entity *(79)*. The most feared complication of GCA is blindness resulting from involvement of the posterior ciliary and opthalmic arteries. Involvement of the vertebral arteries may result in ischemia of the CNS and involvement of the subclavian and axillary artery resulting in limb claudication occurs in about 15% of patients *(80)*.

The etiology of GCA is unknown though the disease appears to commence in the adventitial layers of the vessel wall where CD4 T cells are recruited and activated and direct macrophage activation with the end result being production of a variety of growth factors and cytokines leading to myofibroblastic proliferation, stenosis of the lumen, and the development of ischemia *(81)*.

Physical examination is notable for tenderness or nodularity over the temporal or facial arteries. Elevation of acute-phase reactants such as the sedimentation race, CRP, alkaline phosphatase, or platelets are noted in most cases but in some cases, such markers will be absent. Diagnosis should be confirmed by temporal artery biopsy, which typically shows an inflammatory infiltrate composed of lymphocytes and multinucleated giant cells, although giant cells are not required to confirm the diagnosis. In cases where biopsy is negative (and the contralateral temporal artery is also negative), it still may be appropriate to treat if the clinical suspicion for the disease is high.

Treatment for GCA involves glucocorticoids in doses of 40 to 60 mg per day for 1 month and then a slow taper over a period of 1 to 2 years, although some patients require a longer duration of therapy because relapse is not uncommon. In the case of threatening visual loss, some clinicians will use high-dose methylprednisolone (1 g intravenously for 3 days) although data supporting this approach is limited *(82)*. The use of methotrexate and s steroid-sparing agents has been met with variable results *(83,84)*. Low-dose aspirin may reduce the risk of cranial ischemic complications *(85)*. Trials examining the use of tumor necrosis factor (TNF) antagonists in GCA are underway at present. Morbidity associated with the disease beyond visual loss mostly involves side effects of corticosteroids including weight gain, glucose intolerance, and also a higher risk of thoracic aortic aneurysm and rupture *(86)*.

10. OTHER VASCULITITES

Takayasu's arteritis (TA) is a large-vessel granulomatous vasculitis that affects the aortic arch and branches, affecting mostly women age 40 or below. Patients frequently present with constitutional symptoms such as weight loss, fatigue, and myalgias. Development of inflammation within blood vessels can result in vessel stenosis and aneurysm, leading to symptoms such as claudication caused by subclavian artery occlusion and stroke owing to occlusion of the carotids and vertebral arteries *(87,88)*. Physical examination is notable for decreased or absent pulses, bruits, carotid tenderness, and heart murmurs most frequently related to aortic regurgitation owing to proximal dilatation of the aortic root. Uncontrolled hypertension, which may be difficult to monitor as a result of diminished peripheral pulses, is a significant source of morbidity in TA *(89)*. The sedimentation rate may be elevated, but not in all patients and diagnosis are confirmed utilizing MRI, computed tomography angiography, conventional angiography and most recently, positron emission tomography *(90,91)*.

Corticosteroids are used initially in high doses and there is some evidence to support the use of methotrexate and anecdotal evidence utilizing TNF antagonists as potentially useful. Stenosis that remains symptomatic despite medical treatment may be amenable to vascular intervention with varying degrees of success *(92–94)*.

Behcet's syndrome is characterized by apthous ulceration of the oral and genital areas that can sometimes present with a systemic vasculitis that can affect any size blood vessels, including portal veins, pulmonary arteries, and CNS vessels *(95,96)*. Thrombosis of blood vessels is common. Other important manifestations include a variety of skin lesions which include erythema nodosum, pustular lesions and a characteristic pathergy phenomenon. Corticosteroids are useful during the acute phases of severe disease and treatment with colchicine, azathiporine, cyclosporine, and TNF antagonists are utilized for chronic management *(97)*.

11. NUTRITIONAL VALUES AND VASCULITIS

In reviewing nutrition and vasculitis, the most overwhelming observation is how sparse research has been in this area, with almost no studies looking at even the prevalence of malabsorption or nutritional deficiency in this group of patients. There are, however, nutritional factors that should be considered in managing these patients.

GI involvement is common in systemic vasculitis with 23 to 70% of patients with PAN reporting abdominal pain *(98)*. At its most severe, bowel infarction caused by mesenteric vascular thrombosis may occur with diarrhea, pain, GI bleeding, or malabsorption occurring in less fulminant cases.

Weight loss is also a common feature of any systemic inflammatory state and is frequently seen in systemic vasculitis. Up to 35% of patients with WG have weight loss of more than 10% of their initial body weight *(99)*, despite the fact that bowel involvement is rare in this disease.

Immunosuppressive medications used to treat vasculitis may also produce GI toxicity with nausea and anorexia frequently seen with cyclophosphamide therapy. Corticosteroids, the mainstay of almost all treatment strategies, frequently lead to truncal obesity, decreased muscle mass, and decreased bone density. Concomitant treatment with calcium and vitamin D supplementation is now standard in patients being treated with corticosteroids with prophylactic bisphosphonate therapy also being used in most patients to decrease bone loss. Methotrexate use is associated with folate deficiency through its inhibition of dihydrofolate reductase. Supplementation with folic acid 1 mg daily is standard in these patients with some requiring higher doses or the addition of folinic acid given 12 hours before and/or after their weekly dose of methotrexate.

Recent research on the pathophysiology of systemic inflammatory disease has highlighted the role of superoxide production and its possible role in tissue damage. One study has examined the potential role of antioxidant supplementation in decreasing neutrophil superoxide production in vasculitis. Harper et al. showed decreased *in vitro* respiratory burst and superoxide production by neutrophils isolated from patients with ANCA-associated vasculitis following treatment with vitamins C and E when compared with neutrophils from normal controls *(100)*. *In vivo* studies are still lacking to determine if vitamin C and E supplementation could lead to any clinical response.

11.1. Summary

Despite the lack of data in this area, the natural history of the vasculitic syndromes can clearly result in a wide variety of nutritional challenges either caused by the clinical manifestations of the disease itself or the infectious complications related to treatment. It is imperative that all clinicians that participate in the care of these patients be cognizant of the catabolic effect due to vasculitis and the prompt need for treatment. Monitoring nutritional status may help to avoid the infectious complications that sometimes result from the immunosuppressive effects of treatment.

REFERENCES

1. Frankel SK, Sullivan EJ, Brown KK. Vasculitis: Wegener's granulomatosis, Churg-Strauss syndrome, microscopic polyangiitis, polyarteritis nodosa and Takayasu's arteritis. Crit Care Clinics 2002;18: 855–879.

2. Saleh A, Stone JH. Classification and diagnostic criteria in systemic vasculitis. Best Pract Res Clin Rheumatol 2005;19(2):209–221.
3. Buhaescu I, Covic A, Levy J. Systemic vasculitis: still a challenge. Am J Kidney Dis 2005;46: 173–185.
4. Hellmich B, Gross WL. Difficult to diagnose manifestations of vasculitis: Does an interdisciplinary approach help? Best Pract Res Clin Rheumatol 2005;19(2):243–262.
5. Lie JT. Vasculitis simulators and vasculitis look-alikes. Curr Opin Rheumatol 1992;4:47.
6. O'Keefe ST, Woods BO, Breslin DJ, et al. Blue toe syndrome. Causes and management. Arch Intern Med 1992;152:2197.
7. Guillevin L, Lhote F, Gayraud M, et al. Prognostic factors in polyarteritis nodosa and Churg-Strauss syndrome: a prospective study of 342 patients. Medicine 1996;75:17–28.
8. Griffin J. Vasculitis neuropathies. Rheum Dis Clin North Am 2001;27:751–760.
9. Moore PM, Fauci AS. Neurologic manifestations of systemic vasculitis: a retrospective and prospective study of clinicopathologic features and responses to therapy in 25 patients. Am J Med 1981;71:517–524.
10. Said G, Lacroi-Ciaudo C, Fujimura H, et al. The peripheral neuropathy of necrotizing arteritis: a clinical pathologic study. Ann Neurol 1988;23:461–465.
11. Levine SM, Hellman DB, Stone JH. Gastrointestinal involvement in polyarteritis nodosa (1986–2000); presentation and outcomes in 24 patients. Am J Med 2002;112:386–391.
12. Holsinger DR, Osmundson PJ, Edwards JE. The heart in periarteritis nodosa. Circulation 1962;25: 610–618.
13. Schrader ML, Hochman JS, Bulkley BH. The heart in polyarteritis nodosa: a clinicopathologic study. Am Heart J 1985;109:1353–1359.
14. Lhote F, Guilliven L. Polyarteritis nodosa, microscopic polyangiitis, Churg Strauss syndrome: clinical aspects and treatment. In Hunder GG, ed. Rheum Dis Clinics of North America, Saunders, Philadelphia, PA, 1995, pp. 911–947.
15. Fye KH, Becker MJ, Theofilopoulos AN, et al. Immune complexes in hepatitis B antigen-associated periarteritis nodosa: detection by antibody independent cell-mediated cytotoxicity and the Raji cell assay. Am J Med 1977;62:783–791.
16. Tsukada N, Koh C, Owa M, et al. Chronic neuropathy associated with immune complexes of hepatitis B virus. J Neurol Sci 1983;61:193–211.
17. Carson CW, Conn AJ, Czaja AJ, et al. Frequency and significance of antibodies to hepatitis C virus in polyarteritis nodosa. J Rheum 1993;20:304–309.
18. Cid MC, Grau JM, Casademont J, et al. Immunohistochemical characterization of inflammatory cells and immunologic activation markers in muscle and nerve biopsy specimens from patients with polyarteritis nodosa. Arthritis Rheum 1994;37:1055–1061.
19. Gayraud M, Guillevin L, Toumelin P, et al. Long-term follow-up of Polyarteritis nodosa, microscopic polyangiitis, and Churg-Strauss syndrome. Arthritis Rheum 2001;44(3):666–675.
20. Guillevin L, Mahr A, Cohen P, et al. Short term corticosteroids then lamivudine and plasma exchanges to treat Hepatitis B virus-related polyarteritis nodosa. Arthritis Rheum 2004;51(3):482–487.
21. Guillevin L, Fain O, Lhote F, et al. Lack of superiority of steroids plus plasma exchange to steroids alone in the treatment of polyarteritis nodosa and Churg-Strauss syndrome. A prospective randomized trial in 78 patients. Arthritis Rheum 1992;35:208–215.
22. Citron BP, Halpern M, McCarron M, et al. Necrotizing angiitis associated with drug abuse. N Engl J Med 1970;1003:283.
23. Luqmani R, Watts RA, Scott DGI, et al. Treatment of vasculitis in rheumatoid arthritis. Ann Intern Med 1994;145:566–576.
24. Mertz LE, Conn DL. Vasculitis associated with malignancy. Curr Opin Rheumatol 1992;4:39–46.
25. Somer T, Finegold SM. Vasculitides associated with infections, immunizations, and antimicrobrial drugs. Clin Inf Dis 1995;20:1010–1036.
26. Falk RJ, Nachman PH, Hogan SL, et al. ANCA glomerulonephritis and vasculitis: a Chapel Hill perspective. Semin Nephrol 2000;20(3):233.
27. Guillevin L, Durand-Gasselin B, Cevallos R, et al. Microscopic polyangiitis. Arthritis Rheum 1999;42:421–430.

28. Gaskin G, Jayne D. Adjunctive plasma exchange is superior to methylprednisolone in acute renal failure due to ANCA-associated glomerulonephritis. J Am Soc Nephrol 2002;13(suppl:S2A–S3A.
29. Jayne DRW, Chapel H, Adu D, et al. Intravenous immunoglobulin for ANCA-associated systemic vasculitis with persistent disease activity. Q J Med 2000;93:433–439.
30. Guillevin L, Guittard T, Bletry O, et al. Systemic necrotizing angiitis with asthma: causes and precipitating factors in 43 cases. Lung 1987;165:165–172.
31. Guillevin L, Cohen P, Gayraud M, et al. Churg- Strauss syndrome: clinical study and long-term follow-up in 96 patients. Medicine (Baltimore) 1999;78:26–37.
32. Guillevin L, Visser H, Noel LH, et al. Antineutrophilic cytoplasm antibodies in systemic polyarteritis nodosa with and without hepatitis B virus infection and Churg-Strauss syndrome-62 patients. J Rheumatol 1993;20:1345–1349.
33. Solans R, Bosch JA, Perez-Bocanegra C, et al. Churg-Strauss syndrome: outcome and longterm follow-up of 32 patients. Rheumatology 2001;40:763–771.
34. Sable-Fourtassou, Cohen P, Mahr A, et al. Antineutrophil cytoplasmic antibodies and Churg-Strauss syndrome. Ann Intern Med 143:632–638, 2005.
35. Tarantino A, Campise M, Banfi G, et al. Long-term predictors of survival in essential mixed cryoglobulinemic glomerulonephritis. Kidney Int 1995;47:618–623.
36. Bombardieri S, Paoletta P, Ferri C, et al. Lung involvement in essential mixed cryoglobulinemia. Am J Med 1979;66:748–756.
37. Caniatti LM, Tugnoli V, Eleopra R, et al. Cryoglobulinemic neuropathy related to hepatitis C virus infection. Clinical, laboratory, and neurophysiological study. J Periph Nerv Syst 1996;1:131–138.
38. Gomez-Tello V, Onoro-Canaveral JJ, de la Casa Monje RM, et al. Diffuse recidivant alveolar hemorrhage in a patient with hepatitis C virus related mixed cryoglobulinemia. Intensive Care Med 1999;25(3):319.
39. Agnello V, Ghung RT, Kaplan LM. A role for Hepatitis C virus in type II cryoglobulinemia. N Engl J Med 1992;327:1490.
40. Lamprecht P, Moosig F, Gause A, et al. Immunologic and clinical follow-up of hepatitis C virus associated cryoglobulinemic vasculitis. Ann Rheum Dis 2001;60:385–390.
41. Guillevin L, Pagnoux C. Indications of plasma exchanges for systemic vasculitides. Ther Apher Dial 2003;7(2):155–160.
42. Rieu V, Cohen P, Andre MH, et al. Characteristics and outcome of 49 patients with symptomatic cryoglobulinemia. Rheumatology (Oxford) 2002;41:290–300.
43. Godman GC, Churg J. Wegener's granulomatosis: pathology and review of the literature. Arch Pathol 1954;58:533–553.
44. Fauci AS, Wolff SM. Wegener's granulomatosis: studies in eighteen patients and a review of the literature. Medicine 1973;52(6):535–561.
45. Wolff SM, Fauci AS, Horn RG, et al. Wegener's granulomatosis. Ann Intern Med 1974;81(4):513–525.
46. Popa ER, Tervaert JW, et al. The relationship between Staphylococcus aureus and Wegener's granulomatosis: current knowledge and future directions. Int Med 2003;42(9):771–780.
47. Kerr GS, Fleisher TA, Hallahan CW, et al. Limited prognostic value of changes in antineutrophil cytoplasmic antibody titer in patients with Wegener's granulomatosis. Arthritis Rheum 1993;36(3):365–371.
48. Boomsa MM, Stegeman CA, van der Leij MJ, et al. Prediction of relapses in Wegener's granulomatosis by measurement of antineutrophil cytoplasmic antibody levels: a prospective study. Arthritis Rheum 2000;43(9):2025–2033.
49. Falk RJ, Jennette JC. ANCA are pathogenic—oh yes they are! J Am Soc Nephrol 2002;13(7):1977–1979.
50. Fauci AS, Haynes BF, Katz P, et al. Wegener's granulomatosis: prospective clinical and therapeutic experience with 85 patients for 21 years. Ann Intern Med 1983;98(1):76–85.
51. Schramm VL Jr, Myers EN, Rogerson DR. The masquerade of vasculitis: head and neck diagnosis and management. Laryngoscope 1978;88(12):1922–1934.
52. Goldenberg DL, Goodman ML. Case 26–1985. Case records of the Massachusetts General Hospital: weekly clinicopathological exercises. N Engl J Med 1985;312:1695–1697.

53. Harrington JT, McCluskey RT. Case 24–1979. Case records of the Massachusetts General Hospital: weekly clinicopathological exercises. N Engl J Med 1979;300:1378–1380.
54. McDonald TJ, DeRemee RA: Wegener's granulomatosis. Laryngoscope 1983;93(2):220–231.
55. Langford CA, Sneller MC, Hallahan CW, et al. Clinical features and therapeutic management of subglottic stenosis in patients with Wegener's Granulomatosis. Arthritis Rheum 1996;39(10): 1754–1760.
56. Bernhard JD, Mark EJ. Case 17–1986. Case records of the Massachusetts General Hospital: weekly clinicopathological exercises. N Engl J Med 1986;314:1170–1173.
57. Hoffman G, Kerr G, Leavitt R. Wegener's Granulomatosis: An analysis of 158 patients. Ann Intern Med 1992;116:488–498.
58. Lynch JP, Matteson E, McCune WJ. Wegener's granulomatosis: evolving concepts. Medical Rounds 1989;2:67.
59. Regan M, Hellmann D, Stone J. Treatment of Wegener's Granulomatosis. Rheum Dis Clinics of North America 2001;27(4):863–886.
60. Reinhold-Keller E, Beuge N, Latza U, et al. An interdisciplinary approach to the care of patients with Wegener's granulomatosis. Long-term outcome in 155 patients. Arthritis Rheum 2000;43:1021–1032.
61. Ognibene, FP, Shelhamer JH, Hoffman, GS, et al. Pneumocystis carinii pneumonia: A major complication of immunosuppressive therapy in patients with Wegener's granulomatosis. Am J Respir Crit Care Med 1995;151:795–799.
62. Calabrese LH, Michel BA, et al. The American College of Rheumatology 1990 criteria for the classification of hypersensitivity vasculitis. Arthritis Rheum 1992;33(8):1108–1113.
63. Merkel P. Drug-induced vasculitis. Rheum Dis Clinics of North America 2001;27(4):849–862.
64. Bonilla MA, Dale D, et al. Long-term safety of treatment with recombinant human granulocyte colony-stimulating factor in patients with severe congenital neutropenias. Br J Hematol 1994;88(4):723–730.
65. Blumberg S, Bienfang D, et al. A possible association between influenza vaccination and small vessel vasculitis. Arch Intern Med 1980;140(6):847–848.
66. Ascherio A, Zhang SM, et al. Hepatitis B vaccination and the risk of multiple sclerosis. N Engl J Med 2001;344(5):327–332.
67. Alexander EL. Neurologic disease in Sjogrens syndrome: mononuclear inflammatory vasculopathy affecting the central/peripheral nervous system and muscle. Rheum Dis Clin North Am 1993;19: 869–908.
68. Neamtu L, Belmont M, Miller DC, et al. Rheumatoid disease of the central nervous system with meningeal vasculitis presenting with seizure. Neurology 2001;56(6):814–815.
69. Ellis SG, Verity MA. Central nervous system involvement in systemic lupus erythematosus: a review of neuropathologic findings in 57 cases. Semin Arthritis Rheum 1979;8:212–221.
70. Siva A. Vasculitis of the nervous system. J Neurol 2001;248:451–468.
71. Younger DS, Calabrese LH, Hays AP. Granulomatous angiitis of the nervous system. Neurol Clin 1997;15:821–834.
72. Calabrese LH, Furlan AJ, Gragg LA, et al. Primary angiitis of the central nervous system (PACNS): a reappraisal of diagnostic criteria and revised clinical approach. Cleve Clin J Med 1992;293–306.
73. Duna GF, Calabrese LH. Limitations of invasive modalities in the diagnosis of primary angiitis of the central nervous system. J Rheumatol 1995;222:662–667.
74. Harris K, Tram D, Skekels W, et al. Diagnosing intracranial vasculitis: the roles of MRI and angiography. Am J Neuroradiol 1994;15:317–330.
75. Vanderzant C, Bomberg M, MacGuire A, et al. Isolated small vessel angiitis of the central nervous system. Arch Neurol 1988;45:683–687.
76. Lie JT. Primary (granulomatous) angiitis of the central nervous system: a clinical pathologic analysis of 15 new cases and a review of the literature. Hum Pathol 1992;23:164–1717.
77. Hajj-Ali RA, Ghamande S, Calabrese LH, et al. Central nervous system vasculitis in the intensive care unit. Crit Care Clin 2002;18:897–914.
78. Weyand CM, Goronzy JJ. Giant cell arteritis and polymyalgia rheumatica. Ann Int Med 2003; 139(6):505–515.
79. Calamia KT, Hunder GG. Clinical manifestations of giant cell (temporal) arteritis. Clin Rheum Dis 1980;6:389–403.

80. Brack A, Martinez-Taboada V, Stanson A, et al. Disease pattern in cranial and large-vessel giant cell arteritis. Arthritis Rheum 1999;42(2):311–317.
81. Kaiser M, Weyand C, Bjornsson J, Goronzy JJ. Platelet derived growth factor, intimal hyperplasia and ischeamic complications in GCA. Arthritis Rheum 1998;41:623–633.
82. Chan CC, O'Day J. Oral and intravenous steroids in giant cell arteritis. Clin Experiment Ophthalmol 2003;31(3):179–182.
83. Jover JA, Hernandez-Garcia C, Morado IC, et al. Combined treatment of giant cell arteritis with methotrexate and prednisone. A randomized, double-blind, placebo-controlled trial. Ann Intern Med 2001;134(2):106–114.
84. Hoffman GC, Cid MC, Hellman DB, et al. A multicenter, randomized, double- blind placebo-controlled trial of adjuvant methotrexate treatment for giant cell arteritis. Arthritis Rheum 2002;46(5):1309–1318.
85. Nesher G, Berkun Y, Mates M, et al. Low-dose aspirin and prevention of cranial ischemic complications in giant cell arteritis. Arthritis Rheum 2004;50(4): 1332–1337.
86. Evans JM, Bowles CA, Bjornsson J, et al. Thoracic aortic aneurysm and rupture in giant cell arteritis. Arthritis Rheum 1994;37(10):1539–1547.
87. Kerr GS, Hallahan CW, Giordana J, et al. Takaysu arteritis. Ann Int Med 1994;120:919–929.
88. Vanoli M, Daina E, Salvarani C, et al. Takaysu's arteritis: A study of 104 Italian patients. Arthritis Rheum 2005;15(1):100–107.
89. Chugh KS, Sakhuja V. Takayasu's arteritis as a cause of renovascular hypertension in Asian countries. Am J Nephrol 1992;12:1–8.
90. Andrews J, Al-Nahhas A, Pennell DJ, et al. Non-invasive imaging in the diagnosis and management of Takayasu's arteritis. Ann Rheum Dis 2004;63(8):995–1000.
91. Schmidt WA, Blockmans D. Use of ultrasonography and positron emission tomography in the diagnosis and assessment of large-vessel vasculitis. Curr Opin Rheumatol 2005;17(1):9–15.
92. Hoffman GS, Leavitt RY, Kerr GS, et al. Treatment of glucocorticoid-resistant or relapsing Takayasu arteritis with methotrexate. Arthritis Rheum 1994;37(4):578–582.
93. Hoffman GS, Merkel PA, Brasington RD, et al. Anti-tumor necrosis factor therapy with difficult to treat Takayasu arteritis. Arthritis Rheum 2004;50(7):2296–2304.
94. Liang P, Hoffman GS. Advances in the medical and surgical treatment of Takayasu arteritis. Curr Opin Rheumatol 2005;17(1):16–24.
95. Marshall SE. Behcet's disease. Best Pract Res Clin Rheumatol 2004;18(3):291–311.
96. Suzuki Kurokawa M, Suzuki N. Behcet's disease. Clin Exp Med 2004;4(1):10–20.
97. Pipitone N, Oliveri I, Cantini F, et al. New approaches in the treatment of Adamantiades-Behcet's disease. Curr Opin Rheumatol 2006;18(1):3–9.
98. Guillevin L, Lhote F, Gallais V, et al. Gastro-intestinal tract involvement in polarteritis nodosa and Churg Straus syndrome. Ann Med Interne 1995;146: 260–267.
99. Hoffman G. Wegener's granulomatosis. In: Klippel JL, Dieppe PA, eds. Rheumatology 2nd ed. Mosby, London, 1998, p. 7:22.4.
100. Harper L, Nuttall SL, Martin U, et al. Adjuvant treatment of patients with ANCA associated with vitamins E and C reduces superoxide production by neutrophils. Rheumatology 2002;41: 274–278.

14 Sjögren's Syndrome and Its Implications for Diet and Nutrition

Carole A. Palmer and Medha Singh

Summary

- Sjögren's syndrome is a chronic autoimmune disorder, most common in adult women.
- There is no known etiology or cure for Sjögren's syndrome.
- Sjögren's syndrome is characterized by debilitating ocular and oral manifestations.
- Early diagnosis and palliation are critical.
- Nutrition implications are similar to those for patients undergoing oral cancer and head and neck radiation.
- Omega-3 fatty acids have been implicated as a potential therapeutic agent.

Key Words: Autoimmune disease; dental caries; ocular dryness; Sjögren's syndrome; xerostomia

1. INTRODUCTION

Sjögren's syndrome (SS) is a chronic autoimmune rheumatic disorder that can have devastating multiple organ systems effects, yet is often under-diagnosed and its effects often trivialized [1]. In SS, lymphocytes invade the exocrine (secretory) glands, leading to severe xerostomia (dry mouth), xeropthalmia (dry eyes), and internal organ damage. In its earliest or mildest stages, SS can cause eye discomfort owing to lack of lacrimation, and difficulty in mastication as a result of a lack of oral saliva. If untreated, complications can become severe, and multiple organ damage (kidneys, liver, pancreas, lungs, blood vessels, and brain) can result [2,3].

SS is the second most common autoimmune rheumatic disorder [4]. It is most common in middle-aged white women, but can occur in anyone, including children. Although the causes of SS are unknown, early diagnosis and treatment is essential to provide palliation and prevent debilitating conditions [5,6].

The oral effects are similar to those resulting from head and neck radiation therapy, and include dry mouth from lack of saliva, diminished taste, decreased appetite, great difficulty masticating and swallowing food, decreased nutrient intake, and subsequent weight loss. Figure 1 describes the consequences of salivary hypofunction.

The cause(s) and prevention of SS are unknown to date. However, early diagnosis and management are essential to prevent oral, ocular, and internal organ damage. This

From: *Nutrition and Health: Nutrition and Rheumatic Disease*
Edited by: L. A. Coleman © Humana Press, Totowa, NJ

Consequences of Saliva Hypofunction

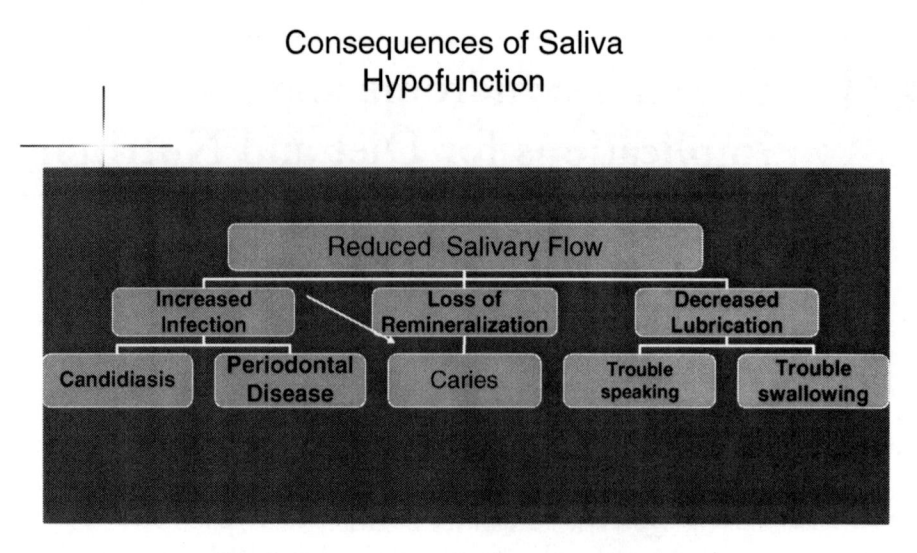

Fig. 1. Consequences of salivary hypofunction.

chapter provides an overview of SS with emphasis on strategies for early intervention, palliation, and nutritional intervention.

2. SJÖGREN'S SYNDROME DEFINED

2.1. History

In 1933, the Swedish ophthalmologist Henrik Samuel Conrad Sjögren (1899–1986) recognized ocular dryness in 19 patients, including 13 who also had rheumatoid arthritis (RA). He called the condition keratoconjunctivitis sicca (KCS *(7)*), where sicca refers to dryness of the eyes and mouth. The syndrome was renamed Sjögren's syndrome in 1953 and was redefined in 1956 as a condition in which at least two of the following three findings are present: KCS, xerostomia (dry mouth), and RA or other connective tissue disease *(8)*.

2.2. Epidemiology

SS is the second most common rheumatic disease in the United States, after RA. It affects between 1 and 4 million people in the United States *(9)* and about 500,000 in the United Kingdom *(10)*. However, the true prevalence may be much higher as many researchers believe that about half the cases are undiagnosed *(10,11)*. SS typically begins in the fourth to sixth decade of life *(11)*. Most (90%) of SS sufferers are middle-aged white, perimenopausal females, but SS has been seen in men, children, and the aged as well. The prevalence ratio of women to men is 9:1.

2.3. Types of Sjogren's Syndrome

There are two types of *SS*—primary and secondary *(11)*. *Primary SS* is so named because it occurs independently of any other associated conditions or precipitating factors *(12)*. *Secondary SS* occurs in association with another connective tissue disease such as systemic lupus erythematosus (SLE), RA, scleroderma, or relapsing polychondritis. SS secondary to an accompanying autoimmune disorder accounts for approx 60% of patients with the disease. Conversely, approx 25% of patients with RA or SLE have histological evidence of having syndromes *(13)*.

2.4. Pathophysiology

SS is a chronic autoimmune disorder in which the lymphocytes invade and destroy the exocrine (secretory) glands (especially the salivary and lacrimal glands), resulting in chronic dysfunction of these glands *(14*; Fig. 2). Tissues involved may include the mouth, salivary glands, eyes, nose, throat, lungs, and vagina. SS can also affect blood vessels, the nervous system, muscles, skin, and other organs such as the liver and pancreas *(3*; Fig. 3).

The processes that begin the humoral and cellular autoimmune reaction in patients with SS are not known, but both B- and T-lymphocytes are involved *(11,15)*. These lymphocytes invade and destroy target organs. B-cell hyperreactivity is manifest through hypergammaglobulinemia and circulating autoantibodies. Approximately 60% of patients with SS are found to have non-organ-specific autoantibodies including rheumatoid factor (RF), antinuclear antibody (ANA), and antibodies to the small RNA protein complexes Ro/SSA and La/SSB *(16,17)*. Organ-specific antibodies include antibodies to the cellular antigens of the thyroid gland, salivary ducts, gastric mucosa, erythrocytes, pancreas, prostate, and nerve cells. It is believed that these autoantibodies can contribute to tissue dysfunction prior to any evidence of inflammation *(16,18)*.

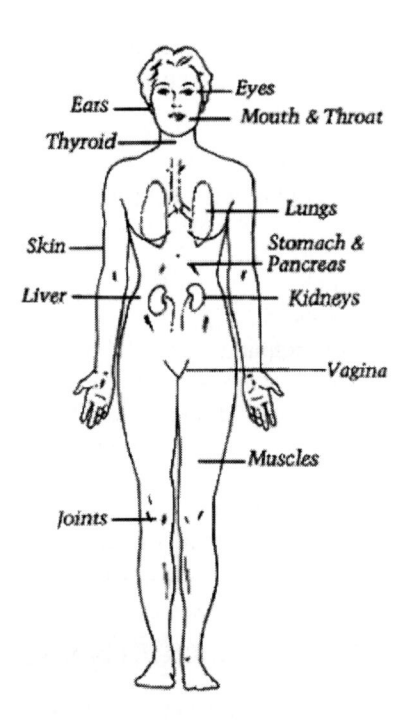

Fig. 2. Locations of Sjogren's syndrome effects in the body. (http://www.orthop.washington.edu/uw/sjogrenssyndrome/tabID__3376/ItemID__55/PageID__5/Articles/Default.aspx).

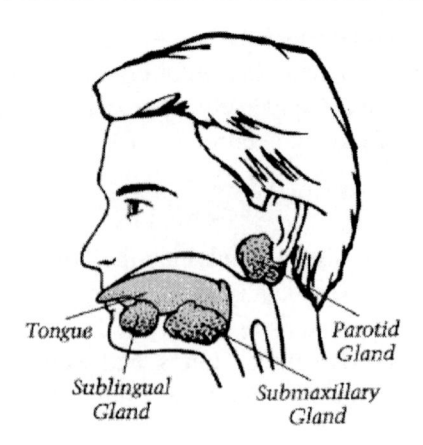

Fig. 3. Salivary gland locations in the oral cavity (http://www.orthop.washington.edu/uw/sjogrenssyndrome/tabID__3376/ItemID__55/PageID__4/Articles/Default.aspx).

Histopathological findings in SS include lymphocytic infiltration primarily around glandular ducts such as salivary and lacrimal glands, and exocrine glands of the gastrointestinal, vaginal, and respiratory tracts. The infiltrates contain T, B, and plasma cells. Activated CD4+helper T cells predominate and produce interleukins (IL)-2, -4, -6, and -1α, and tumor necrosis factor (TNF)-α *(19,20)*.

The inflammatory processes of SS occur via glandular epithelial cells that express antigen-presenting proteins and promote adhesion and co-stimulate T-lymphocytes. Cytokines such as interferon (INF)-α and TNF-α enhance the antigen-presenting function of epithelial cells. INF-α can induce apoptosis of epithelial cells through the up-regulation of Fas protein, which is a cell-surface receptor *(21)*.

2.5. Etiology

Although the etiology of SSn is unknown, multiple factors are thought to be involved in its development: *(8,22,23)*

- Environment: various viruses such as Epstein-Barr virus and cytomegalovirus are under scrutiny as possible inciting agents.
- Sex hormones: the majority of individuals with SS are female, suggesting that sex hormones may play a role in the autoimmune response.
- Genetics: genetic factors are considered likely to play a role, as there is a higher incidence of SS in families of SS sufferers, and along with increased incidence of certain human leukocyte antigens.Increased autoantibodies: the presence of certain antibodies is assnociated with increased SSn symptoms.
- Inflammatory reactivity: several proinflammatory factors are produced in the salivary glands and may play a role in perpetuating the disease process.

3. PHYSIOLOGICAL EFFECTS OF SJÖGREN'S SYNDROME

The symptoms of SS are many and diverse and are summarized in Table 1. Sufferers primarily report mild to extreme discomfort from dry eyes and/or dry mouth, but may have a variety of other signs and symptoms as well. The hallmark symptoms are

Table 1
Possible Effects of Sjogren's Syndrome

Dry eyes

- Pain in the eyes or the feeling that a piece of sand is in the eyes
- Rarely: blindness

Dry mouth

- Trouble chewing and swallowing
- Sore mouth
- Tooth decay
- Swollen salivary glands

Dry skin, dry nose

- Dryness of the upper respiratory system, causing nose bleeds, hoarseness, dry cough, or sinus or lung infections

Vaginal dryness, kidney, blood vessels, lung damage

Involvement of joints, muscles, glands, nerves, liver, pancreas, stomach, and brain

- Fatigue

xeropthalmia (dry eye), and xerostomia (dry mouth *(24)*). General fatigue is also a common complaint *(25)*.

3.1. Ocular Effects (11)

Xeropthalmia (KCS) is a common side effect of SS. Xeropthalmia results from a fluid deficiency of the tear film of the eye. The tear film consists of the mucin, aqueous, and lipid layers. The aqueous layer produces 90% of tear volume. As the tear volume diminishes, the ocular symptoms occur. Individuals with SS often report that their eyes feel extremely dry, "gritty," or "sandy," and they may experience a reduction in tearing as well *(26)*. The patient may report that the eyes "burn" and/or itch, and may look red. A thick substance may accumulate in the inner corner of the eyes during sleep. The eyes may be more sensitive to sunlight than usual as well. If not treated properly and early enough, ulcers of the cornea can result, which may lead to blindness.

3.2. Oral Effects of SS and Their Influence on Diet and Nutrition

SS affects the oral cavity in several ways *(27)*. A primary effect is salivary deficiency (known as xerostomia), which leads to dry mouth. Xerostomia can have far-reaching effects on oral health *(28)* and on diet and nutrition *(29)*.

Dry mouth (xerostomia) is caused by the abnormal reduction in salivary secretions that results from autoimmune diseases such as SS, medications, irradiation of the head and neck, or surgery *(30)*. The oral effects of xerostomia include difficulty swallowing, speaking, chewing, and wearing dentures; changes in taste; burning or soreness of oral

Table 2
Functions of Saliva

- Lubrication to aid in chewing and swallowing
- Maintaining the integrity of the mucous membranes, which are the first lines of defense in innate immunity
- Aiding in remineralization of the teeth
- Buffering acids and maintaining the pH near neutral
- Antimicrobial effect on bacterial growth
- Cleansing the mouth
- Dissolving food to allow the sensations of sweet, sour, salty, and bitter tastes
- Aiding in swallowing and speaking

mucosa; increased susceptibility to oral candidiasis; and an increase in the incidence of severe caries *(4)*. About half of individuals with SS also have swollen and tender parotid, submandibular, and sublingual glands, and may also have fever. Xerostomia, in turn, leads to a variety of oral problems (discussed later) with nutritional implications.

Saliva is an important protective constituent of the oral cavity, and has many functions (Table 2 *(23)*). It aids in the mastication and swallowing of food, lubricates the oral mucosa, facilitates taste bud function, and protects teeth by providing important remineralizing, antibacterial, and lavage functions. Saliva also provides physical and chemical protection to the oral and pharyngeal mucous membranes.

3.2.1. Effects of Xerostomia on the Dentition

Xerostomia increases the risk of developing dental caries (tooth decay). Dental caries is a multifactorial infectious (preventable) disease. It occurs when acids are formed from the bacterial fermentation of dietary carbohydrates in the dental plaque coating teeth. The acid causes the tooth enamel demineralization that initiates the caries process (Fig. 4). Rampant caries is common in patients with SS because of the common presence of xerostomia (Fig. 5).

In the absence of saliva, the oral cavity loses these important protective elements, and the risk of developing dental caries increases significantly. With xerostomia, the soft tissue (gingiva) surrounding the teeth are more susceptible to bacterial infection. If the gingiva recede and newly expose the neck of the tooth, root caries may result (Fig. 6). Saliva plays an important role in buffering acids in the oral cavity. In the absence of saliva, acids from foods and beverages as well as from bacterial fermentation can cause severe tooth enamel demineralization (Fig. 7).

3.2.2. Other Oral Effects

As a result of xerostomia, patients with SS often complain of other oral problems. They may develop a burning sensation in the tongue, and develop tongue fissures and cracks at the corner of the mouth. The loss of the immunity provided by saliva may result in increased incidence of candidiasis and other fungal infections (Fig. 8). The loss of the antimicrobial protection of saliva can result in increased bacterial plaque and associated gingival inflammation and recession, and mild to moderate periodontal disease (disease of the soft tissue and bone surrounding and supporting the teeth).

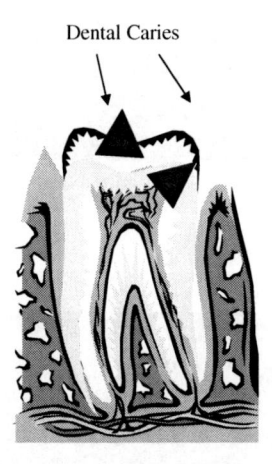

Chapter 14 / Sjögren's Syndrome and Its Implications for Diet and Nutrition   233

Fig. 4. The process of dental caries: 1. Acids are produced on tooth surfaces as an end product of dental plaque bacterial fermentation of simple sugars; 2. acids demineralize dental enamel and dentin, and bacteria invade dentin resulting in carious lesion.

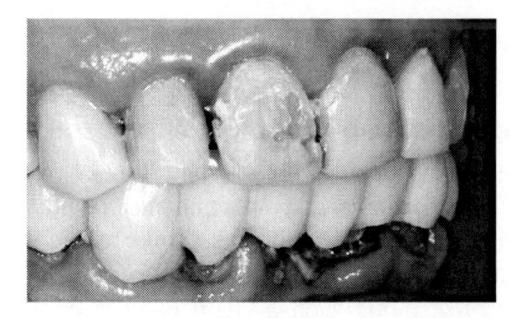

Fig. 5. Rampant caries in adults (photos courtesy of Dr. Athena Papas).

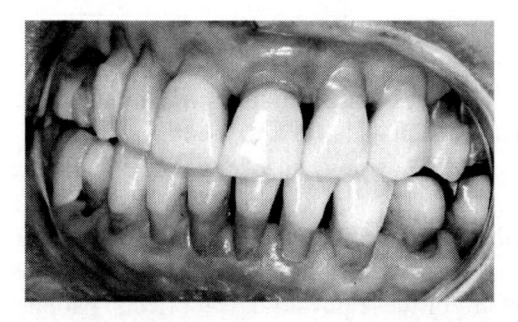

Fig. 6. Generalized gingival recession and root caries adults (photos courtesy of Dr. Athena Papas).

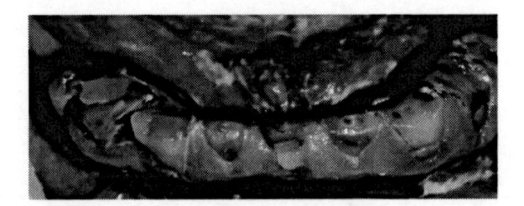

Fig. 7. Acid erosion due to fruit drinks in a xerostomic patient with Sjogren's syndrome (photo courtesy of Dr. Athena Papas).

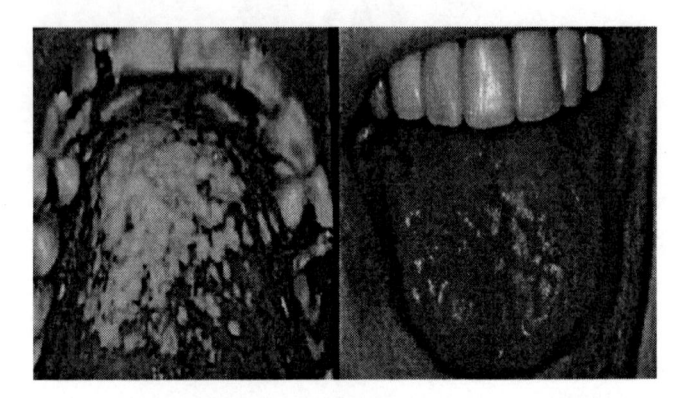

Fig. 8. Candidiasis (photo courtesy of Dr. Athena Papas).

3.2.3. EFFECTS OF XEROSTOMIA ON DIET AND NUTRITION

In the absence of saliva, it becomes a challenge to chew, swallow, and even taste food *(31)*. As a result, dysgeusia and dysphagia may result. Difficulty masticating and lubricating food may make it difficult to eat solid foods. Patients may adapt to a primarily liquid diet that may be low in nutritional value. It is also common that people experiencing dry mouth use items such as hard candies or other slowly dissolving lozenges in an effort to increase salivation. If these items are used frequently and contain sugars, they can be major contributors to increased dental caries incidence. Frequent eating or snacking is a major risk factor for dental caries development that is increased when the oral cleansing effects of saliva are lost.

3.3. Other Physiological Effects

SS may also result in dryness of all mucous membranes, including mouth, throat, lungs, and vagina. Sufferers may have a dry cough, hoarseness, a decreased sense of smell, and nose bleeds. They may also develop pneumonia, bronchitis, and ear problems.

SS can also affect the blood vessels, the nervous system, muscles, skin *(32)*, heart *(33)*, and other organs such as the kidney *(34)*. Lymphomas are seen in 6% of people *(18,35)*. As a result of these physiological effects, patients may develop muscle weakness, confusion and memory problems, dry skin, and feelings of numbness and tingling in the extremities *(36)*. People may also report having joint or muscle pain *(37)*, low-grade fever, increased fatigue *(25)*, and vasculitis.

4. DIAGNOSIS OF SJÖGREN'S SYNDROME

Salivary gland biopsy is considered the "gold standard" for diagnosing SS. However, with newer criteria, patients may be diagnosed as having SS without a biopsy. The new criteria states that a person may be diagnosed as having Sjogren's syndrome if he has at least four of the following six diagnostic tests results (Table 3), including one objective measure (ie, by histopathologic examination or antibody screening) as positive *(16,38)*. Table 4 summarizes the techniques for performing the diagnostic tests:

1. Salivary function test: Salivary function tests are used to determine the actual severity of xerostomia *(39)*. Sialometry measures unstimulated salivary flow rate into a calibrated tube for 15 minutes. The normal salivary flow rate is 1.5 mL for 15 minutes. If the unstimulated salivary gland flow rate is less than 1.5 mL per minute for 15 minutes then it is positive for SS.
2. Salivary gland biopsy: Lip biopsy involves performing biopsy of minor salivary glands in the lower lip. For SS, the biopsy report should have a focus score of 1 or more. Minor salivary gland biopsy remains a highly specific test for the salivary component of SS *(40)*.
3. Dry eye test: The Schirmer's test assesses tear formation. Filter paper is placed in the lower conjunctival sac. If less than 5 mm of paper is wetted in 5 minutes then the test result is positive for SS. Another test that could be performed for dry eye is the Rose Bengal staining test. This test determines the inflammation of the cornea.
4. Laboratory test abnormalities: Serological and laboratory findings associated with SS include diffuse hypergammaglobulinemia, which is found in approx 80% of patients with the disease. Several autoantibodies are among the immunoglobulin's whose levels are elevated, including FF, ANAs, and antibodies to the extractable cellular antigens Ro/SSA, and La/SSB. The following laboratory findings are associated with SS:
   - positive for SSA (Ro) antibodies;
   - positive for SSB (La) antibodies;
   - positive for ANA;
   - positive for RF;
   - elevated immunoglobulin G (IgG);
   - Elevated erythrocyte sedimentation rate (ESR);
   - low albumin levels; and
   - anemia.
5. Symptom for dry mouth: Patient reports of symptoms of dry mouth are also used to help diagnose SS. (However, dry eyes and xerostomia may exist in the absence of patient-recognized symptoms.) A positive response to all of the following is considered diagnostic for salivary hypofunction *(22)*:
   - Do you sip liquids to aid in swallowing dry foods?
   - Does your mouth feel dry when eating a meal?
   - Do you have difficulties swallowing any foods? *(41)*
   - Does the amount of saliva in your mouth seem to be too little?
   - Does your nose or throat feel dry and tickly?
   - Do you have a dry cough, hoarseness, nosebleeds or a decreased sense of taste or smell?

Table 3
Diagnostic Test Performed to Diagnose Sjogren's Syndrome

Salivary function test
Lip biopsy
Dry eye test
Blood test
Symptoms for dry mouth
Symptoms for dry eyes

Table 4
Techniques for Performing Diagnostic Tests for Sjogren's

Salivary function test: Sialometry measures unstimulated salivary flow rate into a calibrated tube for 15 min. The normal salivary flow rate is 1.5 ml for 15 min. If the un-stimulated salivary gland flow rate is less than 1.5 ml/min for 15 min then it is positive for Sjogrens syndrome.

Lip biopsy: a small amount of salivary tissue is removed from inside the lip and examined under a microscope for evidence of Sjogrens syndrome

Schirmer test for dry eyes: helps determine the dryness of eyes. A small piece of filter paper is placed under the lower eyelid to determine the quantity of tear production

Symptom for dry eyes: Patient reports of symptoms of dry eyes are also used to help diagnose Sjogren's syndrome. A positive response to all of the following is considered diagnostic for dry eyes *(22)*:
- Do you Do your eyes feel dry, "gritty" or "sandy" or burn
- Do you use tear substitutes more than 3x/day?

6. Physical Examination: In addition to the routine physical examination, clinical signs such as redness of the eyes, dry cracked tongue, swollen salivary glands, and enlarged lymph glands in the neck may assist in the diagnosis of syndromes *(6)*.

5. MANAGING SJÖGREN'S SYNDROME

There is no known approach to prevent or cure SS. Nevertheless, in addition to early diagnosis, aggressive symptom-based treatment will help alleviate much of the discomfort, retard the progression of the disorder, and promote comfort and productivity *(42)*. Because the treatment is tailored to the symptoms, each patient's management plan will be different *(43)*. The following are examples of the potential menu of management strategies.

5.1. Minimizing Aggravating Factors

The first step in the management plan for patients with SS should be to minimize any factors that may exacerbate the symptoms. Because the eyes and mouth are the most commonly involved, eliminating oral and ocular irritants is important. People with eye involvement should avoid smoke, either active or passive. This includes avoiding smoking and locations where smoking is prevalent. Avoiding outdoor grills and fireplaces may also help. Additionally, a humidifier in the house can be a tremendous help to avoid low humidity conditions.

Caregivers should check to see what medications patients with SS may be taking that may contribute to xerostomia. There are hundreds of common medications that cause xerostomia and can compound the discomfort of the xerostomia already resulting from the SS. If possible, alternative, non-xerostomic medications should be used as substitutes.

Patients should be shown how to avoid any products that can contribute to oral dryness or irritation. Alcohol has a drying effect and should be avoided in both beverages and in oral products such as mouthwashes. Tartar control toothpastes and tooth whitening products should also be avoided as they can be irritating to friable oral tissues. If patients tend to breathe through their mouths, it is often helpful to encourage them to try to increase nasal breathing and check with an otolaryngology specialist if there are impediments to normal nasal breathing. In the presence of xerostomia and decreased immunity, there is often an increase in fungal infections such as oral candidiasis. If present, these should be treated appropriately. Table 5 summarizes these risk factors.

5.2. Eye Palliatives

A variety of lubricants are available over the counter and by prescription to lubricate the eyes and minimize eye itching and burning. Examples are Ristasis™ ; another is TheraTears™ .These palliatives are helpful and seem to be well tolerated *(44)*.

5.3. Oral Palliatives and Therapies (Table 6 (45))

A multitargeted approach is needed for oral care to palliate existing conditions and more importantly, protect oral soft and hard tissues from further damage. Patients should see the dentist at least four times a year for diagnostic evaluations and preventive and palliative treatments. Radiographs should be taken yearly to check for new carious lesions in the dentition.

Every effort should be made to manage the xerostomia and its effects *(30)*. The oral mucosa is often dry and sore as a result of the loss of protective saliva. Oral

Table 5
Environmental Risk Factors To Reduce or Eliminate

- Substitute non-xerostomic medications
- Avoid alcohol and other oral irritants
- Avoid smoking and smoke
- Avoid low-humidity conditions
- Correct mouth breathing
- Treat oral candidiasis
- Avoid tartar control toothpastes

Table 6
Oral Palliatives and Therapies

Goal	Approach
Diagnosis and overall management	• Dental visits four times a year and periodontal prophylaxsis (dental cleaning) on these visits. • Dental X-rays once a year to check for any dental caries

Palliate oral soft tissues	• Saliva substitutes various brands provide limited relief
	• Oral lubricants for soothing effects
	    ∗ Vitamin E, mineral oil
	    ∗ Oral Balance®

Protect dentition and reduce dental caries risk	• Fluoride
	    ∗ Fluoride varnish four times to start and then every 3 months
	    ∗ Prescription strength 1.1% neutral sodium fluoride
	    ∗ Other remineralization
	    ∗ Calcium-containing toothpaste (Mentadent replenishing White®)
	    ∗ Caphasol® remineralizing rinse use twice per day
	    ∗ Remineralizing products
	    ∗ adjunctive treatment (e.g., Mouth Kote®)
	• Sonic tooth brush
	    ∗ Use for plaque removal and stimulation of salivary flow by placing brush on tongue and roof of mouth after brushing for 1 minute
	• Antibacterial Solutions
	    ∗ Chlorhexidine, Triclosan

Promote Salivary Flow	• Sialogogues
	    ∗ Cevimeline(Evoxac®) 30 mg three or four times a day
	    ∗ Pilocarpine HCl (Salagen®) 5 to 7.5 mg four times a day

lubricants such as vitamin E, mineral oil, or a product entitled Oral Balance® are effective in soothing these irritated tissues. A saliva substitute can also be used before eating to mimic the effects of actual saliva. Sialogogues may be prescribed for some patients to promote salivary function. Sialogogues are drugs that work by stimulating the M3 receptors stimulating moisture production throughout the body. They should

Table 7
Management of Oral Candidiasis

Topical agents
- Nystatin oral suspension 100,000 U/mL four times a day
- Clotrimazole troche five per day
- Clotrimazole 1% cream three times a day for angular cheilitis

Systemic agents
- Fluconazole 100 to 200 mg daily
- Itraconazole oral suspension 10 mg/10 mL
- Sporanox 100 mg/10 mL twice per day (liquid swish and swallow)

be taken with food. No serious side effects have been seen but care must be taken if used with concomitant medication or by patients with cardiovascular disease or hypertension *(46)*.

Because the loss of protective saliva in xerostomia increases the vulnerability of tooth enamel surfaces, extra effort must be made to protect teeth from demineralization and dental caries. Fluoride is a mineralizing agent that has several dentally protective effects. It helps mineralize the outer surfaces of tooth enamel, thereby making enamel destruction more difficult, and impedes the function of the oral bacteria that initiate dental caries. Fluoride is available from a variety of sources from fluoridated drinking water and fluoride dentifrices to over-the-counter and prescription concentrated strength forms. Patients with SS need aggressive fluoride therapy in the form of professionally applied concentrated fluoride varnishes and prescription strength 1.1% neutral sodium fluoride applied topically.

Calcium also has a remineralizing effect on dental enamel and a calcium-containing toothpaste or remineralizing oral rinse may be recommended as well. Antibacterial solutions such as Chlorhexidine and Triclosan are indicated in an effort to reduce the growth of dental caries causing oral bacteria.Because the oral tissues and gums may be sore, the use of a normal soft-bristled toothbrush may be uncomfortable. If this is the case, a sonic tooth brush may be recommended *(47)*. Table 7 shows the management strategies for patients who develop oral candidiasis.

5.4. Dietary and Nutritional Management

The goals for nutritional management of patients with SS are as follow:

1. Help these patients to maintain good nutriture despite oral impairment by providing diet suggestions that are well tolerated and high in nutritional value and by providing diet suggestions that do not further irritate oral tissues.
2. Ensure that their dietary habits and patterns do not increase dental caries risk
3. Offer any other nutritional therapies that might be helpful in preventing, retarding, or managing SS.

5.4.1. MAINTAIN GOOD NUTRITURE DESPITE ORAL IMPAIRMENT

Good nutrition is important to assure the consumption of the nutrients known to be essential for good eye and oral health as well as general health. The antioxidant vitamins A, C, and E are important protectors of eye health. Zinc is important in retinal metabolism and tissue regeneration. The essential fatty acid, γ-linolenic acid (GLA) may be helpful in SS and other dry eye conditions *(48)*.

Many of the oral conditions listed previously conspire to limit food choices for these individuals. The lack of saliva makes it difficult to chew food and move it easily through the mouth in preparation for swallowing. Swallowing itself may be difficult with dry foods. If the oral tissues are sore, the physical form of the food may make it painful to bite or chew. Highly spicy foods or hot foods may be painful to eat. In the face of these impediments, it is natural to shy away from offending foods. However, when faced with the inability to eat the usual nutritious diet, people may adapt to a soft diet, which can be low in nutritional value. The therapeutic challenge is to provide food choices that help patients overcome the oral impediments while maintaining optimum nutriture. Table 8 provides food choice suggestions from each of the recommended food groups that will be nutritious and yet will help overcome specific oral impediments. For example, liberal use of fluids is important to help overcome oral dryness. These could include soothing beverages with meals, gravies on foods, soups, and soothing smooth deserts like ice cream and gelatin.

5.4.2. Ensure That Dietary Habits and Patterns Do Not Increase Risk for Dental Caries

The primary focus of dietary prevention of dental caries is to decrease the caries-promoting properties of the diet and enhance its protective qualities. Impaired oral clearance of food is the major factor contributing to increased caries in the patient with xerostomia. A dry mouth has a slower oral clearance, allowing carbohydrates prolonged contact with plaque bacteria, and increasing acid production. This effect is enhanced by the absence of saliva to buffer these acids. The important dietary factors include the following:

- frequency of meals and snacks;
- oral retentiveness of the diet;
- length of time between meal/snacks; and
- sequence of food consumption.

Each time a carbohydrate is consumed, the salivary pH drops below the critical *(49)* level for 20 to 30 minutes, and in those with xerostomia, the pH may remain low for an extended period with little saliva available to help buffer the acids. If meals/snacks are frequent, the rate of demineralization will exceed the rate of remineralization and caries will result. Nutrition counseling should stress having fewer simple carbohydrate-containing snacks between meals to reduce caries risk and allow for dental enamel remineralization.

Chewing provides a strong mechanical stimulus for saliva production and may help in alleviating dry mouth. When consumed at the end of a meal or snack, some foods help increase saliva, buffer or neutralize the acid challenge from bacteria, and help remineralize the tooth surface. These food sialagogues include cheese, sugar-free gum, and sugar-free artificially sweetened hard candy *(50)*. A summary list of diet recommendations for patients is provided in Table 9.

Table 8
Food Choice Suggestions for Patients With Oral Complications of Sjogren's Syndrome

Food Group	Xerostomia and Mucositis	Weight Loss	Dysphagia
Dairy Products			
At least two servings (Double-strength milk Mix: 1 c. non-fat dry milk powder and 1 qt. whole milk Provides twice the protein, vitamins, and minerals and 1.5 times the calories.)	Instant breakfast, egg-nogs, frappes, custards, puddings, hot cereal, creamed soups, cheese sauces (all made with double-strength milk. When possible) ice cream, cottage cheese, plain or fruited yogurt. Tilt head or use straw to swallow	*See* xerostomia plus: Cheese used liberally (sandwiches, sauces, toppings and in baking), cream, cream cheese, When not contraindicated	*See* xerostomia, Avoid hard, unmelted cheese
Protein Sources			
At least two servings. No raw eggs.	Hearty meat, fish, poultry, beans, tofu, peanut butter stews, soups, and chowders, meat, sauces, pot roasts. Gravies and sauces added to most, fish and poultry. Eggs added to soups, sauces and hot cereal. Avoid spicy, highly seasoned foods.	*See* xerostomia Peanut butter added to frappes, fruit, and bread. **Fruit**	*See* xerostomia Pureed or blenderized meat, fish poultry, beans and tofu, added to soups and added to mashed or pureed vegetables.
Two to three servings as tolerated.	Soft, ripe fruits and fruit juices, applesauce, cooked and canned fruits, chopped meat mixed with fruit juices', frozen fruit/fruit juice popsicles. Avoid all citrus fruits, tomatoes, and acid fruits.	All fruit, especially bananas, grapes and pineapple juice, cooked fruit with cream or liquid supplement.	Pureed fruits, all fruit and vegetable juices as tolerated, apple-sauce or banana blended with tofu, frozen fruit juice Popsicles.

(*Continued*)

Table 8
(Continued)

Food Group	Xerostomia and Mucositis	Weight Loss	Dysphagia
Vegetables Three to five servings, as tolerated	Soft, cooked vegetables, hearty vegetable soups, stews, vegetable juices.	All vegetables with sauces and gravies, starchy vegetables such as potatoes, winter squash, creamed corn.	Pureed or mashed potatoes and all vegetables (carrots, beets, corn, etc.) vegetable juices as tolerated.
Grain Products 6-11 servings	Creamy, hot cereals, noodles, pasta, bread, Dry cereals added to soups and sauces Wheat germ added to cereals, breakfast drinks, custards, frappes, yogurt etc. French toast, pancakes, bread pudding. Avoid dry toast and hard crusty bread unless soaked in beverage or soup.	All breads (sandwiches, bread puddings, cereals, cakes, cookies, pies) Caution: instruct patient to brush thoroughly after eating sweets.	Same as xerostomia column
Fats For added calories use as tolerated, if not contraindicated by obesity or diarrhea.	Oil, cream, margarine or butter used liberally in hot cereals, soups, sauces, gravies, and on vegetables; cream cheese; sour cream, mayonnaise and avocados. Use liberally except when contraindicated by heart or weight issues.	*See* xerostomia column	*See* xerostomia column

Sweets

Cakes, cookies, pies, candies, other sweet desserts and snacks.	Use artificially sweetened deserts such as flavored diet gelatin or puddings. Have sweets only as deserts when oral hygiene procedures can follow. Any sweet desserts should be minimally retentive in the mouth such as ice cream, sherbet, frozen yogurt, etc. Avoid foods sweetened with natural sugars of any type between meals. Never use slowly dissolving hard candies, lozenges, cough drops, or breath mints as they promote dental caries. Artificially sweetened hard candies are permitted.	Have more portions of nutritious foods at and between meals. If sweet snacks are needed, they should be in liquid form such as ice cream sodas or nutritional supplements and followed by oral hygiene procedures	*See xerostomia column*
Complete Nutritional Supplements (for added calories, protein, vitamins and minerals). Powdered breakfast beverage • Readily available • Inexpensive • Many flavors • About 280 calories. with whole milk • Use lactose-free milk if needed Ensure, Sustacal, Boost • More expensive • Lactose and milk free • Average 250 calories per can	All supplements are high in sugar, therefore stress toothbrushing after eating Add to, or use to replace milk in beverages, French toast, puddings, sodas, etc.	Use as needed.	Use as needed.

Adapted from Palmer Carole ed. Diet and Nutrition in Oral Health, NJ, PrenticeHall, 2006, table 11–8

Table 9
Summary: Dietary Recommendations To Reduce the Effects of SS

- Drink plenty of fluids with meals to aid in chewing, tasting, and swallowing.
- Have liberal intake of low fat dairy products such as low-fat milk, cheese, and yogurt. Dairy products can have anti-caries effects.
- Avoid dry crunchy foods that are difficult to swallow and may cause oral abrasion or choking.
- Avoid acidic foods and beverages that can irritate oral tissues and contribute to dental enamel demineralization
- Avoid frequent intake of sugar-containing foods.
- Eliminate the use of any slowly dissolving sugar-containing candy, mint, or lozenge use of sugarless candies, chewing gum (xylitol doesn't promote caries).
- Avoid alcohol because it can cause dessication of the oral mucous membranes
- Avoid alcohol and caffeinated beverages because they can cause dehydration and increase dryness.
- Eat foods at moderate temperatures to avoid burning or freezing sensitive oral tissues
- If a liquid diet is indicated, see a registered dietitian to find ways to ensure nutritional adequacy.
- Have fatty fish like salmon a few times a week for the omega-3 fatty acids.
- Enjoy tea as a beverage for the beneficial polyphenols.
- Take a daily multivitamin-mineral supplement if you think that your diet may not be optimal.

5.4.3. OTHER NUTRITIONAL THERAPIES FOR PREVENTING, RETARDING, OR MANAGING SS

Evidence suggests that dietary factors may contribute to the etiology and/or progression of SS, and nutritional interventions may help modify the severity of the pathological effects of the disorder *(29,51)*.

Diets rich in various essential fatty acids have shown some clinical benefit in patients with RA, and may be helpful to patients with SS as well *(52)*. Recent research has found a possible association between intake of omega-3 (n-3) fatty acids and dry eye syndrome *(53)*. In a study of 32,470 women in the Women's Health Study, it was found that frequent eaters of fish such as tuna and salmon had a 17% lower risk of developing dry eye syndrome than those who ate little of these fish. Women who ate tuna or salmon at least five times a week had a 68% lower risk of developing dry eye. Conversely, dry eye syndrome was 2.5 times more common in women who ate the least n-3 fatty acids and the most n-6 fatty acids*(54)*.

Although this data does not pertain directly to Sjogren's syndrome, it may be helpful to people suffering from dry eye to recommend that they increase their consumption of foods high in n-3 fatty acids *(49)*. A randomized, prospective, placebo-controlled clinical trial to determine possible effects of an n-3 fatty acid supplement on dry mouth and dry eye in patients with SS found that salivary flow was improved in the intervention group as was the perception of oral and ocular improvement *(55)*.

Dietary intake may also affect the lipid profiles of patients with SS *(56)*. GLA has been used experimentally to treat fatigue *(57)*.

There have also been suggestions that green tea may be associated with the incidence of SS. In China and Japan, both leading green tea-consuming countries, the incidence of SS and xerostomia are considerably lower than in the United States and England *(58–60)*. Green tea contains polyphenols that possess anti-inflammatory and anti-apoptotic properties in normal human cells. It may be that these polyphenols could provide protective effects against autoimmune reactions in salivary glands and skin as well. However, caution must be exercised, as too much tea can provide excessively high amounts of caffeine as well *(58)*.

6. SUMMARY

SS is an autoimmune condition that results in dryness in many of the body's tissues. The condition is rarely fatal, but its symptoms can severely compromise health and quality of life. The disease course of SS can vary from very mild to faintly significant. Individuals with secondary SS seem to have milder disease, as compared with those with primary SS.

Early diagnosis and treatment are extremely important in trying to prevent damage to major organs. Ocular and oral care is particularly important to prevent serious harm to eyes and teeth. The oral side effects of SS can result in dietary and nutritional problems, which can then further compromise health. Many effective strategies are available to help patients manage their symptoms. A variety of support resources are available to people with SS. Several are summarized in Table 10. Routine follow-up care with the physician and the dentist is important *(16)*. With early intervention and good individualized care, people with SS should be able to lead full and comfortable lives.

Table 10
Selected SS Resources

Newsletter

"The Moisture Seekers"
Sjogren's Syndrome Foundation Inc
333 No Broadway
Jerico, NY, 11753
Phone: 516-933-6365 or 1-800-4-sjogren
Fax: 516-933-6368

Related Organizations and Websites

National Institute of Neurological Disorders and Stroke NIH Neurological Institute
P.O. Box 5801
Bethesda, MD 20824

Voice: (800) 352-9424 or (301) 496-5751
TTY (for people using adaptive equipment): (301) 468-5981

http://www.ninds.nih.gov/disorders/sjogrens/sjogrens.htm

(Continued)

Table 10
(Continued)

National Organization for Rare Disorders (NORD)
P.O. Box 1968
(55 Kenosia Avenue)
Danbury, CT 06813-1968
orphan@rarediseases.org
http://www.rarediseases.org
Tel: 203-744-0100 Voice Mail 800-999-NORD (6673)
Fax: 203-798-2291

National Eye Institute (NEI)
National Institutes of Health, DHHS
31 Center Drive, Rm. 6A32 MSC 2510
Bethesda, MD 20892-2510
2020@nei.nih.gov
http://www.nei.nih.gov
Tel: 301-496-5248

National Institute of Arthritis and Musculoskeletal and Skin Diseases (NIAMS)
National Institutes of Health, DHHS
31 Center Dr., Rm. 4C02 MSC 2350
Bethesda, MD 20892-2350
NIAMSinfo@mail.nih.gov
http://www.niams.nih.gov
Tel: 301-496-8190 877-22-NIAMS (226-4267)

National Institute of Dental and Craniofacial Research (NIDCR)
National Institutes of Health, DHHS
31 Center Drive, Room 5B-55
Bethesda, MD 20892
nidcrinfo@mail.nih.gov
http://www.nidcr.nih.gov
Tel: 301-496-4261

Sjogren's Syndrome Foundation
8120 Woodmont Ave.
Suite 530
Bethesda, MD 20814-1437
tms@sjogrens.org
http://www.sjogrens.org
Tel: 301-718-0300 800-4-SJOGREN (475-6473)
Fax: 301-718-0322

Arthritis Foundation
1330 West Peachtree Street
Suite 100
Atlanta, GA 30309

help@arthritis.org
http://www.arthritis.org
Tel: 800-568-4045 404-872-7100 404-965-7888
Fax: 404-872-0457

Sjogren's Syndrome Association, Inc. / Association du Syndrome de Sjogren Inc.

Address:
1650 de Maisonneuve West
Suite 401
Quebec, H3H 2P3
Canada

Phone: 514-934-3666
Fax: 514-934-1241

REFERENCES

1. Petruzzi LM, Vivino FB. Sjogren's syndrome– implication for perioperative practice. The Association of Perioperative Registered Nurse 2003;77(3):611–628.
2. Venables PJ. Sjogrens syndrome. Best Pract Res Clin Rheumatol 2004;18(3):313–329.
3. University of Washington. About Sjogren's syndrome. http:/www.orthop.washington.edu/uw/tabID_3376, accessed 12/19/06.
4. Delaleu N, Jonsson R, Koller MM. Sjogren's syndrome. Eur J Oral Sci 2005;113(2):101–113.
5. Chamber MS. Sjogren's syndrome. ORL Head Neck Nurs 2004; 22(4):22–30.
6. Mignogna SF, et al. Sjogren's syndrome: the diagnostic potential of early oral manifestations preceding hyposalivation/xerostomia. J Oral Pathol Med 2005;34:1–6.
7. Gentric A. Sicca syndromes in the elderly. Rev Prat 2001;51(2):177–180.
8. Fox RI. Sjogren's syndrome: controversies and progress. Clin Lab Med 1997;1(3):431–444.
9. National Institute of Neurological Illnesses and Stroke. NINDS Sjogren's Syndrome Information Page. http://www.ninds.nih.gov/disorders/sjogrens/sjogrens.htm, accessed June14, 2006.
10. British Sjogren's Syndrome Association. What is Sjogren's syndrome? a clinical overview. http://www.rheumatology.org.uk/link/patient_support_links/britishsjogrenssyndromeassoc, Accessed July 12, 2006 7/12.
11. Kassan SM. Moutsopoulos H. Clinical manifestations and early diagnosis of Sjogren syndrome. JAMA 2004;164:1275–1284.
12. Sawyer S. Primary Sjogren's syndrome. Nurs Stand 2004;18(23):33–36.
13. Dafni UG, Tzioufas AG, Staikos P et al. Prevalence of Sjogrens syndrome in a closed rural community. Ann Rheum Dis 1997;56:521–525.
14. Kitagawa S, et al. Abundant IgG4-positive plasma cell infiltration characterizes chronic sclerosing sialadenitis (Kuttner's tumor). Am J Surg Pathol 2005;29(6):783–791.
15. Hansen A, Lipsky PE, Dorner T. Immunopathogenesis of primary Sjogren's syndrome: implications for disease management and therapy. Curr Opin Rheumatol 2005;17(5):558–565.
16. Robinson C, Yamachika S. A Novel NOD derived murine model of primary Sjogren's syndrome. Arthritis Rheum 1998;41:150–156.
17. Gottenberg JE, et al. Tolerance and short term efficacy of rituximab in 43 patients with systemic autoimmune diseases. Ann Rheum Dis 2005;64(6):913–920.
18. Haga HJ, et al. Reproduction and gynaecological manifestations in women with primary Sjogren's syndrome: a case–control study. Scand J Rheumatol 2005;34(1):45–48.
19. Moutsopoulos H. Sjogren's syndrome: autoimmune epithelitis. Clin Immunol Immunopathol 1994;74:162–165.

20. Oxholm P, Asmussen K, Wiik A, Horrobin DF. Essential fatty acid status in cell membranes and plasma of patients with primary Sjogren's syndrome. Correlations to clinical and immunologic variables using a new model for classification and assessment of disease manifestations. Prostaglandins Leukot Essent Fatty Acids 1998:59(4):239–245.
21. Abu-Helu R, Dimitriou ID. Induction of salivary gland epithelial cell injury in Sjogren's syndrome: in vitro assessment of T cell derived cytokines and Fas protein expression. J Autoimmune 2001;17: 141–153.
22. Muscal E, Morales de Guzman M, Jung LK, Flaitz C. Sjogren's syndrome. 2004 (cited 2006 8/06/06). http://www.emedicine.com/ped/topic2811.htm
23. Dodds MWJ, Johnson DA, Yeh C-K. Health benefits of saliva: a review. J Dent 2005; 33(3):223–233.
24. Al-Hashimi I. Xerostomia secondary to Sjogren's syndrome in the elderly: recognition and management. Drugs Aging 2005;22(11):887–899.
25. Lwin CEA. The assessment of fatigue in primary Sjogren's syndrome. Scand J Rheumatol 2003;32(1):33–37.
26. Morozova RP, et al. The normal tear fluid and decreased tearing in patients with Sjogren's disease and Sjogren's syndrome. II. The lipid content. Ukr Biokhim Zh 1996;68(2):82–87.
27. Soto-Rojas A, Villa AR, Sifuentes-Osornio J, Alarcon-Segovia D, Kraus A. Oral manifestations in patients with Sjogren's syndrome. J Rheumatol 1998;25(5):906–910.
28. Atkinson J. Sjogren's syndrome: oral and dental considerations. J Am Dent Assoc 1993;124:74–86.
29. Cermak JM, et al. Nutrient intake in women with primary and secondary Sjogren's syndrome. Eur J Clin Nutr 2003;57(2):328–334.
30. Porter S, Scully C, Hegarty AM. An update of the etiology and management of xerostomia. Oral Surg Oral Med Oral Pathol Oral Radiol Endod. 2004; 97(1):28–46.
31. Hay KD, Morton RP, Wall CR. Quality of life and nutritional studies in Sjogren's syndrome patients with xerostomia. N Z Dent J 2001;97(430):128–131.
32. Yoneyama K, et al. Primary localized cutaneous nodular amyloidosis in a patient with Sjogren's syndrome: a review of the literature. J Dermatol 2005:32(2):120–123.
33. Schumann C, et al. Autoimmune polyglandular syndrome associated with idiopathic giant cell myocarditis. Exp Clin Endocrinol Diabetes 2005;113(5):302–307.
34. Terai C, Sakurai T. Renal lesions related to Sjogren's syndrome. Nippon Naika Gakkai Zasshi 2005;94(5):871–875.
35. Kassan SS, Thomas TL, Moutsopoulos HM, et al. Increased risk of lymphoma in sicca syndrome. Ann Intern Med. 1978;89(6):888–892.
36. Michowitz Y, et al. Transient lower limbs paralysis—a rare presenting symptom of Sjogren's syndrome. Harefuah 2005;144(4):241–242.
37. Seve P, et al. Cricoarytenoid arthritis in Sjogren's syndrome. Rheumatol Int 2005;25(4):301–302.
38. Longman L, Highan SM, Bucknall R, Kaye SB, Edgar WM, Field EA. Signs and symptoms in patients with salivary gland hypofunction. Postgrad Med J 1997;73(856):93–97.
39. Dawes C. How much saliva is enough for avoidane of xerostomia? Caries Res 2004;38(3):236–240.
40. Hocevar A, et al. Ultrasonographic changes of major salivary glands in primary Sjogren's syndrome. Diagnostic value of a novel scoring system. Rheumatology 2005;44(6):768–772.
41. Turk T, et al. Manometric assessment of esophageal motility in patients with primary Sjogren's syndrome. Rheumatol Int 2005;25(4):246–249.
42. Scagliusi P, et al. New therapeutic perspectives in Sjogren syndrome: leflunomide. Recenti Prog Med 2005;96(4):194.
43. Derk CT, Vivino FB. A primary care approach to Sjogren's syndrome. Helping patients cope with sicca symptoms, extraglandular manifestations. Postgrad Med 2004;116(3):49–54.
44. Papas A, Sherrer YS, Charney M, et al. Successful treatment of dry mouth and dry eye symptoms in Sjogren's syndrome patients with oral pilocarpine. A randomized placebo-controlled, dose-adjustment study. J Clin Rheumatol 2004;10:169–177.
45. Fox P. Management of dry mouth. Dent Clin North Am 1997;41(4):863–875.
46. Papas A. The Clinicians Guide to the Diagnosis and Treatment of Salivary Gland Disorders and Chemosensory Disorders. Tufts University School of Dental Medicine, Boston, MA.

47. Martuscelli G, Singh M, Papas AS, Cohen J. Use of a power toothbrush in a high risk population. J Dent Res 2004;83(special issue A):2435.
48. Brown NA, et al. Nutrition supplements and the eye. Eye 1998;12(Pt 1):127–133.
49. Dry eyes? Eat more fish. Health News 2006;12(4):11.
50. Edgar W. Sugar substitutes, chewing gum and dental caries: a review. Br Dent J 1998;184:29–32.
51. Muthukumar AR, et al. Calorie restriction decreases proinflammatory cytokines and polymeric Ig receptor expression in the submandibular glands of autoimmune prone (NZB x NZW)F1 mice. J Clin Immunol 2000;20(5):354–361.
52. Belch JJ. Hill A. Evening primrose oil and borage oil in rheumatologic conditions. Am J Clin Nutr 2000;71(1 suppl):352S–356S.
53. Aragona P, et al. Systemic omega-6 essential fatty acid treatment and pge1 tear content in Sjogren's syndrome patients. Invest Ophthalmol Vis Sci 2005;46(12):4474–4479.
54. Miljanovic B, Trivedi KA, Dana MR, Gilbard JP, Buring JE, Schaumberg DA. Relation between dietary n-3 and n-6 fatty acids and clinically diagnosed dry eye syndrome in women. Am J Clin Nutr 2005;82(4):887–893.
55. Singh M, Singh ML, Papas AS. The Effect of an Omega-3 supplement on Dry Mouth and Dry Eyes in Sjogren's Patients. IXth International Symposium on Sjögren's Syndrome. Washington DC. Abstract #: 87: April 2006.
56. Sullivan BD, et al. Correlations between nutrient intake and the polar lipid profiles of meibomian gland secretions in women with Sjogren's syndrome. Adv Exp Med Biol 2002;506(Pt A):441–447.
57. Theander E, et al. Gammalinolenic acid treatment of fatigue associated with primary Sjogren's syndrome. Scand J Rheumatol 2002;31(2):72–79.
58. Aizaki T, et al. Hypokalemia with syncope caused by habitual drinking of oolong tea. Intern Med 1999;38(3):252–256.
59. Hsu S. Dickinson D. A new approach to managing oral manifestations of Sjogren's syndrome and skin manifestations of lupus. J Biochem Mol Biol 2006;39(3):229–239.
60. Hsu S., et al. Inhibition of autoantigen expression by (-)-epigallocatechin-3-gallate (the major constituent of green tea) in normal human cells. J Pharmacol Exp Ther 2005;315(2):805–811.

15 Chronic Arthritides of Childhood

Basil M. Fathalla and Donald Goldsmith

Summary

- The juvenile idiopathic arthritides are a group of heterogeneous disorders characterized by chronic arthritis with frequent extra-articular manifestations.
- Differences in nomenclature and terminology require care in the interpretation of the medical literature.
- Nutritional impairment is common in children with rheumatic diseases and assessment of nutritional status is a pivotal part of each child's evaluation.
- Growth delay occurs in patients with juvenile idiopathic arthritis as a result of several factors such as early epiphyseal fusion, chronic steroid use, increased energy expenditure, and malnutrition.
- Restriction of salt intake or supplemental vitamins such as vitamin D and folic acid are often required in patients who are receiving certain medications such as corticosteroids and methotrexate.

Key Words: Growth delay; juvenile chronic arthritis; juvenile idiopathic arthritis; juvenile rheumatoid arthritis; nutritional impairment

1. INTRODUCTION

The chronic arthritides of childhood are a group of disorders characterized by persistent arthritis. Each arthritis subtype has a distinct constellation of clinical manifestations and laboratory features. Chronic arthritis is the most common pediatric rheumatic disease and represents one of the most frequent causes of chronic illness and disability in children. Its clinical spectrum is variable and ranges between arthritis affecting a single joint to a severe systemic inflammatory disease involving multiple joints. Although the etiology of the various types of chronic arthritis in children largely remains unknown, recent advances in the basic understanding of the inflammatory response has led to several breakthroughs in the treatment and management of this group of disorders *(1,2)*.

Nutritional impairment is common in patients with rheumatic disease. Weight loss can develop as a result of severe inflammatory cachexia, and malnutrition can occur secondary to poor oral intake as a result of temporomandibular joint (TMJ) involvement, anorexia, and gastrointestinal (GI) side effects of medications. Assessment of nutritional status is a pivotal part of each patient's evaluation *(2)*. In this chapter we present an overview of the subtypes of the chronic arthritides in children

From: *Nutrition and Health: Nutrition and Rheumatic Disease*
Edited by: L. A. Coleman © Humana Press, Totowa, NJ

along with a historic review that highlights the evolution of each of the known classification systems. A detailed clinical description of all subtypes of juvenile idiopathic arthritis (JIA) and an overview of the medications used in management with a special emphasis on nutritional status are discussed.

2. HISTORICAL BACKGROUND

The earliest reference of childhood arthritis in the English literature dates back to 1545 in *The Boke of Chyldren* by Thomas Phaer from Wales. He included a section on *stiffenes of the limmes* a condition that he attributed to exposure to the cold *(3–5)*. Aside from acute rheumatic fever, previously known as acute rheumatism, only a few case reports of chronic arthritis in children were described before the year 1900. Two reports of a relatively large number of patients with chronic arthritis were published at the end of 19th century; the first, in 1891 authored by Diamant-Berger, a French physician and the second in 1897 by George Fredric Still. The latter is considered by many to be a landmark publication in the history of pediatric rheumatology *(3–7)*. Both reports emphasized that chronic arthritis in children was different from adults and that it included several subtypes, perhaps suggesting that various disorders could be operative.

Only a few but important benchmark events took place during the first half of the 20th century. The association between Group A β hemolytic streptococcal and acute rheumatic fever was established in 1930 *(8)*. The synthesis of cortisone paved the way for the use of corticosteroids in treating several rheumatic conditions including chronic arthritis *(3,9)*. In 1910, Ohm described a child with arthritis who developed chronic iridocyclitis *(3,5)*. However, the association of antinuclear antibodies (ANAs) with chronic iridocyclitis was described many decades later in 1974 by Jane Schaller and colleagues *(10)*. As more cases of children with chronic arthritis were identified, several published reports appeared during the early decades of the 20th century.

It soon became apparent that the wide spectrum of the presentation of chronic arthritis of children implied that the disorder was quite heterogeneous. This led to a divergence in nomenclature between reports coming out of Europe versus reports from North America. The initial classification criteria were assembled by the American College of Rheumatology (ACR) and the disorder was labeled juvenile rheumatoid arthritis (JRA *(11–13)*). The European League Against Rheumatism (EULAR) reclassified the disease juvenile chronic arthritis (JCA *(5)*). Several years later, in 1994, the pediatric task force of the International League of Associations for Rheumatology (ILAR) proposed the third classification system with the newer term, JIA *(14)*, which has been subsequently revised twice in 1997 *(15)* and 2001 *(16)*.

3. TERMINOLOGY AND CLASSIFICATION

These differences in nomenclature require care in the interpretation of the medical literature because JRA, JCA, and JIA are not interchangeable owing to major differences in inclusion and exclusion criteria. As noted previously, the JRA was preferred in North America, whereas JCA was advocated in the European literature. Accordingly, most of the reported case series and studies done before 1993 have used either of these two terms. However, in recent years, ILAR classification criteria have been preferred and most centers now use the JIA and its different subtypes for their research and publications. Accordingly, we use the term JIA as per the ILAR for the remainder of this text.

It is important to note that the primary purpose for establishing uniform classification criteria is to delineate a relatively homogenous group of patients, which will facilitate accurate collection of clinical data between research centers. However, in clinical practice, these classification criteria often provide the framework for a proper diagnosis. The following is a brief review of the main features of each classification system.

3.1. The ACR Classification Criteria for JRA

The ACR classification criteria include an age limit for onset (<16 years), the presence of arthritis in one or more joints, and duration of disease of at least 6 weeks. There are three major subtypes: pauciarticular onset (arthritis involving four or less joints), polyarticular onset (arthritis involving five or more joints), and systemic onset (arthritis with characteristic systemic features such as double quotidian fever and classic rash). Diagnosis requires the exclusion of other forms or causes of juvenile arthritis. These criteria have been widely used, validated, and are easy to apply in clinical practice. It does, however, require the exclusion of other forms of juvenile arthritis that do not have validated classification criteria.

3.2. The EULAR Classification Criteria for JCA

According to this classification, the age limit remains 16 years of age but the duration of the disease should extend for 3 months or more. Another major difference is the particular application and use of the term *rheumatoid*. In the ACR classification this term is used to cover all subtypes, whereas the term *rheumatoid* was selected for only one particular subtype of JCA (polyarticular disease and positive rheumatoid factor [RF]), then called *juvenile rheumatoid arthritis (17)*. Therefore, these terms are not interchangeable.

The European classification system includes six major subtypes: systemic onset (arthritis with characteristic systemic features such as quotidian fever and classic rash), pauciarticular onset (arthritis involving four or less joints), polyarticular onset (arthritis involving five or more joints without a positive RF test), *juvenile rheumatoid arthritis* (arthritis involving five or more joints with a positive RF test), and two added categories: juvenile psoriatic arthritis and juvenile ankylosing spondylitis (JAS).

3.3. The ILAR Classification Criteria for JIA

In 1993, the pediatric task force of the ILAR proposed a new classification format for the chronic juvenile arthritides. Utilizing the term *juvenile idiopathic arthritis* several subtypes were identified including an "undifferentiated" category *(14)*. This international classification was subsequently revised twice, in 1997 *(15)* and 2001 *(16)*. Those patients who fulfilled more then one subtype criteria or did not fulfill any subtype criteria were categorized under the subtype of undifferentiated arthritis. Tables 1 and 2 provide a summary of the three main classification systems and delineate their major differences.

The ILAR classification encompasses seven categories: systemic disease; oligoarticular onset (arthritis involving four or less joints), which is further subdivided into

Table 1
Subtypes of Chronic Arthritis in Children According to the Three Classifications of the Chronic Juvenile Arthritides

Juvenile Rheumatoid Arthritis (ACR Classification)	Juvenile Chronic Arthritis (EULAR Classification)	Juvenile Idiopathic Arthritis (ILAR Classification)
1. Systemic onset JRA	1. Systemic onset JCA	1. Systemic onset JIA
2. Pauciarticular JRA	2. Pauciarticular JCA	2. Oligoarticular JIA • Persistent • extended
3. Polyarticular JRA	3. Polyarticular JCA	3. Polyarticular RF negative
	4. Juvenile rheumatoid arthritis	4. Polyarticular RF positive
	5. Juvenile psoriatic arthritis	5. Psoriatic arthritis
	6. Juvenile ankylosing spondylitis	6. Enthesitis related arthritis
		7. Undiffrentiated: • Fit neither category • Fit more than one category

ACR, American College of Rheumatology; EULAR, European League Against Rheumatism; ILAR, The International League of Associations for Rheumatology; JCA, juvenile chronic arthritis; JIA, juvenile idiopathic arthritis; JRA, juvenile rheumatoid arthritis; RF, rheumatoid factor

Table 2
Comparison of the ACR, EULAR, and ILAR Classifications of Chronic Juvenile Arthritides

	ACR	EULAR	ILAR
Age of onset	< 16 years	< 16 years	< 16 years
Onset types	3	6	7
Duration of arthritis	> 6 weeks	> 3 months	> 6 weeks
Includes JPsA	No	Yes	Yes
Includes JAS	No	Yes	Yes
Includes IBD	No	Yes	Yes
Exclude other diseases	Yes	Yes	Yes

ACR, American College of Rheumatology; EULAR, European League Against Rheumatism; IBD, inflammatory bowel disease; ILAR, The International League of Associations for Rheumatology; JAS, juvenile ankylosing spondylitis; JPsA, juvenile psoriatic arthritis

either persistent (the number of joints involved remains four or less after 6 months of disease onset) or extended (the number of joints involved becomes more then four joints 6 months after disease onset); polyarticular onset with both RF-negative and RF-positive subgroups; juvenile psoriatic arthritis; enthesitis-related arthritis (arthritis seen in the context of inflammatory bowel disease [IBD] and JAS), and an undifferentiated category for patients who either do not fit any of the above categories or fit more than one category. Each of the above seven subgroups has detailed inclusion and exclusion criteria *(14–16)*.

4. CLINICAL FEATURES

Chronic arthritis in children is not rare, however, the exact incidence and prevalence is not known and varies considerably based on gender, race, and geographic areas. Based on analysis of 34 reported epidemiological studies from 1966 to 2002*(18)*, the incidence varies from 0.008 to 0.226 per 1,000 children and prevalence from 0.07 to 4.01 per 1,000 children. Of the 34 reported studies, 17 used the JCA criteria, 13 used the JRA criteria, 3 reported JRA and spondyloarthropathy cases, and 1 report described arthritis in children without using specific terminology. The major factors contributing to the wide variations included diagnostic difficulties, the use of different definitions, differences in case ascertainment (community-based vs case studies), and definition of the study population.

4.1. Oligoarticular JIA

Patients with oligoarticular JIA develop chronic articular inflammation in four or less joints. The most commonly affected joints are the knees and ankles. Its most common presentation is monoarthritis affecting one knee, which occurs in almost half of all affected patients. These patients do not usually complain of any significant pain and most often remain quite functional *(19,20)*.

Patients who continue with arthritis in no more than four joints after the first 6 months are said to have persistent oligoarticular JIA, whereas those who eventually develop arthritis in more than four joints are said to have an extended oligoarticular JIA. Patients with an extended course have a worse prognosis. Risk factors for developing extended disease include hand changes, wrist or ankle involvement, symmetric disease, elevated erythrocyte sedimentation rate (ESR) and positive ANA *(21,22)*.

Extra-articular manifestations are extremely rare with the exception of chronic uveitis. The onset of uveitis is usually insidious and completely asymptomatic *(23)*. Sometimes, uveitis may precede the development of arthritis. Some children will develop change in vision, photophobia, or pain and redness in the eyes later in the course. Uveitis is usually bilateral but unilateral involvement may occur. Risk factors for developing uveitis include oligoarticular disease (in comparison to polyarticular disease or systemic disease), female gender, and a positive ANA test. The risk is never absent but uveitis usually develops in the first 5 to 7 years after onset. Patients require regular ophthalmological evaluations so early treatment may be implemented, usually with glucocorticoid ophthalmic drops with or without mydriatic agents. Chronic uveitis is considered to be the most serious consequence of oligoarticular disease, sometimes also requiring systemic glucocorticosteroid therapy, methotrexate or tumor necrosis factor (TNF) blockers *(10,23–26)*.

Localized growth disturbance is one of the important complications that require special attention in both this variety and other forms of arthritis. Arthritis of the lower extremities, most often the knee, may lead to accelerated growth, early epiphyseal maturation, and subsequent leg-length discrepancy, particularly with unilateral involvement.

4.2. Polyarticular JIA

Patients with polyarticular JIA develop chronic inflammation in five or more joints. Two types of polyarticular JIA are identified; RF- positive and RF- negative polyarticular JIA. Both are more often seen in females with the former being more common during late childhood and adolescence, whereas the latter is more common during early childhood. Patients with RF-positive polyarticular disease usually have symmetrical arthritis of the small and large joints and often have severe erosive disease *(27–29)*. These children may also develop subcutaneous nodules and exhibit some systemic manifestations such as low-grade fever, anorexia, weight loss, and growth delay *(30,31)*. Chronic uveitis may occur but is less frequent than with oligoarticular JIA *(23–26)*.

Inflammation of TMJs may be seen in all subtypes of juvenile arthritis; however, it is more common in polyarticular disease *(32–34)*. Micrognathia and retrognathia may occur as a result of chronic inflammation of the TMJs and are considered to be additional examples of localized growth disturbance. Other cosmetic effects such as facial asymmetry or bird face deformity can be seen in chronic disease. Persistent inflammation of the TMJs may affect oral intake secondary to pain and dysfunction; contributing to nutritional impairment.

4.3. Systemic-Onset JIA

This form of arthritis is characterized by unique extra-articular manifestations such as quotidian or double quotidian fever and a characteristic rash *(6,7,30)*. However, the initial presentation is often nonspecific and the child is considered to have a fever of unknown origin. Systemic features usually precede the development of arthritis, which prompts extensive assessment to rule out a malignancy or an infectious disease. This form of arthritis is the least common of the chronic arthritides of childhood. It has no definite age peak at onset and in contrast to other forms of arthritis is seen equally in both males and females *(17,35)*.

Almost all patients present with fever and are usually ill at onset with systemic features overshadowing articular symptomatology. Systemic features include the classic rash, lymphadenopathy, hepatosplenomegaly, pericarditis, and pleuritis. Several weeks, often even months, may pass before arthritis develops and then dominates the clinical picture. Arthritis can develop in many joints, but most commonly affected are the knees, wrists and then the hips, cervical spine, and small joints of the fingers and toes.

The fever and rash are the most characteristic systemic features. The fever is classically quotidian or double quotidian (two peaks daily) and the temperature rises to 39°C or higher with a rapid decline to baseline or below. The fever may be noted at any time during the day but most often occurs toward late afternoon and early evening and is often accompanied by the typical rash. This rash, initially described by Boldero in 1933 *(36)* consists of evanescent discrete salmon-pink polymorphous macules measuring 2 to 5 mm in size. It is most often not pruritic and usually occurs on the trunk and proximal extremities but may also be seen on the face. Typical lesions (usually linear) are elicited by rubbing the skin (Koebner phenomenon) or by exposure to heat *(35,37,38)*. Other systemic features include symmetrical enlargement of the cervical, axillary, and inguinal lymph nodes, and hepatosplenomegaly sometimes causing abdominal distention. Nonspecific hepatitis can be seen in the context of active systemic disease but chronic changes are rare. Pericarditis and pleuritis may cause chest pain and dyspnea, but asymptomatic pericardial effusions are most common.

Laboratory features include striking increases in acute phase reactants such as white blood cells, platelet count, ESR, C-reactive protein, ferritin, and fibrinogen levels. Often, patients have anemia and hypoalbuminemia. The ANA and RF are absent.

Two complications of systemic JIA may lead to serious consequences: secondary amyloidosis resulting from chronic inflammation and macrophage activation syndrome (MAS [*(35)*]). Secondary amyloidosis refers to tissue deposition of amyloid protein secondary to chronic inflammatory disorders such as familial Mediterranean fever, systemic JIA, and chronic infections. This complication has been reported in European patients with chronic arthritis but it is rarely reported in North America. It is characterized clinically by proteinuria, hepatosplenomegaly, anemia, and diarrhea and laboratory tests usually reveal elevated CRP and serum amyloid A levels. The diagnosis is usually confirmed by tissue biopsy.

MAS is characterized clinically by the rapid development of fever, hepatosplenomegaly and/or hepatic failure with encephalopathy, bruising, and mucosal bleeding. Laboratory features include cytopenias, particularly thrombocytopenia, elevated transaminases, hypoalbuminemia, and abnormal coagulation studies suggestive of disseminated intravascular coagulation (prolonged prothrombin time, international normalized ratio, activated partial thromboplastin time, thrombocytopenia and elevated D-dimers, and fibrin degradation products). Blood levels of vitamin K-dependent coagulation factors are also decreased. Paradoxically, the ESR is markedly decreased from its usually markedly elevated levels owing to the consumption of fibrinogen. The condition is rare but life-threatening and its etiology is unknown. It may be triggered by an intercurrent infection or after medication changes but it is not clear if such triggers are just coincidental. Patients with MAS may have a fatal outcome and need to be treated aggressively. Treatment with high-dose mythelprednisolone and cyclosporine is required with intensive medical care *(39–42)*.

4.4. Psoriatic Arthritis

Chronic inflammatory arthritis associated with psoriasis in the juvenile age group is known as psoriatic arthritis. This diagnosis is challenging when the arthritis precedes the development of the skin lesions (*psoriatic arthritis sine psoriasis*). Arthritis most often presents in an asymmetrical pattern involving only a few joints, making it difficult to distinguish from oligoarticular JIA. Sometimes a polyarticular pattern may be seen at onset or later in the course. Other characteristic features include involvement of the distal interphalangeal joints and the presence of dactylitis. Skin changes include the typical rash of psoriasis, and less commonly guttate psoriasis, pustular psoriasis or diffuse generalized psoriasis. Nail changes entail pitting and onycholysis. As with other patients with chronic arthritis, these patients may develop constitutional features such as anorexia, decreased activity, anemia, and poor growth. Chronic uveitis, clinically similar to what is seen in oligoarticular JIA may occur *(43–45)*.

4.5. Enthesitis-Related Arthritides

The spondyloarthropathy concept accommodates a group of chronic arthritides, which predominantly affect the axial skeleton and are characterized by the presence of HLA-B27 antigen and the absence of RF or other autoantibodies. Such disorders include JAS, the arthritis of IBD, reactive arthritis, and psoriatic arthritis. Recently, the term *enthesitis-related arthritis* was introduced as part of the ILAR criteria as a subtype of JIA. Reactive arthritis was excluded because the trigger is usually identified (e.g., Group A β hemolytic streptococcus, Yersinia, etc.) and therefore not idiopathic. Additionally, psoriatic arthritis is considered to be a separate subtype as noted earlier *(14–16)*.

4.5.1. Juvenile Ankylosing Spondylitis

The age of onset of JAS is usually late childhood or adolescence with a much higher frequency in males than females. Onset is usually insidious with vague arthralgias, musculoskeletal pain and stiffness, then followed by peripheral arthritis with or without enthesitis. There may be mild systemic signs such as fatigue and low-grade fever. On occasion, the onset may be more abrupt, with oligoarticular disease. Axial skeletal involvement is a late manifestation in children in contrast to adult-onset disease *(46–48)*. Enthesitis (inflammation of enthesis) is an early characteristic manifestation of the disease but may also be seen in other forms of arthritis. It often causes significant pain and discomfort, with the most common sites being at the knees, ankles, and feet. Peripheral arthritis is the most common earlier form of arthritis seen in JAS, particularly in the lower extremities, whereas axial involvement is rarely present at onset. Eventually, the majority of patients develop sacroiliac joint and lumbosacral spine involvement *(46–50)*. Extra-articular manifestations seen in JAS include acute iritis and cardiac disease (aortic insufficiency) *(51,52)*.

4.5.2. Arthritides of IBD

Arthritis is considered to be one of the most frequent extraintestinal manifestations of IBD. Two patterns of arthritis are described: a polyarticular distribution involving the peripheral joints (non-HLA-B27-associated) and arthritis involving the sacroiliac joints and the axial skeleton (HLA-B27-associated). The first pattern is more common and usually affects the joints of the lower extremities. It presents as brief episodes of acute arthritis that tend to recur and severity and duration usually correlates with GI disease flares. However, severe joint damage is unusual. The second pattern is primarily associated with the presence of the HLA-B27 antigen and resembles the course of enthesitis-related arthritis. The course of the disease in the latter pattern does not correlate with underlying IBD disease activity. These two patterns resemble the IBD types described in adults *(53,54)*. In addition to arthritis, generalized skeletal pain as a result of osteopenia and/or osteoporosis may be associated with chronic glucocorticosteroid administration or as part of the primary disease *(55,56)*. Other extraintestinal manifestations of IBD include vasculitis, uveitis, and skin changes such as erythema nodosum and pyoderma gangrenosum.

GI symptoms of IBD include anorexia, abdominal pain, and diarrhea. Skin tags and fistulas are suggestive of Crohn's disease, whereas hematochezia is more often seen in ulcerative colitis. Poor nutrition and growth delay are major complications of poorly controlled disease. Accordingly, careful assessment of growth parameters and accompanying nutritional deficiencies is an essential part of the management of patients with IBD *(56,57)*.

5. MANAGEMENT AND TREATMENT

Management of patients with JIA is challenging and multidimensional. Issues include choice of medications; attention to physical and occupational therapy needs; and guidance with nutrition, psychosocial development, and appropriate immunization *(58,59)*. In this section we review the different categories of medications used in the treatment of the juvenile arthritides and discuss nutritional status and growth-related issues.

Medications used in treating children with chronic arthritis may be categorized into five groups: nonsteroidal anti-inflammatory drugs (NSAIDs), disease-modifying antirheumatic drugs (DMARDs), glucocorticosteroids (GCS), immunosuppressive agents, and biologic immunomodulators. Drugs in each category may cause significant side effects and/or adverse events. Most often, the safest and simplest drugs are used initially, but recently, more potent medications may be introduced earlier in the disease course in order to rapidly control the inflammatory process and thereby minimize the development of permanent sequelae. Risks of drug toxicity, however, must always be balanced with the benefits of more aggressive treatment. There are no medications currently available that are effective for every child and all medications have potential side effects. Care providers are obligated to consider all these issues while attempting to improve the quality of life and limit deformities and disabilities *(58–60)*.

The relationship between administration of medications and food intake is noteworthy. Whereas NSAIDs are given on a full stomach to avoid GI side effects such as gastritis and/or ulcer formation, other medications such as methotrexate are preferably given on an empty stomach to improve bioavailability. Children with chronic arthritis often take multiple medications and the practitioner must be aware of potential drug interactions. The treatment plan is individualized for each patient based on the JIA subtype, and disease course and severity. A recent review of the medical treatment of JIA indicates that many drugs have not been studied completely or definitely proven to be helpful *(61)*.

5.1. NSAIDs

NSAIDs are in general the first-line medications used for the treatment of JIA. They possess good analgesic and antipyretic properties with a relatively mild toxicity profile. Mechanisms of action primarily include inhibition of prostaglandin (PG) and leukotriene synthesis. NSAIDs inhibit cyclooxygenase enzymes responsible for the metabolism of arachchidonic acid to PGs, thromboxanes, and prostacyclin. Several NSAIDs are commonly used in the juvenile age group such as naproxen, ibuprofen, indomethacin, and tolmetin. Historically, aspirin was the primary NSAID; however, its use has significantly declined because of concerns about toxicity, particularly Reye syndrome *(60,62)*.

In general, the simultaneous use of more than one NSAID is discouraged. A trial of 6 to 8 weeks of each NSAID is generally required prior to declaring lack of efficacy;

however, a majority of patients usually feel some benefit within 2 weeks. Patients should be monitored carefully for evidence of effectiveness and/or toxicity. Several side effects have been described including GI, renal, hepatic, and cutaneous *(60)*.

5.2. DMARDs

This group is often referred to as slow-acting anti-rheumatic drugs and includes methotrexate, sulfasalazine, leflunomide, D-penicillamine, antimalarials, and gold compounds. These medications are often associated with some toxicity and historically this led to delay in their use in the juvenile age group. However, there is now more appreciation of the potential irreversible damage that may result from uncontrolled disease, improved knowledge of the mechanisms of action of each preparation, and a better ability to monitor for toxicity, and several of these medications are now being used much earlier in the course of the disease. Although some of the DMARDs, such as gold compounds, are no longer in use, several newer medications such as biologic immunomodulators are now emerging as one of the most important treatment categories in children with chronic arthritides *(60,61)*.

Methotrexate is most often considered to be the first choice of the second-line medications to be used for chronic arthritis. It is one of the few medications that has been proved to be efficacious in a randomized controlled trial and has been in use for several decades with a very good safety profile *(63)*. Methotrexate has anti-metabolitic, anti-inflammatory and immunomodulatory properties. Methotrexate exerts its anti-metabolitic effects through its role as a folic acid analogue, which leads to potent competitive inhibition of dihydrofolate reductase with subsequent interference of purine synthesis. Its anti-inflammatory effects result from the inhibition of adenosine deaminase, which leads to accumulation and enhanced release of adenosine, which is an inhibitor of neutrophil adherence. Methotrexate's effects on the immune system include modulation of inflammatory cell function, cytokine production, as well as inhibition of synovial cell proliferation *(64)*. Several potential toxicities, although rare in children, include hepatic, renal, and hematological effects that require frequent clinical and laboratory evaluation. Oral ulcers, nausea, and vomiting are the most commonly reported side effects. This may lead to chronic decreased oral intake and occasionally contribute to the overall poor nutritional status of some children.

Other DMARDs used for the treatment of JIA include sulfasalazine, used commonly in enthesitis-related arthritis, and thalidomide, which seems to be helpful in some children with systemic-onset disease. Gold compounds and D-penicillamine are no longer regularly used for JIA.

5.3. Glucocorticosteroids

Glucocorticoids are very potent anti-inflammatory and immunosuppressive agents with both physiological and pharmacological effects. Glucocorticoids do not usually alter the natural history of rheumatic disorders, however, their discovery several decades ago was considered to be one of the major therapeutic advances in the history of rheumatology *(9,60)*. They remain as the treatment of choice for life-threatening complications of several rheumatic disorders including systemic JIA, but routine use is hindered by the severity and frequency of adverse effects. GCS may be also administered locally as ophthalmic drops or intra-articular injections. GCS are usually administered during peak disease activity until second-line agents (DMARDs) become effective. The overall goal is to limit the dose and duration of GCS to the lowest possible level while still achieving disease control. High-dose and prolonged glucocorticosteroid therapy leads to adrenal axis dysfunction, growth suppression, osteoporosis, avascular necrosis of bone, cardiovascular effects such as hypertension and dyslipoproteinemia, metabolic effects such as impaired carbohydrate tolerance and protein wasting, myopathy, central nervous system changes such as psychosis and mood disturbance, and immunosuppression *(58,60)*.

Secondary or iatrogenic Cushing's syndrome is the term used to describe the systemic adverse effects of chronic glucocorticosteroid use and is characterized by truncal obesity, thinning of the subcutaneous tissues, osteoporosis, cataracts and glaucoma, psuedotumor cerebri, and hypertension. Weight gain reflects both fluid retention and increased caloric intake caused by increased appetite. Minimizing weight gain by limiting salt and caloric intake is an important part of the therapeutic regimen but is often difficult to achieve. Growth suppression is a well-described long-term adverse effect in children with rheumatic diseases who receive long-term glucocorticosteroid therapy *(65–67)*. Whether growth suppression is directly related to chronic glucocorticosteroid use or is a consequence of the underlying disease process remains unclear*(66,68)* . Growth retardation is most likely the net result of both these factors as well as malnutrition. Growth retardation in children with JRA (ACR criteria) may be more severe than in those with systemic lupus erythematosus, suggesting a more prominent role of the underlying process *(66)*. Growth suppression may vary in patients with similar disease and similar regimens, which suggests interindividual variability and susceptibility. It is mandatory in clinical practice to carefully monitor growth velocity and weight gain. When appropriate, growth hormone therapy may be considered because recent data suggest potential benefit *(69–71)*.

Osteoporosis is another serious and worrisome consequence of chronic glucocorticosteroid therapy. Several other factors also contribute to the development of osteoporosis including active inflammatory disease, inadequate intake of vitamin D and calcium, decreased exposure to sunlight, reduced physical activity, and pubertal delay *(58,60,72–75)*. GCS have profound effects on both the developing and mature skeleton, which are related to both dose and duration of therapy. The pathogenesis of glucocorticosteroid-induced osteoporosis is multifactoral and includes decreased numbers of bone-forming cells owing to impaired osteoblastic-cell differentiation and increased apoptosis, decreased absorption of calcium from the GI tract, increased urinary calcium excretion leading to secondary hyperparathyroidism, and decreased synthesis of insulin-like growth factor-1 with subsequent decreased collagen I production, and reduced bone matrix available for mineralization *(73,75)*. Prevention and treatment of secondary osteoporosis is discussed later.

The administration of GCS directly into an inflamed joint was shown to be effective in resolving symptoms and signs in children with arthritis. Intra-articular GCS are now most commonly used in patients with oligoarticular onset JIA or targeted joints in polyarticular JIA. Additionally, several advantages can be achieved including minimizing localized muscle wasting, joint contractures, and localized growth discrepancies *(76,77)*. Adverse effects include skin atrophy and localized calcifications.

5.4. Cytotoxic and Immunosuppressive Drugs

This category includes several preparations such as azathioprine, mycophenolate mofetil, cyclophosphamide, cyclosporine, and chlorambucil *(58,60,61)*. The use of these medications is usually reserved for active disease that is resistant to other regimens. Accordingly, patients are usually more severely ill and at risk for development of adverse effects and acquisition of severe infections. Possible drug interactions should be monitored carefully to avoid toxicity or diminished efficacy.

5.5. Biological Immunomodulators

The use of biological agents, such as intravenous immunoglobulin (IVIG), for the treatment of rheumatic disorders such as juvenile dermatomyositis and Kawasaki disease is not new. Unraveling the intricacies of the inflammatory response has led to the development of drugs that target one or more steps in the proinflammatory pathway. There are many obstacles, however. A single mediator may have more than one biological function and therefore targeting that molecule may lead to suppression of the undesired function but may also lead to alteration of other biological processes as well. Two distinct mediators may have similar biological function and targeting one molecule may not lead to the desired effect because the other is not targeted. Biological function assessed *in vitro* also may not be relevant *in vivo*. The transition from bench to bedside is not always successful because the mechanisms of the disease process may not be completely understood. The potential long-term effects on a child's relatively immature immune system are unknown. Studies in adults may not be generalizable to children and long-term monitoring for growth, development, and immune function is required.

Biological immunomodulators may ameliorate the inflammatory response through changes in cellular function, cell–to-cell interaction, or interference with cytokines. Biological immunomodulators available for use in children include etanercept and infliximab (TNF blockers *(78,79)*), and anakinra (interleukin [IL]-1 receptor antagonist *(80)*). Recent data suggests that the anti-IL-6 receptor antibody is promising in systemic JIA but it is not yet approved for clinical use *(81)*.

6. NUTRITIONAL STATUS

Nutritional impairment is a common problem in patients with JIA but is often overlooked during the routine medical care of these patients *(2,82)*. Physicians caring for children with chronic arthritis are usually more attentive to the acute and chronic articular manifestations with a focus on pharmacological issues. Nutritional status should be considered to be a pivotal part of each child's care. Dietary issues and GI side effects from medications should be regularly discussed with the patient and parents. Documentation of growth parameters such as body weight and height, with careful monitoring of growth velocity should be part of each visit and a dietician should be consulted when there is concern about nutritional deficits *(2)*. Nutritional impairment in patients with JIA varies considerably according to JIA subtype, severity of disease, and medications used. Manifestations of nutritional dysfunction may also include obesity. In this section we discuss the factors leading to, as well as the specific manifestations of nutritional impairment.

6.1. Oral Health in Patients With JIA

Oral health problems may contribute to nutritional impairment in patients with JIA through several circumstances. Significant TMJ involvement interferes with oral intake caused by painful mastication, limited oral opening, and malocclusion *(33,34,83)*. Various degrees of condylar head distraction and poor mandibular growth can lead to various deformities depending on the severity, chronicity, and symmetry of disease (e.g., unilateral vs bilateral). Radiographic changes such as bony erosions are most severe in patients with polyarticular course, particularly with early-onset, long-standing, and bilateral TMJ involvement *(33,34,83)*.

Patients with JIA are also at risk to develop dental carries and periodontal disease. Limited oral opening and systemic disease may complicate operative procedures, with the need for nasotracheal intubation rather than through the oropharynx. Regular dental check-ups, plaque control, and oral exercises are important in preventing complications *(83,84)*. Some medications may cause dental erosions (chewable aspirin), gingival overgrowth (cyclosporine), or pose a risk for prolonged bleeding (NSAIDs), which may then possibly complicate planned surgical procedures *(83)*.

Other problems that may lead to feeding difficulties in patients with JIA include painful oral ulcers, which may be part of the underlying disorder such as Crohn's disease or as a side effect from medications such as methotrexate. Folic acid supplementation minimizes the evolution of oral ulcerations in those children taking methotrexate.

6.2. Risk Factors for Developing Nutritional Impairments

Mechanical feeding difficulties are often encountered in patients with JIA particularly at an age when the child is approaching independence. Arthritis of the upper extremities may interfere with meal preparation and utensil mastery. Affected children should be allowed additional time for meals particularly during school hours. Occupational therapy interventions are often useful *(82)*.

Anorexia, nausea, and vomiting often interfere with nutritional intake. Anorexia, a common constitutional symptom seen with inflammation, is most likely related to increased levels of proinflammatory cytokines, and is one of the major factors that contribute to nutritional impairment in patients with JIA. Patients often need to be in intensive care settings particularly during severe flares of systemic disease or for management of life-threatening MAS. Total parenteral nutrition is then essential to deliver the daily requirement of calories and nutrients. Patients with the JIA subtype related to IBD are at high risk for nutritional deficiencies particularly with small bowel involvement typically seen in Crohn's disease.

Medications used in the treatment of JIA often have nutritional implications. Side effects such as anorexia and nausea may develop with cytotoxic and immunosuppressive drugs. NSAIDs may cause nausea, vomiting, gastritis, and GI ulcerations. All NSAIDs should be administered after meals. On the other hand, medications such as methotrexate and penicillamine should be given on an empty stomach to maximize absorption. Almost all DMARDs may cause GI side effects such as nausea, oral ulcerations, vomiting, and hepatic toxicity. Penicillamine may alter taste sensation, whereas cyclosporine may cause gingival hyperplasia and dysphagia. Patients often take combinations of medications and drug interactions are common. For example, antacid preparations containing aluminum and magnesium decrease absorption of mycophenolate mofetil *(60,82,85)*.

Patients taking GCS have several nutritional vulnerabilities. As noted earlier, patients often develop a markedly increased appetite and limiting salt and caloric intake is difficult. Chronic glucocorticosteroid use may also lead to other adverse effects such as inducing catabolic muscle wasting, negative calcium balance and osteoporosis, inhibition of cell growth and division, which may contribute to the already existing risk of growth delay characteristic of the underlying disease process *(66,72–75,82,85)*.

Decline in physical activity related to severe arthritis may contribute to altered body composition resulting in obesity; those on chronic GCS are particularly burdened. These children should be encouraged to increase physical activity (swimming and biking are good choices) to facilitate weight loss, increased lean body mass, improve cardiovascular fitness, and enhance muscle tone. Most children with JIA have a tendency to gain weight as a result of decreased activity resulting from specific physical limitations or activity restrictions. The appropriate level of participation and form of exercise should be tailored for each patient according to disease extent and severity *(82)*.

6.3. Nutritional Impairments in Patients With JIA

Nutritional and growth abnormalities are common in patients with JIA as a result of one or more of the above risk factors. Nutritional impairments in patients diagnosed with subtypes of JIA include those cited here.

6.3.1. Growth Abnormalities

Generalized and localized growth disturbances have been described in patients with JIA *(82,86,87)*. The pattern of growth disturbance depends primarily on the JIA subtype. Children with oligoarticular disease are at risk for localized growth retardation, whereas patients with severe polyarticular or systemic disease often experience both localized and generalized growth delay depending on the pattern of joint involvement. Localized growth disturbances may have minimal functional impact such as shortening of one digit; but significant dysfunction may result from chronic arthritis involving major joints such as the knees. Leg-length discrepancy affects gait and exerts stress on the hips and back. Poor growth of the mandible as a result of chronic TMJ involvement is another example of localized growth retardation, which may exert significant impact on overall well-being. Intra-articular glucocorticosteroid injections of involved joints are beneficial in preventing or reducing localized growth disturbances *(32–34,76,77)*.

Generalized growth suppression in patients with JIA likely results from multiple factors, including the underlying disease, chronic glucocorticosteroid use, increased energy expenditure, and malnutrition *(65,66,68,88,89)*. There is growing evidence that abnormal growth patterns in patients with JIA may be modulated by proinflammatory cytokines through systemic effects and local effects acting directly at the level of the growth plates *(90)*. The role of the underlying disease was suggested in one of the earliest studies to address this issue in JRA (ACR criteria) *(66)*. Growth suppression was more severe in patients with JRA than systemic lupus and more severe in systemic-onset JRA when compared to polyarticular or pauciarticular disease, although patients with systemic JRA had received more GCS than the other groups. These findings infer that the underlying disease and JRA subtype play a primary role in determining the severity of growth retardation. This was also supported by the fact that almost one-third of the patients in that study was below the third percentile for height at the time of diagnosis *(66)*. Early epiphyseal fusion of the knees contributes largely to the net final height. Several studies have suggested a decline in linear height during periods of active arthritis. The final height of affected patients is closely dependent on the severity of growth suppression during active disease and on subsequent linear growth achieved after remission *(66,68,89)*. Accordingly, introduction of GH therapy may be beneficial if begun early. Several studies have shown improvement in final height with early use of GH *(69,70)*. A double-blind, placebo-controlled follow-up study showed that human recombinant GH was effective in reversing severe growth retardation in patients with JCA (EULAR criteria) with the response noted following 6 months of therapy *(71)*.

6.3.2. MALNUTRITION AND NUTRIENT DEFICIENCIES

Malnutrition contributes to poor growth, weight loss, osteoporosis, and chronic anemia in patients with JIA. In a random sample of 33 patients with JRA (ACR criteria), all had caloric intake less then 50% of estimated needs *(82)*. In another study, 123 patients with JIA showed undernutrition in 16%. This study also suggested that a younger age and five or more active joints are factors that correlate with a lower body mass index *(91)*. Weight loss in patients with JIA is secondary to several factors such as decreased caloric intake, increased caloric requirement and severity of inflammation. Proinflammatory cytokines such as IL-1, TNF, and IL-6 play a major role in mediating the inflammatory response in most subtypes of JIA *(57,86,87,92)*. The role of such cytokines in inflammatory cachexia has been studied in human models such as RA and animal models such as adjuvant arthritis *(93–96)*. Loss of body cell mass in adjuvant arthritis is not attributed to anorexia alone. It also correlated with elevated production of TNF-α and IL-1β by spleen cells *(93)*.

Laboratory evaluation of patients with JIA exhibit several abnormalities. Protein stores such as prealbumin and albumin are frequently decreased *(82)*. Children with JIA often develop anemia of chronic disease reflected by mild to moderate normocytic hypochromic anemia, low serum iron, low total iron-binding capacity, but adequate or elevated hemosiderin stores *(82,97)*. Precise pathophysiology causing the anemia in chronic inflammatory disease is not fully understood, however, increased production of IL-6 and TNF-α appear to be pivotal. These cytokines inhibit erythroid progenitor proliferation, which blunts the expected erythropoietin response to anemia, reducing the flow of iron from reticuloendothelial cells to the bone marrow and thus impairing iron uptake by erythroblasts *(96,98,99)*. Microcytic hypochromic iron-deficiency anemia may also be seen in JIA secondary to malnutrition and/or GI blood loss. Anemia of chronic disease is often difficult to distinguish from iron-deficiency anemia and both forms may sometimes coexist *(82,97–99)*. Anemia is seen in all subtypes of JIA but children with systemic and polyarticular JIA are most often affected *(97,98)*.

There is a paucity of studies addressing other nutrient abnormalities such as vitamin and mineral deficiencies in patients with JIA. In one study of 34 children with JRA (ACR classification), one-third of all patients were below the 10th percentile for height, particularly in children with systemic-onset or polyarticular disease *(100)*. This study also evaluated several biochemical nutritional indices including proteins (transferrin, albumin, prealbumin, retinol binding protein, and ceruloplasmin), vitamins (A, C, and E), minerals (calcium, phosphorous, iron, zinc, copper, and selenium), and other metabolic markers including alkaline phosphatase, aspartate aminotransferase (AST), somatomedin, cholesterol, and glutathione peroxidase. Overall, the mean dietary intake for calories and essential nutrients reported by patients was found to be adequate with few exceptions for all subtypes. The pauciarticular group (12 patients) most closely matched normal expectations for dietary intake. The systemic disease group (8 patients) was found to be short for age and above average in the weight for height index. There was a less than the recommended caloric intake for age and low circulating levels of albumin, retinol binding protein, vitamin C, and zinc. Many children in the polyarticular group (14 patients) were short for age with accompanying deficiencies in vitamin A, C, and E levels and lowered zinc levels. Influence of chronic inflammation on these findings is not fully understood and discrepancies between intake and certain nutrient levels may reflect alterations in the requirements, absorption, or utilization of these nutrients in the presence of chronic inflammation *(100)*.

Another report evaluated oral intake and serum levels of copper and zinc in patients with JRA (ACR criteria) in view of each mineral's role in the activation of several key cellular metabolic enzymes *(101)*. HERE Mean intakes of both copper and zinc were below the recommended daily requirements but did not differ from the control group. Also, the mean daily intake of zinc and copper did not differ between patients with active or inactive disease. Serum zinc levels in patients with JRA did not differ from the control group or disease characteristics, whereas, serum copper levels in the JRA group were greater than the control group and its variation was related to the number of inflamed joints. While these studies are interesting and may shed more light on the nutritional status of patients with JRA or JIA, the practical and clinical implementations are not clear.

6.3.3. BODY COMPOSITION ABNORMALITIES

Despite limited data, it is well known that anthropometric measurements are a simple and effective tool to assess nutritional status in patients with JIA. Measurements include height for age, weight for age, weight for height, mid-arm circumference (an index of body energy stores and protein mass), triceps skinfold circumference (an index of body fat), and calculating mid-arm muscle circumference (an index for lean muscle mass *(87,102–104)*). Some parameters are difficult to obtain accurately in patients with JIA. As an example, flexion contractures of the lower extremities make accurate height measurement difficult to obtain, which will then affect the weight-to-height index. One study assessed these measurements in 33 patients with JRA (8 patients with pauciarticular JRA, 16 with polyarticular JRA, and 9 with systemic JRA; ACR criteria *(102)*). Results indicated a tendency for patients with JRA to be more height retarded than weight retarded when compared with the normal population. Of these patients, 18% had height at or below the fifth percentile for age, 15% had weight at or below the fifth percentile for age, and 9% had weight for height at or below the fifth percentile. Triceps skinfold circumferences were increased in all JRA groups when compared with normal standards suggesting increased fat stores, whereas the mean mid-arm circumference was below the 25th percentile in patients with pauciarticular and systemic subtypes. The mean mid-arm muscle circumference for patients in the study was below the mean for a normal population with all those with systemic diseases measuring at or below the fifth percentile. Lower heights, weights, weight-for-height; greater fat stores; and a decreased lean muscle mass were seen in the patients with JRA versus a normal population. It was undetermined whether these findings were the result of undernutrition or disease activity.

Truncal obesity occurs in iatrogenic Cushing's syndrome as a result of the redistribution of fat predominantly to subcutaneous tissues of the abdomen, upper back (buffalo hump), and the face (moon facies). Weight gain in patients receiving prolonged courses of GCS reflects both fluid retention and increased oral intake secondary to increased appetite. Limiting salt intake while observing a healthy diet may help to reduce weight gain but in reality this is often difficult to achieve. Combined with characteristic purple striae, hirsutism and acne, the body appearance changes dramatically and these cosmetic changes often become a major issue, particularly in the adolescent. Counseling for depression and eating disorders is often needed.

6.3.4. OSTEOPENIA AND OSTEOPOROSIS

Patients with JIA are at risk for localized and/or generalized osteopenia and osteoporosis. Osteopenia is defined as low bone mass for skeletal age and stage of sexual maturation. In young adults, a bone mineral density between 1 and 2.5 standard deviations below the mean for age and gender indicates osteopenia. Osteoporosis is the parallel loss of bone mineral content and matrix and is defined in young adults as a bone mineral density less than 2.5 standard deviations below the mean for age and gender. However, there are no accepted definitions for osteopenia and osteoporosis in childhood *(74,75)*. Localized osteopenia is commonly identified with plain X-ray studies early in the disease process, whereas generalized osteopenia and osteoporosis develop later as disease progresses and results in an increased risk for the development of pathological fractures in the vertebrae and long bones *(29,74,75)*.

Osteopenia and osteoporosis develop in patients with JIA as a result of malnutrition, chronically active inflammatory disease, decreased physical activity, decreased sun exposure, and medications. Adequate vitamin D and calcium intake and weight-bearing physical activities reduce the risk for developing both conditions, whereas active inflammatory disease and chronic glucocorticosteroid use increase the risk, particularly in children with early-onset disease. Other factors contributing to the risk are the subtype of JIA, polyarticular disease, and duration of disease (decreased bone formation may be detected early in the course *(74,105–107)*). Limited physical activity, low functional class, tobacco use, and lowered calcium intake during adolescence may contribute to the risk of developing osteopenia in adults with a history of JRA (ACR criteria *(108)*).

7. DIETARY MANAGEMENT

There are no specific studies that address the Recommended Dietary Allowances (RDAs) for children with JIA. The daily caloric requirement for patients with JIA is likely to be higher than healthy individuals because of active inflammation, higher metabolic rate, and increased resting energy expenditure, particularly in patients with systemic disease *(87,88,91)*. Nearly one-third of the patients with JRA (ACR criteria) have been reported to develop protein-energy malnutrition according to one study *(104)*. The mean caloric intake in patients with pauciarticular and polyarticular JRA (ACR criteria) in another report was 74% of the RDA in healthy children of comparable age and gender. Decreased iron and calcium intake was also noted *(103)*.

Patients with JIA should receive at a minimum, a daily caloric requirement similar to that of healthy child with subsequent adjustments to the daily intake then addressed based on the nutritional status of each patient. Dietary counseling is needed if patients do not meet the RDA or to help with other issues such as excessive or inadequate weight gain, food allergies or intolerance, and/or the presence of other medical disorder that require dietary modifications (e.g., diabetes). Occasionally, a nasogastric tube is needed for enteral feeding of the malnourished child or total parenteral nutrition for the medically unstable patient. Other factors that need to be considered in patients with decreased intake include depression, eating disorders, neglect and abuse, and socioeconomic factors.

Parents often implement unconventional dietary regimens without consulting a physician. Not only do such practices cause an economic burden, they also may be injurious and interfere with standard therapy *(82,109)*. In one survey, 70% of patients with JRA or JCA (ACR or EULAR criteria) admitted to using unconventional remedies. Such remedies include copper bands; acupuncture and patent medicines such as seaweed extracts, cod liver oil, megavitamins and herbal preparations; and/or diet alterations such as restricting certain vegetables, fasting, and increased fish intake and fish-oil supplements *(109)*. There are no scientific studies to date indicating that dietary restrictions or special unconventional dietary regimens have a role in management of patients with JIA. Increased fish intake and fish-oil supplement has shown potential benefits in adult patients with RA *(110)*. Accordingly, fish-oil supplementation may have potential role in patients with JIA but more studies are required. Sometimes, parents implement such regimens in combination with conventional therapy, but on occasion these remedies are the only therapy provided to the child, and then lead to significant adverse effects *(109)*. The role of food allergies as inducers of any subtype of JIA is unknown. Other than scattered case reports, there are no published population-based studies that estimate the prevalence of food-related chronic arthritis in the pediatric age group *(82)*. Educating patients and parents about healthy nutritional habits (e.g., avoiding excessive consumption of fast food), ensuring adequate caloric and nutrients intake, and monitoring growth parameters remain the essential aspects of management.

Vitamins and other nutrient supplements are often required in patients with JIA. Ensuring adequate daily calcium intake for age and daily vitamin D of at least 400 IU per day may play a role in prevention of the development of osteopenia and osteoporosis *(111–113)*. Behavioral interventions such as providing nutritional information to parents along with behavioral child management skills to assist in motivating their children to increase calcium-rich foods in their daily intake was shown to be beneficial in increasing both dietary calcium intake and bone mineral content in children with JRA *(112,114)*. Several therapeutic options have been used to treat established osteopenia or osteoporosis and treatment selection should be individualized based on severity and presence of active disease, subtype of JIA, and presence of fractures. There is limited data regarding the medical treatment of osteoporosis in children, which currently includes calcium, vitamin D, and bisphosphonates. The efficacy and safety of bisphosphonates in children are unknown and require further evaluation with randomized, controlled, long-term trials. GI side effects such as nausea, dyspepsia, esophagitis, and abdominal pain may be encountered in patients taking bisphosphonates. Musculoskeletal adverse effects include transient skeletal pain, epiphyseal and metaphyseal radiologic sclerosis in growing bones, and mandibular osteonecrosis. Possible feared but not confirmed adverse effects include irreversible effect on bone remodeling, impaired healing and non-union of fractures, damage to growth plates, and impairment to linear growth, and fetal abnormalities *(74,75,115)*.

Other supplements that provide clear benefits include multivitamins and folic acid. Patients receiving methotrexate require folic acid supplementation to minimize the occurrence of oral ulcers. Nutrient deficiencies should be corrected. Control of underlying chronic inflammation usually corrects the anemia of chronic disease, however, iron supplementation may be beneficial if iron-deficiency anemia coexists (i). Occasionally, recombinant human erythropoietin is considered for the treatment of anemia in rheumatic diseases *(116)*.

8. RECOMMENDATIONS

In summary, JIA is a group of heterogeneous disorders characterized by chronic arthritis with frequent extra-articular manifestations. Nutritional impairment is common in the various subtypes of JIA owing to several risk factors including mechanical feeding difficulties, anorexia and GI symptoms, medications, increased energy expenditure, decreased caloric intake, decreased physical activity, and severe inflammatory cachexia related to the severity and chronicity of the underlying disease process. Examples of nutritional impairment seen in the context of JIA include cachexia and malnutrition, growth delay, osteoporosis, anemia, and obesity. Several recommendations are helpful in preventing some aspects of the nutritional impairment seen in patients with JIA and/or help to treat some aspects of its complications.

Careful nutritional history and anthropometric assessment such as body weight, height, body mass index, leg-length discrepancy, and monitoring of growth velocity should be part of the evaluation of each child with JIA. A dietician should be part of the rheumatology team and should be consulted when there is concern about nutritional deficits or the presence of other medical disorders that require dietary modifications. Regular prophylactic dental examinations are essential to promote oral health.

Adequate daily caloric intake is essential to ensure a healthy nutritional status. Special considerations exist for patients with IBD depending on the extent and location of intestinal involvement. Patients with JIA should receive the RDAs for healthy children of comparable age and gender. Further studies are needed to establish the RDAs for patients with each subtype of JIA. To date, no special diet or dietary restrictions have been shown to provide any major benefit for the management of the child with JIA. However, there may be potential benefits for increased fish intake and fish-oil supplements but further studies are needed. Supplementation with daily requirements of vitamins or other nutrients may be required to ensure adequate intake of the daily age recommendations.

Patients with JIA should be encouraged to participate in age-appropriate physical activities taking into consideration the actual physical limitations and severity of their underlying disease. Swimming and nonweight-bearing exercises can improve range of motion and function of joints, restore cardiovascular fitness, facilitate weight loss in overweight patients, and enhance muscle tone and facilitate increased lean body mass.

Discussing medication comprehensively with patients and parents helps them to anticipate and minimize side effects. Every effort should be made to minimize the dose and duration of GCS as mandated by the disease activity. Folic acid supplementation is useful to decrease the side effects of methotrexate such as oral ulcerations, nausea, and vomiting.

Limiting the development of osteoporosis in patients receiving high-dose corticosteroids may be accomplished by ensuring the needed daily requirements of vitamin D and calcium. Early diagnosis of osteopenia and osteoporosis is essential for treatment and prevention of morbid complications such as vertebral compression fractures. Patients with JIA should be monitored and treated for the anemia of chronic disease. Anemia may be corrected with adequate treatment of the underlying disorder but iron supplementation for coexisting iron-deficiency anemia should be considered.

Early referral to an endocrinologist for possible implementation of growth hormone therapy should be considered early in patients with growth retardation or those at risk for growth suppression (systemic-onset disease and chronic use of GCS). Counseling for depression and eating disorders should be considered in patients with anorexia or obesity. It is vital to address the risk of unconventional dietary remedies, socioeconomic status, and/or issues of child neglect or abuse.

Finally, there is a need for further clinical investigations to examine the various aspects of nutritional impairment in patients with JIA and establish more specific guidelines for RDAs, routine nutrient supplementation, monitoring of nutrient deficiency, and treatment of osteopenia and osteoporosis.

REFERENCES

1. Schneider R, Passo MH. Juvenile rheumatoid arthritis. Rheum Dis Clin North Am 2002;28:503–530.
2. Weiss JE, Ilowite NT. Juvenile idiopathic arthritis. Pediatr Clin N Am 2005;52:413–442.
3. Bywaters EG. The history of pediatric rheumatology. Arthritis Rheum 1977;20(2 suppl):145–152.
4. Schaller JG. The history of pediatric rheumatology. Pediatr Res 2005;5:997–1007.
5. Hofer M, Southwood T. Classification of childhood arthritis. Best Pract Res Clin Rheumatol 2002;16(3):379–396.
6. Still GF. On a form of chronic joint disease in children. R Med Chir Soc London 1897;80:47–59. Reprinted in Clin Orthop 1990;259:4–10.
7. Still GF. On a form of chronic joint disease in children. Medico-Chirurgical Trans 1897;80:47–59.Reprinted in Am J Dis Child 1978;132:195–200.
8. Schlesinger B. The relationship of throat infection to acute rheumatism in childhood. Arch Dis Child 1930;5:411–430.
9. Lundberg IE, Grubdtman C, Larsson E, Klareskog L. Corticosteroids—from an idea to clinical use. Best Pract Res Clin Rheumatol 2004;18(1):7–19.
10. Schaller JG, Johnson GD, Holborow EJ, Ansell BM, Smiley WK. The association of antinuclear antibodies with the chronic iridocyclitis of juvenile rheumatoid arthritis (Still's disease). Arthritis Rheum 1974;17:409–416.
11. Brewer EJ, Bass JC, Cassidy JT, et al. Criteria for the classification of juvenile rheumatoid arthritis. Bull Rheum Dis 1972;23:712–719.
12. Brewer EJ, Bass J, Baum J, et al. Current proposed revision of JRA criteria. Committee of the American Rheumatism Section of The Arthritis Foundation. Arthritis Rheum 1977;20:195–199.

13. Cassidy JT, Levinson JE, Brewer EJ. The development of classification criteria for children with juvenile rheumatoid arthritis. Bull Rheum Dis 1989;38:1–7.
14. Fink C. Proposal for the development of classification criteria for idiopathic arthritides of childhood. J Rheumatol 1995;22:1566–1569.
15. Petty RE, Southwood TR, Baum J, et al. Revision of the proposed classification criteria for juvenile idiopathic arthritis: Durban, 1997. J Rheumatol 1998;25:1991–1994.
16. Petty RE, Southwood TR, Manners P, et al. International League of Associations for Rheumatology Classification of Juvenile Idiopathic Arthritis: Second Revision, Edmonton, 2001. J Rheumatol 2004;31:390–392.
17. Cassidy JT, Petty RE. Chronic arthritis in childhood. In: Cassidy JT, Petty RE, Laxer RM, and Lindsley's CB. The Text Book of Pediatric Rheumatology, 5th ed. Elsevier Saunders, Philadelphia, PA, 2005, pp. 206–260.
18. Manners RJ, Bower C. Worldwide prevalence of Juvenile arthritis—why does it vary so much? J Rheumatol 2002;29(7):1520–1530.
19. Sharma S, Sherry D. Joint distribution at presentation in children with pauciarticular arthritis. J Pediatr 1999;134:642–643.
20. Huemer C, Malleson PN, Cabral DA, et al. Patterns of joints involvement at onset differentiate oligoarticular juvenile psoriatic arthritis from pauciarticular juvenile rheumatoid arthritis. J Rheumatol 2002;29:1531–1535.
21. Al-Matar MJ, Petty RE, Tucker LB, Malleson PN, Schroeder ML, Cabral DA. The early pattern of joint involvement predicts disease progression in children with oligoarticular (pauciarticular) juvenile rheumatoid arthritis. Arthritis Rheum 2002;46(10):2708–2715.
22. Ravelli A, Felici E, Magni-Manzoni S, et al. Patients with antinuclear antibody-positive juvenile idiopathic arthritis constitute a homogeneous subgroup irrespective of the course of joint disease. Arthritis Rheum 2005;52(3):826–832.
23. Schaller J, Kupfer C, Wedgwood RJ. Iridocyclitis in juvenile rheumatoid arthritis. Pediatrics 1969;44(1):92–99.
24. Chylack LT Jr. The ocular manifestations of juvenile rheumatoid arthritis. Arthritis Rheum 1977;20 (suppl):217–223.
25. Weiss AH, Wallace CA, Sherry DD. Methotrexate for resistant chronic uveitis in children with juvenile rheumatoid arthritis. J Pediatr 1998;133:266–268.
26. Carvounis PE, Herman DC, Cha S, Burke JP. Incidence and outcomes of uveitis in juvenile rheumatoid arthritis, a synthesis of the literature. Graefe's Arch Clin Exp Ophthalmol 2006;244:281–290.
27. Ansell BM. Joint manifestations in children with juvenile chronic polyarthritis. Arthitis Rheum 1977;20 (suppl):204–206.
28. Cassidy JT, Martel W. Juvenile rheumatoid arthritis: clinicoradiologic correlations. Arthritis Rheum 1977;20 (suppl):207–211.
29. Mason T, Reed AM, Nelson AM, et al.. Frequency of abnormal hand and wrist radiographs at time of diagnosis of polyarticular juvenile rheumatoid arthritis. J Rheumatol 2002;29(10):2214–2218.
30. Calabro JJ. Other extraarticular manifestations of juvenile rheumatoid arthritis. Arthritis Rheum 1977;20 (suppl):237–240.
31. Bernstein BH, Stobie D, Singsen BH, Koster-King K, Kornreich HK, Hanson V. Growth retardation in juvenile rheumatoid arthritis (JRA). Arthritis Rheum 1977;20 (suppl):212–216.
32. Pedersen TK, Jensen JJ, Melsen B, Herlin T. Resorption of the temporomandibular candela bone according to subtypes of juvenile chronic arthritis. J Rheumatol 2001;28(9):2109–2115.
33. Twilt M, Mobers S, Arends LR, Cate Rt. Temporomandibular involvement in juvenile idiopathic arthritis. J Rheumatol 2004;31(7):1418–1422.
34. Twilt M, Schulten AJM, Nicolaas P, Dülger A, Van Suijlekom-Smit LWA. Facioskeletal changes in children with juvenile idiopathic arthritis. Ann Rheum Dis 2006;65:823–825.
35. Cassidy JT, Petty RE. Systemic arthritis. In: Cassidy JT, Petty RE, Laxer RM, and Lindsley's CB. The Text Book of Pediatric Rheumatology, 5th ed. Elsevier Saunders, Philadelphia, PA, 2005, pp. 291–303.
36. Boldero HEA. A case of Still's disease. Trans Med Soc London 1933;16:55.

37. Schaller J, Wedgwood RJ. Pruritis associated with the rash of juvenile rheumatoid arthritis. Pediatrics 1970;45:296–298.
38. Calabro JJ, Marchesano JM. Fever associated with juvenile rheumatoid arthritis. N Engl J Med;1967;276(1):11–18.
39. Scott JP, Gerber P, Maryjowski MC, Pachman LM. Evidence for intravascular coagulation in systemic onset, but not polyarticular juvenile rheumatoid arthritis. Arthritis Rheum 1985;28(3): 256–261.
40. Hadchouel M, Prieur A-M, Griscelli C. Acute hemorrhagic, hepatic, and neurologic manifestations in juvenile rheumatoid arthritis: possible relationship to drugs or infection. J Pediatr 1985;106:561–566.
41. Sawhney S, Woo P, Murray KJ. Macrophage activation syndrome: a potentially fatal complication of rheumatic disorders. Arch Dis Child 2001;85:421–426.
42. Mouy R, Stephan JL, Pillet P, Haddad E, Hubert P, Prieur A–M. Efficacy of cyclosporine A in the treatment of macrophage activation syndrome in juvenile arthritis: a report of five cases. J Pediatr 1996;128:750–754.
43. Singsen BH. Psoriatic arthritis in childhood. Arthritis Rheum 1977;20:: 408–410.
44. Southwood TR, Petty RE, Malleson PM, et al. Psoriatic arthritis in children. Arthritis Rheum 1989;32:1007–1013.
45. Huemer C, Malleson PN, Cabral DA, et al. Patterns of joint involvement at onset differentiate oligoarticular juvenile psoriatic arthritis from pauciarticular juvenile rheumatoid arthritis. J Rheumatol 2002;29:1531–1535.
46. Hofer M. Spondyloarthropathies in children—are they different from those in adults? Best Pract Res Clin Rheumatol 2006;20(2):315–326.
47. Schaller JG, Bitnum S, Wedgwood RJ. Ankylosing spondylitis with childhood onset. J Pediatr 1969;74:505–516.
48. Schaller JG. Ankylosing spondylitis of childhood onset. Arthritis Rheum 1977;20: 398–401.
49. Baek HJ, Shin KC, Lee YJ, Kang SW, Lee EB, Yoo CD. Juvenile onset ankylosing spondylitis (JAS) has less severe spinal disease course than adult onset ankylosing spondylitis (AAS): Clinical comparison between JAS and AAS in Korea. J Rheumatol 2002;29:1780–1785.
50. Sherry DD, Sapp LR. Enthesalgia in childhood: Site specific tenderness in healthy subjects and in patients with seronegative enthesopathic arthropathy. J Rheumatol 2003;30:1335–1340.
51. Monnet D, Breban M, Hudry C, Dougados M, Brézin AP. Ophthalmic findings and frequency of extraocular manifestations in patients with HLA-B27 uveitis. Ophthalmology 2004;111:802–809.
52. Huppertz HI, Voigt I, Müller-Scholden J, Sandhage K. Cardiac Manifestations in patients with HLA-B27-associated juvenile arthritis. Pediatr Cardiol 2000;21:141–147.
53. Lindsley CB. Arthritis in inflammatory bowel disease in children. Arthritis Rheum 1977;20: 411–413.
54. Orchard TR, Wordsworth BP, Jewell DP. Peripheral arthropathies in inflammatory bowel disease: their articular distribution and natural history. Gut 1998;42:387–391.
55. Boot AM, Bouquet J, Krenning EP, Keizer-Schrama SMPF. Bone mineral density and nutritional status in children with chronic inflammatory bowel disease. Gut 1998;42:188–194.
56. Thearle M, Horlick M, Bilezikian JP, et al. Osteoporosis: An unusual presentation of childhood Crohn's disease. Endocrinol Metab 2000;85:2122–2126.
57. Kleinman RE, Baldassano RN, Caplan A, et al. Nutrition support for pediatric patients with inflammatory bowel disease: A clinical report of the North American society for pediatric gastroenterology, hepatology, and nutrition. J Pediatr Gastroenterol Nutr 2004;36(1):15–27.
58. Milojevic DS, Illowit NT. Treatment of rheumatic diseases in children: special considerations. Rheum Dis Clin North Am 2002;28:461–482.
59. Wallace CA. Current management of juvenile idiopathic arthritis. Best Pract Res Clin Rheumatol 2006;20(2):279–300.
60. Giannini EH, Cawkwell GD. Drug treatment in children with juvenile rheumatoid arthritis: Past, present and future. Pediatr Clin North Am 1995;42(5):1099–1125.
61. Hashkes PJ, Laxer RM. Medical treatment of juvenile idiopathic arthritis. JAMA 2005;294(13): 1671–1684.
62. Illowit NT. Current treatment of juvenile rheumatoid arthritis. Pediatrics 2002;109(1):109–115.
63. Giannini EH, Brewer EJ, Kuzmina N, et al., for the Pediatric Rheumatology Collaborative Study Group and the Cooperative Children's Study Group. Methotrexate in resistant juvenile rheumatoid arthritis.

Results of the USA–USSR Double-Blind Placebo-Controlled Trial. N Engl J Med 1992;326(16): 1043–1049.
64. Cronstein BN. The mechanism of action of methotrexate. Rheum Dis Clin North Am 1997;23: 739–751.
65. Hyams JS, Carey DE. Corticosteroids and growth. J Pediatr 1988;113(20):249–254.
66. Bernstein BH, Stobie D, Singsen BH, Koster-King K, Kornreich HK, Hanson V. Growth retardation in juvenile rheumatoid arthritis. Arthritis rheum 1977;20(suppl):212–216.
67. Wang SJ, Yang YH, Lin YT, Yang CM, Chiang BL. Attained adult height in juvenile rheumatoid arthritis with or without corticosteroid treatment. Clin Rheumatol 2002;21:363–368.
68. Saha MT, Verronen P, Laippala P, Lenko HL. Growth of prepubertal children with juvenile chronic arthritis. Acta Pediatr 1999;88:724–728.
69. Bechtold S, Ripperger P, Häfner R, Said E, Schwartz P. Growth hormone improves height in patients with juvenile idiopathic arthritis: 4-year data of a controlled study. J Pediatr 2003;143:512–519.
70. Simon D, Lucidarme N, Prieur AM, Ruiz JC, Czernichow P. Effects of growth and body composition of growth hormone treatment in children with juvenile idiopathic arthritis requiring steroid therapy. J Rheumatol 2003;30:2492–2499.
71. Saha MT, Haapasaari J, Hannula S, Sarna S, Lenko HL. Growth hormone is effective in the treatment of severe growth retardation in children with juvenile chronic arthritis. Double blind placebo-controlled followup study. J Rheumatol 2004;31:1413–1417.
72. Pepmueller PH, Cassidy JT, Allen SH, Hillman LS. Bone mineralization and bone mineral metabolism in children with juvenile rheumatoid arthritis. Arthritis Rheum 1996;39(5):746–757.
73. Canalis E. Mechanisms of glucocorticoid action in bone: implications to glucocorticoid-induced osteoporosis. J Clin Endocrinol Metab 1996;81(10):3441–3447.
74. Cassidy JT. Osteopenia and osteoporosis in children. Clin Exp Rheumatol 1999;17:245–250.
75. Rabinovich EC. Bone metabolism in childhood rheumatic disease. Rheum Dis Clin North Am 2002;28:655–667.
76. Sherry DD, Stein LD, Reed AM, Schanberg LE, Kredich DW. Prevention of leg length discrepancy in young children with pauciarticular juvenile rheumatoid arthritis by treatment with intraarticular steroids. Arthritis Rheum 1999;42(11):2230–2334.
77. Arabshahi B, Dewitt M, Cahill AM, Kaye RD, Baskin KM, Towbin RB, Cron RQ. Utility of corticosteroid injection for temporomandibular arthritis in children with juvenile idiopathic arthritis. Arthritis Rheum 2005;52(11):3563–3569.
78. Lovell DJ, Giannini EH, Reiff A, et al., for the Pediatric Rheumatology Collaborative Study Group. Etanercept in children with polyarticular juvenile rheumatoid arthritis. N Engl J Med 2000;342(11):763–769.
79. Gerloni V, Pontikaki I, Gattinara M, et al. Efficacy of repeated intravenous infusions of an anti-tumor necrosis factor α monoclonal antibody, infliximab, in persistent active, refractory juvenile idiopathic arthritis. Arthritis Rheum 2005;52(2):548–553.
80. Pascual V, Allantaz F, Arce E, Punaro M, Banchereau J. Role of interleukin-1 (IL-1) in the pathogenesis of systemic onset juvenile idiopathic arthritis and clinical response to IL-1 blockade. J Exp Med 2005;9:1479–1486.
81. Yokota S. Miyamae T, Imagawa T, Katakura S, Kurosawa R, Mori M. Clinical study of Tocilizumab in children with systemic-onset juvenile idiopathic arthritis. Clin Rev Allergy Immunol 2005;28:231–237.
82. Henderson CJ, Lovell DJ. Nutritional aspects of juvenile rheumatoid arthritis. Rheum Dis Clin North Am 1991;17:403–413.
83. Walton AG, Welbury RR, Foster HE, Thomason JM. Juvenile chronic arthritis: a dental review. Oral Dis 1999;5:68–75.
84. Ahmed N, Bloch-Zupan A, Murray KJ, Calvert M, Roberts GJ, Lucas VS. Oral health of children with juvenile idiopathic arthritis. J Rheumatol 2004;31:1639–1643.
85. Laxer RM. Pharmacology and drug therapy. In: Cassidy JT, Petty RE, Laxer RM, and Lindsley's CB. The Text Book of Pediatric Rheumatology, 5th ed. Elsevier Saunders, Philadelphia, PA, 2005, pp.76–141.
86. Ostrov BE. Nutrition and pediatric rheumatic diseases. Hypothesis: Cytokines modulate nutritional abnormalities in rheumatic diseases. J Rheumatol 1992;19(suppl 33):49–53.

87. Souza L, Machado SH, Bredemeier M, Brenol JCT, Xavier RM. Effect of inflammatory activity and glucorticoid use on nutritional variables in patients with juvenile idiopathic arthritis. J Rheumatol 2006;33:601–608.
88. Knops N, Wulffraat N, Lodder S, Houwen R, Meer K. Resting energy expenditure and nutritional status in children with juvenile rheumatoid arthritis. J Rheumatol 1999;26:2039–2043.
89. Simon D, Fernando C, Czernichow P, Prieur. Linear growth and final height in patients with systemic juvenile idiopathic arthritis treated with longterm glucocorticoids. J Rheumatol 2002;29:1296–1300.
90. MacRae VE, Farquharson C, Ahmed SF. The pathophysiology of the growth plate in juvenile idiopathic arthritis. Rheumatology 2006;45:11–19.
91. Cleary AG, Lancaster GA, Annan F, Sills JA, Davidson JE. Nutritional impairment in juvenile idiopathic arthritis. Rheumatology 2004;43:1569–1573.
92. Mangge H, Kenzian H, Gallistl S, et al. Serum cytokines in juvenile rheumatoid arthritis. Correlation with conventional inflammation parameters and clinical subtypes. Arthritis Rheum 1995;38(2):211–220.
93. Roubenoff R, Freeman L, Smith DE, Abad LW, Dinarello CA, Kehayias J. Adjuvant arthritis as a model of inflammatory cachexia. Arthr Rheum 1997;40: 534–539.
94. Roubenoff R, Roubenoff RA, Cannon JG, et al. Rheumatoid cachexia: cytokine-driven hypermetabolism and loss of lean body mass in chronic inflammation. J Clin Invest 1994;93:2379–2386.
95. Walsmith J, Roubenoff R. Cachexia in rheumatoid arthritis. Int J Cardiol 2002;85(1): 98–99.
96. Tracey KJ, Wei H, Manogue KR, Fet al. Cachectin/ Tumor necrosis factor induces cachexia, anemia, and inflammation. J Exp Med 1988;167:1211–1227.
97. Koerper MA, Stempel DA, Dallman PR. Anemia in patients with juvenile rheumatoid arthritis. J Pediatr 1978;92(6):930–933.
98. Cazzola M, Ponchio L, Benedetti F, et al. Defective iron supply for erythropoiesis and adequate endogenous erythropoietin production in the anemia associated with systemic-onset juvenile chronic arthritis. Blood 1996;87(11):4824–4830.
99. Kivivuori SM, Pelkonen P, Ylijoki H, Verronen P, Siimes MA. Elevated serum transferring receptor concentration in children with juvenile chronic arthritis as evidence of iron deficiency. Rheumatology 2000;39:193–197.
100. Bacon MC, White PH, Raiten DJ, et al. Nutritional status and growth in juvenile rheumatoid arthritis. Semin Arthritis Rheum 1990;20(2):97–106.
101. Amancio OS, Chaud DA, Yanaguibashi G, Hilário MO E. Copper and zinc intake and serum levels in patients with juvenile rheumatoid arthritis. Eur J Clin Nutr 2003;57:706–712.
102. Warady BD, McCamman SP, Lindsley CB. Anthropometric assessment of patients with juvenile rheumatoid arthritis. Top Clin Nutr 1989;4(1):7–14.
103. Miller ML, Chacko JA, Young EA. Dietary deficiencies in children with juvenile rheumatoid arthritis. Arthritis Car Res 1989;2(1):22–24.
104. Henderson C, Lovell DJ. Assessment of protein-energy malnutrition in children and adolescence with JRA. Arthritis Care Res 1989;2(4):108–113.
105. Kotaniemi A, Savolainen A, Kröger H, Kautiainen H, Isomäki H. Weight-bearing physical activity, calcium intake, systemic glucocorticoids, chronic inflammation, and body constitution as determinants of lumbar and femoral bone mineral in juvenile chronic arthritis. Scand J Rheumatol 1999;28:19–26.
106. Lien G, Flato B, Haugen M, et al. Frequency of osteopenia in adolescents with early-onset juvenile idiopathic arthritis. A long term outcome study of one hundred five patients. Arthritis Rheum 2003;48(8):2214–2223.
107. Lien G, Selvaage AM, Flato B, et al. A two-year prospective controlled study of bone mass and bone turnover in children with early juvenile idiopathic arthritis. Arthritis Rheum 2005;52(3):833–840.
108. French AR, Mason T, Nelson AM, et al. Osteopenia in adults with a history of juvenile rheumatoid arthritis. A population based study. J Rheumatol 2002;29:1065–1070.
109. Southwood TR, Malleson PN, Roberts-Thomson PJ, Mahy A. Unconventional remedies used for patients with juvenile arthritis. Pediatrics 1990;85(2):150–154.
110. Stamp LK, James MJ, Cleland LG. Diet and rheumatoid arthritis: A review of the literature. Semin Arthritis Rheum 2005;35:77–94.

111. Sambrook P, Birmingham J, Kelly P, et al. Prevention of corticosteroid osteoporosis. A comparison of calcium, calcitirol, and calcitonin. N Engl J Med 1993;328:1747–1752.
112. Stark LJ, Davis AM, Janicke DM, et al. A randomized clinical trial of dietary calcium to improve bone accretion in children with juvenile rheumatoid arthritis. J Pediatr 2006;148:501–507.
113. Lovel DJ, Glass D, Ranz J, et al. A randomized controlled trial of calcium supplementation to increase bone mineral density in children with juvenile rheumatoid arthritis. Arthritis Rheum 2006;54(7): 2235–2242.
114. Stark LJ, Janicke DM, McGrath AM, Mackner LM, Hommel KA, Lovell D. Prevention of osteoporosis: A randomized clinical trial to increase calcium intake in children with juvenile rheumatoid arthritis. J Pediatr Psychol 2005;30(5):377–386.
115. Bianchi ML. How to manage osteoporosis in children. Best Pract Res Clin Rheumatol 2005;19(6): 991–1005.
116. Fantini F, Gattinara M, Gerloni V, Bergomi P, Cirla E. Severe anemia associated with active systemic-onset juvenile rheumatoid arthritis successfully treated with recombinant human erythropoietin: a pilot study. Arthritis Rheum 1992;35(6):724–726.

III Nutrition and Rheumatic Disease-Related Resources

Appendix A: *Nutrition Resources*

NUTRITION

American Dietetic Association – www.eatright.org
American Society for Nutrition – www.nutrition.org
Center for Science in the Public Interest – www.cspinet.org
Centers for Disease Control and Prevention – www.cdc.gov
Food and Drug Administration – www.fda.gov
National Center for Complementary and Alternative Medicine (National Institutes of Health) – www.nccam.nih.gov
Nutrition.gov – www.nutrition.gov
Office of Dietary Supplements (National Institutes of Health) – www.dietary-supplements.info.nih.gov
United State Department of Agriculture (USDA) Food and Nutrition Service – www.fns.usda.gov/fns
USDA Food Guide Pyramid – www.mypyramid.gov
Tufts University Health and Nutrition Letter – www.healthletter.tufts.edu

EXERCISE

American College of Sports Medicine – www.acsm.org

Appendix B: *Rheumatology Resources*

American College of Rheumatology – www.rheumatology.org
Arthritis Foundation – www.arthritis.org
Lupus Foundation of America – www.lupus.org
National Fibromyalgia Association – www.fmaware.org
National Institute of Arthritis and Musculoskeletal and Skin Diseases (National Institutes of Health) – www.niams.nih.gov
Scleroderma Foundation – www.scleroderma.org
Sjogren's Syndrome Foundation – www.sjogrens.org
The Myositis Association – www.myositis.org
Vasculitis Foundation – www.vasculitisfoundation.org

Index

A

AA, *see* Arachidonic acid (AA)
Activities of daily living (ADLs), 27
Adalimumab, 62
Adenosine triphosphate (ATP), 189
Alfalfa, 164
   harmful for SLE, 164–165
American Heart Association's (AHA) diet recommendation, 176
Anabolic steroids
   risks of, on nonprescription, 203–204
Ankylosing spondylitis (AS), 74
Anthropometry, 17
   edema, 20
   fatness
      skinfolds, 19–20
      waist circumferences, 19
   height/stature, 17
   muscle and bone
      bioelectrical impedance analysis, 20
      dual-energy X-ray absorptiometry, 20
   weight and body mass index, 17–19
Antibodies, against self-antigens, *see* Autoantibodies
Antigen presentation, altered, 4
Antineutrophilic cytoplasmic antibodies (ANCAs), 8
   cytoplasmic (c-ANCA), 9
   perinuclear (p-ANCA), 9
Antinuclear antibodies (ANAs), 5
   detection of, for diagnostic SLE, 5
   in SLEs, 5
   and SS, 7
Anti-Sm antibody, 6
Apoptosis, 4
Apoptotic blebs, 4
Aquatherapy, 80
Arachidonic acid (AA), 59, 134
   metabolism, 60
Arthritic joints, restriction of movement, 73
Arthritis, 28
   frequency of self-reported, 47
   limiting ROM, 28
   modified diet to ameliorate, 90
   preventing symptoms of, 57
Arthritis-attributable activity limitation
   NHIS and, 45–46
Arthritis, Diet, and Activity Promotion Trial, 147
Ascorbic acid, *see* Vitamin C
Aspirin (acetylsalicylic acid), 102
Atkins™, 176
Autoantibodies, 4
   and cryoglobulinemia, 9
   and disease manifestations, 6
   formation in, 4–5
      inflammatory muscle disease, 7–8
      rheumatoid arthritis, 9–10
      scleroderma, 7
      SLE, 5–6
      SS, 6–7
      vasculitides, 8–9
   varied pathogenecity of, 6
Autoimmune rheumatic disorder (Sjögren's syndrome)
   causation, 230
   consequences of saliva hypofunction, 227–228
   effects of, 227, 231, 234
   locations of effects in body, 229
   prevalence of women, 228
   primary SS, 228
   salivary gland locations in oral cavity, 230
   secondary SS, 228–229
Autoimmune thyroid disease, 5
Autoimmunity, 4
Autumn crocus (*Colchicum autumnale*), 176
Avocado/Soybean Unsaponifiables (ASUs), 104–105, 145
   increased basal synthesis of aggrecan, 146
Avoiders, defined, 82

B

Biochemical indices, comorbidities, 23
   anemia of chronic disease, 23
   hyperglycemia, 23
   hyperlipidemia, 23
   markers of inflammation, 23

Biochemical tests, 16, 20–21
  example, 21
Bioelectrical impedance analysis (BIA), 16, 20
Body mass index (BMI), 17–18
  calculation, 18
  limitations, 18, 19
Body weight, 19
Bone mineral density (BMD), 131

C

Calciferol, see Vitamin D
Calcium, 22
Caloric restriction for SLE, 160
  autoimmune-prone NZB/NZW F1 (B/W) as model, 160
CAM, see Complementary and alternative medicine (CAM)
Case-control studies (retrospective), epidemiological study designs, 42
Catastrophizing, 82
  See also Confronters
Celecoxib, (COX-2 inhibitor), 59
Celiac disease, 5
Centers for Disease Control and Prevention (CDC), 89
Central nervous system vasculitides, 219–220
Cherries
  compared with other fruits, 174
  decrease in plasma urate, 175
  role in preventing gout, 174
Childhood-onset type 1 diabetes, 44
Chiropractic care, 90
Chlorella pyrenoidosa, 189
Chondroitin, 99–101
  treatment of OA, 99–101
Chronic arthritides of childhood
  clinical features, 255
    oligoarticular JIA, 255–256
    polyarticular JIA, 256
    psoriatic arthritis, 257
    systemic-onset JIA, 256–257
  dietary management, 267–269
  enthesitis-related arthritides
    arthritides of IBD, 258–259
    juvenile ankylosing spondylitis, 258
  historical background, 252
  management and treatment, 259
    biological immunomodulators, 262
    cytotoxic and immunosuppressive drugs, 262
    DMARDs, 260
    glucocorticosteroids, 260–261
    NSAIDs, 259–260

nutritional impairments in patients with JIA, 264
  body composition abnormalities, 266–267
  growth abnormalities, 264–265
  malnutrition and nutrient deficiencies, 265–266
  osteopenia and osteoporosis, 267
nutritional status, 262
oral health in patients with JIA, 263
recommendations, 269–270
risk factors for developing nutritional impairments, 263–264
terminology and classification, 252–253
  ACR classification criteria for JRA, 253
  EULAR classification criteria for JCA, 253
  ILAR classification criteria for JIA, 253–255
Chronic arthritis, 251
Chronic fatigue syndrome, 185
Chronic inflammation, symptoms of, 195, 199
Chronic joint symptoms
  frequency of, 47
Chronic juvenile arthritides, classifications of
  comparison of ACR, EULAR, and ILAR, 254
  subtypes of chronic arthritis in children, 254
Churg-Strauss syndrome (CSS), 217
  characteristics of, 217
Cohort, epidemiological study designs, 41
Colchicine, 176
  See also Autumn crocus (*Colchicum autumnale*)
Complementary and alternative medicine (CAM), 89
  NCCAM's definition, 89–90
  types, 90
Confronters, 82
  vs avoiders, 83
Coping strategies, 82
Copper bracelets or magnets, 90
Corticosteroids, 57, 221
  as alternative for NSAIDS in RA, 65
  drugs for RA, 65
Corticotrophin-releasing hormone, 185
Creatine supplement, 202–203
Creatinine, 21–22
Crepitus, 126
CREST syndrome, 5
  See also Scleroderma
Cryoglobulinemia, 9
Cryoglobulinemic vasculitides, 217–218
Curcumin (turmeric), 105
Cyclic citrullinated peptides (CCPs), 10
Cyclooxygenase (COX), 59

Cytokines, 12
    beneficial effects of, 198
    and rheumatic diseases, 12
    role of, 62
Cytoplasmic (c-ANCA), 9

D

Daily energy expenditure, total (TEE), 117
Dehydroepiandrosterone (DHEA), 164
    side effects, 164
    and SLE, 163–164
Dental caries, 232
    acid erosion in xerostomic patient, 234
    candidiasis, 234
    gingival recession and root caries, 233
    process of, 233
    rampant caries, 233
    remineralizing agents, 239
Dermatomyositis/polymyositis, 7, 195–208
    balanced diet, intake of, 200–206
    creatine supplement and physical exercise, 201, 202–203
    supplements
        with calcium and vitamin D, 205–206
        to reduce risk of steroid-induced osteoporosis, 205–206
Descriptive studies (cross-sectional), epidemiological study designs, 41, 42
Devil's claw (Harpagophytum Procumbens), 102
    efficacy in OA, 102
Diacerein, 144–145
Diagnosis of SS, 235
Diagnostic tests of SS, 235
Dietary assessment, 16, 24–25
Dietary fat intake and SLE, 161
Dietary intake
    assessment methods
        24-hour recalls, 25
        food-frequency questionnaires, 25–26
        food records, 26
    need for assessment of, 24–25
Dietary management for patients with JIA, 267–269
    benefits of supplements, 267–269
Dietary n-3 fatty acids, 61
Dietary status, 15
Dietary supplementation, fibromyalgia, 191–192
Dietary supplements, 90
    fish oil (omega-3 polyunsaturated fatty acids), 92–93
    γ–tlinolenic acid, 96–97
    herbal supplements, 101–106
    vitamins, 97–101
Diet programs, popular, 176
Diets and SLE, low-protein, 160
Diets, special, 90
Disease incidence, 42
Disease-modifying anti-rheumatic drug (DMARD), 57–58, 114, 260
    drugs for RA, 65
Disease prevalence, 42
Diseases affecting elderly
    OA - most prevalant, 126
Diuretics, 172
DMARD, *see* Disease-modifying anti-rheumatic drug (DMARD)
Double-stranded DNA (dsDNA), 5
Drug absorption and bioavailability, 58
Drug-induced vasculitides, 219
    causative drugs, 219
Drug–nutrient interactions in rheumatic diseases, 57–58
    cytokine antagonists
        anti-TNF-α-based therapies, 62
        modulation of proinflammatory cytokines by n-3 fatty acid supplementation, 62–63
        proinflammatory cytokines in pathogenesis of rheumatic diseases, role of, 62
    disease-modifying anti-rheumatic drugs, 63
        folate status and supplementation in methtotrexate treatment, 63–64
        interaction of glutamine with methotrexate, 64
        nutritional status and dietary management, 64
    importance, 57
    mechanisms of, 58
        biological mediators of rheumatic diseases by nutrients, modulation of, 58
        nutritional status by drugs, change in, 58
        pharmacokinetics by food, alteration of, 58
    nonsteroidal anti-inflammatory drugs, 59
        arachidonic acid metabolism and prostaglandin production, 59–61
        clinical benefits of n-3 fatty acids in rheumatoid arthritis, 61
        concomitant food intake on bioavailability of NSAIDs, effects of, 59
        impact of vitamin E in rheumatoid arthritis, 61–62
    recommendations, 66
Dry eye test of SS, 235
DsDNA antibodies, 6
Dual-energy X-ray absorptiometry (DEXA), 16

E

Echinacea
   harmful for SLE, 165
   treatment for colds, 165
Ecological (correlational) studies, epidemiological study designs, 41, 42
Edema, 20
Electrical stimulators, 90
Energy expenditure profile, 117–118
Enthesitis-related arthritides
   arthritides of IBD, 258–259
   juvenile ankylosing spondylitis, 258
Environmental epidemiology, 43–44
Enzyme-linked immunosorbent assay (ELISA), 9
Epidemiological, study designs, 41
   experimental studies, 42
      randomized controlled trial, 41, 43
   observational studies, 42
      case-control (retrospective), 41
      cohort, 41
      descriptive, 41, 42
      ecological (correlational), 41, 42
Epidemiologist
   study methods, 40
Epidemiology, 39–40
   and definitions of prevention, 40
   subdisciplines, 43–44
      examples of, 43
      social, 43
Essential fatty acids, 161
Etanercept (anti-TNF-based therapy), 62
Exercises
   benefits of, 73
      health, 78–80, 83–85, 86
      improving joint movement, 73, 84, 86
      improving proprioception, 77
      improving strength and endurance, 74–77, 34–85
      modifying risk factors for progression, 77–78
   discomfort during/following, 70, 74–75
   discontinuing, 85
   enhancing self-efficacy, 84
   essentiality, 86
   incorporating strengthening, effective, 75
   initiating, 73
   maintenance, 84–85
   psychosocial effects, 80–85
   rheumatic disease and, 70
   role of, 201
      for patients with myositis, improved performance, 201
   self-monitoring, 71
   stretching and flexibility, 74
      ankylosing spondylitis (AS), 74
      rheumatic conditions, 74
Exercises, recommendations
   assessing cardiovascular risk, 72
   general advice, 71
   muscle strengthening, 75
   NICE guidelines, 78
   pain self-management, 80
   for physical health, 70–72
   psychological theories, 83
   stretching, 71, 74
Exocrine tissues, histopathology of, 7
Extracellular matrix (ECM), 130

F

Fasting, 92
Fatness, anthropometry, 19
   skinfolds, 19–20
   waist circumferences, 19
Fatty acids, 205
   clinical trials of, supplementation, 161
   modulates immune system, 161
   role in energy metabolism, 93
Feverfew (Tanacetum parthenium), 104
   increased bleeding time, 104
Fibromyalgia, 35
   alleviation of symptoms using vegetarian diets, 184
   Chlorella pyrenoidosa for treatment, 189
   diagnosis, 184
   and diet, 183–184
      discussion, 190–191
   dietary recommendations, 191–192
      advice to patients, 191
      dietary supplementation, 191–192
   dietary treatment, 184
   frequency, 90
   gastrointestinal (GI) symptoms and, 183
   higher substance P levels in patients, 185
   increasing incidence with age, 183
   lower growth hormone (GH) in patients, 185
   no effective drug therapy, 185
   nutrition and, 186
      vegetarian diets, 186–190
   overcoming, by consumption of vegetarian foods, 191
   pathophysiology of, 184–185
      theories on, 184
   poor sleep, 185
   symptoms, 183
Fish oil (omega-3 polyunsaturated fatty acids), 92–93

Index 287

advantages and disadvantages, 61
adverse effects of, 95–96
amounts of EPA and DHA, 94
clinical trials of, in RA, 91–92
impact on proinflammatory cytokines, 62–63
inhibitory effect of, 63
low prevalence of rheumatic diseases in Eskimos, 92
supplementation, 161
  anti-inflammatory effects, 161
See also Dietary n-3 fatty acids
Flaxseed and its benefits for SLE, 163
Flurbiprofen (Ansaid), 59
Food-frequency questionnaires (FFQ), 25–26
advantages, 26
types, 26
Framingham Osteoarthritis Study, 133

G

Garlic *(Allium sativum)*, for gout and rheumatism, 176
Gastrointestinal (GI)
physiology, 58
symptoms and fibromyalgia, 183
GCA, *see* Giant cell arteritis
GCS, *see* Glucocorticosteroids (GCS)
Gelling, 126
Genetic (molecular) epidemiological studies, 44
Giant cell arteritis (GCA), 8, 220–221
symptoms and treatment of, 220–221
Ginger (Zingiber officinale), 103
Gliadin, 5
γ-tlinolenic acid (GLA), 96–97
side effects of, 97
source, 97
treatment of RA, 96
Glomerular filtration rate (GFR), 160
Glomerulonephritis, 6
and zinc, 163
Glucocorticoids
combination with immunosuppressants, 199
Glucocorticosteroids (GCS), 260–261
adverse effects of, 260–261
Glucosamine, 99
and chondroitin sulfate, 138–140
  disease-modifying agents, 143–144
  pain and function, 141–143
  sulfate, 140–141
efficiency in OA, 99
Glucosamine/Chondroitin Arthritis Intervention Trial (GAIT), 101
Glutamine, 204–205
Gluten, 202

Glycosaminoglycan (GAG), 128
Gout, 31–32
alcohol as dietary risk factor for, 177, 178
body weight and, 31
Colchicine as treatment for, 176
dairy intake inversely correlated with, 174
food sources protecting against, 175
and gluttony, 169, 170
importance of dietary assessment, 31
link between purine-rich diets and, 173
low meat and high dairy products prevents, 172–173
prevalence of, in relation to BMI, 171
prevention of arthritis, 57
rare among blacks, 172
study on high-protein diet, 176
use of cherries prevents, 174
use of garlic, 176
Gouty arthritis, 39
sustained hyperuricemia, risk factor, 169
Grave's disease, patients with polymyositis, 5
Growth delay, 264

H

Hashimoto's thyroiditis, 4
Herbal supplements, 101–102
avocado and soybean unsaponifiables, 104–105
devil's claw (Harpagophytum Procumbens), 102
  efficacy in OA, 101
feverfew (Tanacetum parthenium), 104
  increased bleeding time, 104
ginger (Zingiber officinale), 102–103
immunostimulatory preparations, 207
polyphenols, 207
thunder god vine (Tripterygium wilfordii), 103
  achievement of therapeutic effect, 103
  beneficial effect, 103
turmeric (Curuma longa), 105
willow bark (salix sp), 102
  refined product of, *see* Aspirin (acetylsalicylic acid)
Herbal therapies, 90
Herbs, 176
High-protein diets, 175–176
popular diet programs, 176
Hormones
growth hormone and insulin-like growth factor-I, 119
insulin, 119–120
Human leukocyte antigen (HLA) class II molecules, 48
location, 48

Hyperglycemia, 23
Hyperlipidemia, 23
Hyperuricemia, 169–170
   and alcohol, 177
   association with MetS, 170
   cause of, 170
   correlation between obesity and, 171
   defined, 170
   dehydration as cause, 172
   and diet, 172
      dairy products, 174
      fruits and vegetables, 174–175
      high-protein diets, 175–176
      purine-rich foods, 172–173
   diuretics, 172
   effect of dairy products against, 174
   food sources protecting against, 175
   hydration for prevention, 172
   metabolic syndrome and, 169
   rare among blacks, 172
   SU level, 170
   surrogate marker of insulin-resistance syndrome, 170
   weight management, 178
Hyperuricemia, gout, and diet, 169, 170, 178–179
   alcohol, 177–178
   dietary supplements
      herbs, 176
      vitamin/mineral supplements, 177
   nutritional status
      dehydration/starvation, 172
      metabolic syndrome and hyperuricemia, 170–171
      obesity, 171–172
Hypocomplementemia, 6

I

Ibuprofen (NSAIDs), 59
Idiotypes, 4
Illness behavior
   coping strategies, 82
   determinants, 82
Immune complexes
   and vasculitides, 8
Immune system
   role in rheumatic diseases, 4
Immunology and rheumatic diseases, 3–4, 12–13
   autoimmunity, 4
   cytokines and rheumatic diseases, 12
   diseases with autoantibodies, autoantibody formation, 4–5
      associated with rheumatoid arthritis, 8–9
      in inflammatory muscle disease, 7–8

      Sjogren's Syndrome, 6–7
      in SLE, 5–6
      in systemic sclerosis (scleroderma), 7
      in vasculitides, 8–9
   MHC and rheumatic diseases, 10–11
      inflammatory myositis, 11
      RA, 12
      SLE, 11
      SS, 11
      systemic sclerosis, 11
      vasculitides, 11–12
Inflammatory cytokines, 116–117
   influence on whole body protein and metabolism, 116
Inflammatory muscle disease, 7
   autoantibody formation in, 7–8
   MHC and, 11
Inflammatory myopathies, 198
   risks of supplements, 198
Infliximab, 62
Instrumental activities of daily living (IADLs), 27
Interleukin (IL)-1β, 116
Intestinal microflora, 190
Intracellular defense, antioxidant enzymes, 127
Iron, 22
   anemia, 23
   harmful for SLE, 164

J

JIA patients, recommendations for, 269–270
Joint effusions, 127
Juvenile chronic arthritis (JCA), 253
Juvenile idiopathic arthritis (JIA), 252, 253
Juvenile rheumatoid arthritis (JRA), 29–31, 253

K

Kashin-Beck disease, 137
Keutel syndrome, 136

L

Laboratory test abnormalities of SS, 235
Limited scleroderma, *see* CREST syndrome
Lip biopsy, 235
Lipooxygenases (LOX), 145
Lipopolysaccharide, 4
Living food diet (LFD), 187
   antioxidants on, 190
   positive effects on serum lipids, 187
   studies with, 187–188
   therapeutic effect of, 188
Lyme disease, 57
   preventing symptoms of arthritis, 57

Index

M

Major histocompatibility complex (MHC), 4
  molecules classes, 10
    class II molecule, 11
    class I molecule, 10
  and rheumatic diseases, 10–11
    inflammatory myositis, 11
    RA, 12
    scleroderma, 11
    SLE, 11
    SS, 11
    vasculitides, 11–12
Malnutrition, 18
Management and treatment
  biological immunomodulators, 262
  cytotoxic and immunosuppressive drugs, 262
  DMARDs, 260
  glucocorticosteroids, 260–261
  NSAIDs, 259–260
Management strategies of SS
  dietary and nutritional management, 239
    dietary prevention of dental caries, 240–243
    dietary recommendations to reduce effects of SS, 244
    food choice suggestions for patients with oral complications of Sjogren's syndrome, 241–243
    good nutriture despite oral impairment, 239–240
    other nutritional therapies for preventing, retarding, or managing SS, 244–245
  eye palliatives, 237
  minimizing aggravating factors, 236–237
  oral candidiasis, management of, 239
  oral palliatives and therapies, 237, 238
Metabolic Equivalent (MET), 79
Methotrexate, 260
  effective in fasting state, 58
  as filate antagonist, 58, 63
  toxic effects, 63
MHC, *see* Major histocompatibility complex (MHC)
Microscopic polyangiitis, 217
Minnesota Leisure Time Physical Activity Questionnaire, 72
Molecular mimicry, 4
Morinda citrifolia, 165
  See also Noni juice (Morinda citrifolia)
Mouse, autoimmune-prone NZB/NZW F1 (B/W), 160
Muscle and bone, anthropometric measurements
  bioelectrical impedance analysis, 20
  dual-energy X-ray absorptiometry, 20

Musculoskeletal pain, 81
Myeloperoxidase (MPO), 9
Myositis, 197, 200
Myositis-specific antibodies (MSA), 8

N

N-3 fatty acids
  beneficial effect
    in cardiovascular disease (CVD), 92
    in rheumatic diseases, 92
  fish contents
    docosahexaenoic acid (DHA), 93
    eicosapentaenoic acid (EPA), 93
  metabolism, 93, 95
  See also Fish oil (omega-3 polyunsaturated fatty acids)
N-3 fatty acids *vs* n-6 fatty acids, 93, 95
N-6 fatty acids
  metabolism, 93, 95
  unhealthy, 93
Nabumetone (NSAIDs), 59
Naproxen (NSAIDs), 59
National Center of Complementary and Alternative Medicine (NCCAM), 89
National Health Interview Survey (NHIS), 45
Necrotizing vasculitides, and serological diagnostic test, 8
NHIS, *see* National Health Interview Survey (NHIS)
Noni juice (Morinda citrifolia)
  effect on C57BL/6 mice, 165
  as harmful for SLE, 165
Nonsteroidal anti-inflammatory drugs (NSAIDs), 23, 59, 259–260
  arachidonic acid metabolism and prostaglandin production, 59–61
  concomitant use, 64
  drugs in RA, 65
  examples, 59
  nutrients influencing production of PGs inhibit, 59
  side effects, 59
    See also Cyclooxygenase (COX)
    See also Iron, anemia
Nonsynonymous single-nucleotide polymorphism (R620W), 49
Norepinephrine, 185
NSAIDs, *see* Nonsteroidal anti-inflammatory drugs (NSAIDs)
Nutrients and drug components
  physicochemical interactions between, 58
Nutritional assessment, overview of, 15
  anthropometric measurements, 17

Nutritional assessment, overview of (*Cont.*)
    fatness, 19–20
    height/stature, 17
    muscle and bone, 20
    weight and body mass index, 17–19
  biochemical indices, 20–21
    comorbidities, 23
    nutritional implications, medications with, 23
    nutritional status, key indicators of, 21–23
  clinical indices, 24
    comorbidities, 24
  dietary intake, 24–26
  dietary status *vs* nutritional status, 15
  environmental factors, 27
  essential components of, 16–17
  functional status
    activities of, 27
    health-related quality of life, 28
    instrumental activities of, 27
    range of motion and difficulties performing everyday tasks, 28
  historical perspective, 16
  various arthritic and rheumatoid diseases, 29
    gout, 31–32
    juvenile rheumatoid arthritis, 29–31
    other rheumatic and arthritic diseases, 34–35
    polymyositis, 33–34
    rheumatoid arthritis, 29
    Sjögren's Syndrome, 34
    systemic sclerosis, 32–33
Nutritional impairment, 251, 262
Nutritional issues in vasculitides
  central nervous system vasculitides, 219–220
  Churg-Strauss syndrome, 217
  cryoglobulinemic vasculitides, 217–218
  drug-induced vasculitides, 219
  giant cell arteritis, 220–221
  microscopic polyangiitis, 217
  nutritional values and vasculitides, 222
  other vasculitides, 221
  polyarteritis nodosa, 215–216
  Wegener's granulomatosis, 218–219
Nutritional status, 15
  ABCDEFs of
    anthropometry, 16
    biochemistry, 16
    clinical evaluation, 16
    dietary history, 17
    environmental assessment, 17
    functional status, 17
  decline of, 17
  dietary management, gluten, 202
  glucocorticoids, 200–201
  muscle metabolism, 200
  nutritional impairments in patients with JIA
    body composition abnormalities, 266–267
    growth abnormalities, 264–265
    malnutrition and nutrient deficiencies, 265–266
    osteopenia and osteoporosis, 267
  oral health in patients with JIA, 263
  risk factors for developing nutritional impairments, 263–264
  role of exercise, 201–202
Nutritional status, key indicators of
  calcium, 22
  iron, 22–23
  serum proteins, 21
    albumin, 21
    creatinine, 21–22
    transthyretin (prealbumin), 21
    urinary 3-methylhistidine, 22
    urinary creatinine, 22
  vitamin D, 22
Nutritional status, supplements
  anabolic steroids, 203–204
  creatine, 202–203
  fatty acids, 205
  glutamine, 204–205
  herbal supplements, 207
  vitamin D, 205–206
  vitamin E, 206
Nutritional values and vasculitides, 222
  toxicity of drugs, 222
Nutrition and polymyositis and dermatomyositis
  clinical features, 197–198
  epidemiology, 196
  etiology, 196
  historical perspectives, 196–197
  laboratory features
    molecules present in muscle tissue in inflammatory conditions, 198–199
    muscle tissue features, 198
    pharmacological treatment, 199
    prognosis, 199
  nutritional status
    dietary management, gluten, 202
    glucocorticoids, 200–201
    muscle metabolism, 200
    role of exercise, 201
    supplements, 202
  nutritional status, supplements
    anabolic steroids, 203–204
    creatine, 202–203
    fatty acids, 205
    glutamine, 204–205

Index

herbal supplements, 207
vitamin D, 205–206
vitamin E, 206

O

OA epidemiology, 52–53
   incidence rates in US, 52
   symptomatic prevalence, 52
Obesity
   correlation between hyperuricemia and, 171
   defined, 171
Observational studies (experimental)
   randomized controlled trial, epidemiological study designs, 41
Ocular effects of SS, 231
Oligoarticular JIA, 255–256
Omega-3 (n-3) fatty acids, 145, 161
   sources, 145
Omega-6 (n-6) fatty acids, 145, 161
   sources, 145
Oral effects of SS and influence on diet and nutrition, 231–232
   functions of saliva, 232
Osteoarthritic process, 131
Osteoarthritis (OA), 4, 27, 34
   affected areas, 126
   Arthritis, Diet, and Activity Promotion Trial, 147
   as consequence of aging, 126
   cross-sectional studies suggesting inverse relationship between osteoporosis and, 131
   diagnostic criteria, 52
   effects of vitamin D deficiency, 132
   efficacy of devil's claw extract, 102
   as example of primordial prevention, 40
   findings on physical examination, 126–127
   frequency, 90
   of hip, risk of incident, 133
   most prevalent, affecting elderly, 126
   overweight people at increased risk of, knee, 146
   primary, 52
   relationship between vitamin D and cartilage loss, 133
   risk for developing
      hand, 53
      hip, 52
      knee, 52
   secondary, 52
   strengthening exercise, 75
   symptom, 126
   TGF in pathophysiology, 130

   vitamin C, beneficial effects of, 129–130
      placebo-controlled case-crossover study, 130
Osteoarthritis, nutrition and nutritional supplements and, 125–126, 149
   clinical features, 126–127
   historical perspective, 126
   nutritional status and dietary management
      antioxidant micronutrients, 127
      avocado/soybean unsaponifiables, 145–146
      diacerein, 144–145
      glucosamine and chondroitin sulfate, 138–144
      nutritional products, 146
      polyunsaturated fatty acids, 145
      selenium and iodine, 137–138
      vitamin C, 127–131
      vitamin D, 131–134
      vitamin E, 134–135
      vitamin K, 135–137
   weight loss, 146–148
Osteopenia, defined, 267
Osteophytes, 126, 130, 131
Osteoporosis, defined, 267

P

PAN, *see* Polyarteritis nodosa
Penicillamine
   effective in fasting state, 58
Perceived exercise, rating of, 73
Perinuclear (p-ANCA), 9
   antigens of, 9
PGE2, 59
Pharmacoepidemiology, 43
Pharmacokinetics, 58
   effect of food on, 58
   effect on ibuprofen, 59
Physical activity, 71–72
   assessment of, 72
      individual's cardiovascular risk, 72, 73
   examples of light and moderate, 79
   exercise, 70
   low levels of, obesity, 77
   misconception regarding, 80
   psychosocial effects, 80–83
   reduced activity and benefits of exercise, 74
Physicochemical interaction, 58
Piascledine, 146
Plant herb and SLE, 163
Polyarteritis nodosa, 215–216
   symptoms and treatment of, 215–216
Polyarticular JIA, 256
Polyclonal activation, 4

Polymyositis, 7, 33–34, 195–208
　antisynthetase antibodies as characteristic of, 8
　prescription of corticosteroids, 34
Polypharmacy, 23
Polyunsaturated fatty acid (PUFA), 145
　metabolized by COX and LOX, 145
　　omega-3 (n-3), 145
　　　sources, 145
　　omega-6 (n-6), 145
　　　sources, 145
Poor sleep, 185
Prevention, epidemiological definitions of, 40
Primary angiitis of CNS (PACNS)
　treatment of, 220
Primary prevention, rheumatic disease, 40
Primordial prevention, rheumatic disease, 40
Proinflammatory cytokines
　role in pathology of rheumatic diseases, 58, 62
Proprioception, 75
Proteinase 3 (pR3), 9
Protein diets and SLE
　high intake accelerates kidney damage, 160
　low, 160
　　improved survival in NZB/NZW mice, 160
　restriction of different, 160
Protein tyrosine phosphatase gene, 49
Psoriatic arthritis, 257
Psychosocial traits, interactions of, 93
Purine-rich foods, 172–173
　cooking techniques, 173
　risk of developing gout, 173
Purpura, 8

Q

Quality-of-life
　arthritis-specific, 28
　questionnaires, disease-specific health-related, 28

R

RA, *see* Rheumatoid arthritis (RA)
RA epidemiology, 46–49
　diagnosed age, 46
　prevalence, 46
　risk of developing
　　rheumatoid factor (RF) proportional to, 46
　　tobacco smoke as, 44
Range of motion (ROM), 28
Rapid Assessment of Physical Activity, 72
Reactive oxygen species (ROS), 127
　chondrocytes as sources, 127
Recreational swimming/water aerobic exercises, 80
Retinol, *see* Vitamin A
Rheumatic diseases, 3
　biopsychosocial model of, 80
　classification of
　　difficulties in, 44
　　restrictive, 45
　effect of nutrients on symptoms of, 58
　epidemiological issues in studying, 44–45
　and folate deficiency, 66
　heterogeneity and variability in, 39
　interactions between patients with, and environment, 81
　limitations
　　complex etiologies of, 45
　　identifying individuals with, 44–45
　pathogenesis of, 4
　people with
　　challenging erroneous ill-health beliefs, 83–84
　　importance of muscle strength, 73
　　prescription of exercises for, 73
　　and psychosocial traits, 83
　　stretching exercises, 74
　prevention, 40
　symptoms leading to low appetites, 64
　varying treatment, 57
　See also individual rheumatic diseases
Rheumatic disease epidemiology, 39
　arthritic conditions, burden of
　　osteoarthritis epidemiology, 52–53
　　rheumatoid arthritis epidemiology, 46–49
　　systemic lupus erythematosus epidemiology, 49–52
　epidemiological issues in studying rheumatic diseases, 44–45
　epidemiological methods, 39–40
　　epidemiology subdisciplines, 43–44
　　primary epidemiological study design, 40–43
　methodological issues in, 45
　R620W in tyrosine phosphatase gene, 49
Rheumatic diseases
　nutritional approach of treatment, misunderstood, 184
　and self-medication, 184
Rheumatic diseases, exercise in, 69–70
　benefits of exercise, 73
　　health benefits, 78
　　improve joint movement, 73
　　improve proprioception, 77
　　improve strength and endurance, 74–77
　　modifying risk factors for progression, 77–78

Index

discontinuing exercise, 85
exercise maintenance, 85
exercise safety, 70–71
initiating an exercise regimen, 71–72
   assessment, 72
   self-monitoring, 73
psychosocial effects of physical activity, 80–83
   education, 83–84
   positive mastery, 84
   traits and symptoms, 83
recommendations, 86
Rheumatic diseases, medications
   anticytokine-based therapies, 58
   corticosteroids, 57
   disease modifying anti-rheumatic drugs (DMARDs), 57
   fasting drugs, 58
   nonsteroidal anti-inflammatory drugs (NSAIDs), 57
   timing of, 58
Rheumatic diseases, therapies, 89–90, 105–106
   categories of, 90
   complementary and alternative medicine, 90
   diets and dietary supplements, 92–93
      diets, 91–92
      hinders, 92–101
Rheumatoid arthritis (RA), 3, 9, 23, 29, 42, 46, 113
   antibodies to CCPs, 10
   autoantibody formation in, 9–10
   body composition of patients with, 115
   cachexia in, 115
   cardiovascular disease and role of n-3 fatty acids, 95
   classification of, 42
   clinical trials of fish oil in, 93
   corticosteroids treatment, 58
   decreased fertility and, 48
   drugs used in, and interactions with nutrients, 65
   elevated levels of (IL)-1β and (TNF)-α, 58
   epidemiology, 46–49
   fish-oil use in, 61
   frequency, 90
   greatest risk of deficiency, 120
   high concentration of TNF-α and IL-1β, 115
   idiopathic, 46
   impact of vitamin E in, 61–62
   incidence in selected cities, 48
   inheritance of, 48
   joint damage, involvement of TNF-α and IL-1β in, 116
   low physical activity, 119
   oral contraceptives and onset of, 48
   patient having Hashimoto's thyroid disease, 5
   during pregnancy, 48
   prevalence, 46
      in Australia, 42
   and progressive resistance, 76
   randomized controlled trials, effect of n-3 fatty acids, 61
   relationship between (TNF)-α production and lean body mass, 116
   RF in, 10
   role of proinflammatory cytokines in, 58, 62
   and sarcopenia, 77
   therapy
      TNF-α as target, 58
   tobacco smoke as increased risk, 44
   treated with dietary fish-oil, meta-analysis, 61
   treating
      pharmacotherapeutic options, 43
   treatment via GLA, 97
   types of anti-TNF antibodies, 62
   See also Adalimumab; Infliximab
Rheumatoid arthritis (RA), patients with
   fasting, 92
   fish- or plant-oil preparations in diet, 91
   prevention of CVD, a key feature, 95
   vegan and lacto-vegetarian diet, placebo-controlled study, 91–92
   and vegetarian diets, 91
Rheumatoid cachexia (RC), 113–114
   clinical features
      pathophysiology of, 116–119
      signs and symptoms, 114–115
   dietary prescription, 120
   exercise prescription, 120–121
   historical perspective, 114
   interactions leading to, 121
   management, recommendations, 120–121
   nutritional status, 119–120
   reduced physical activity, 114
Rheumatoid cachexia, pathophysiology of
   energy expenditure profile, 117–118
   hormones
      growth hormone and insulin-like growth factor-I, 119
      insulin, 119–120
   inflammatory cytokines, 116–117
      interleukin (IL)-1β, 116
      tumor necrosis factor (TNF)-α, 116
   physical activity, 119
   whole-body protein turnover, 118
Rheumatologists
   importance of pharmacoepidemiology, 43
ROM, *see* Range of motion (ROM)
Rose Bengal staining test, 235

S

Salivary function test of SS, 235
Salivary gland biopsy of SS, 235
Sarcopenia, 77
Schirmer test, 235
Scleroderma, 3, 32–33
    autoantibody formation in, 7
    biochemical indices and, 33
    dietary intake, 33
    MHC and, 11
    symptoms, 7
Sclerosis, 131
Secondary prevention, rheumatic disease, 40
Selenium, 137, 162
    clinical trial, 138
    deficiency, 137
    efficacy in treating OA symptoms, 138
    and SLE, 163
    toxicity, 163
Selenium and iodine
    OA and nutritional supplements, 137–138
Self-antigens
    formation of antibodies and, 4
Self-efficacy, 82
Serological diagnostic test
    and necrotizing vasculitides, 8
Serotonin, 185
Serum albumin, 21
Serum urate (SU)
    alcohol and increased, 177
    Chinese vegetarians *vs* omnivores in, 175
    dietary intervention and decreased, 176
    effect of diet on, 171
    effect of vitamin C, 177
    foods that increase, levels, 172
    higher levels in humans, 169
    increased, 170
    milk proteins reduce, 174
    purine-rich foods and increased, 173
Sjögren's syndrome (SS), 5, 6
    and ANAs, 7
    autoantibody formation in, 6–7
    defined, 227, 229
    diagnosis of, 235
    dietary and nutritional management, 239–245
        dietary habits and patterns, 240–244
        good nutriture despite oral impairment, 239–240
        nutritional therapies, 244–245
    dry eyes, 24
    effect on exocrine glands, 6
    efficacy of GLA, 97
    epidemiology, 228
    etiology, 230
    history, 228
    hypergammaglobulinemia in, 7
    immunoglobulin (Ig)G found in, 7
    managing, 236–239
        eye palliatives, 237
        minimizing aggravating factors, 236–237
        oral palliatives and therapies, 237–239
    MHC and, 11
    nonerosive arthritis, 6
    nutritional assessment in, 34
    other adverse effects, 6
    pathophysiology, 229–230
    physiological effects of, 230–234
        effects of xerostomia on dentition, 232
        effects of xerostomia on diet and nutrition, 234
        ocular effects, 231
        oral effects and influence on diet and nutrition, 231–232
        other oral effects, 232–234
        other physiological effects, 234
    types of, 228–229
Skinfold thickness, 19
    measuring, 19
SLE, *see* Systemic lupus erythematosus (SLE)
SLE epidemiology, 49–52
    concordance rates among twins, 52
    different classification criteria in studies, 49
    environmental influences, 49
    incidence by Race and Gender for Selected Studies, 50
    incidence rates in
        African-American females, 49
        age-specific, African-American and white females, 51
        age-standardized rates, in Baltimore, 51
        Europe, 49, 51
        NY males *vs* females, 49
    similar gender- and race-specific rates in studies, 49
    suspected risk factors, 51
Sm, 5
    involvement in RNA processing, 5
Social epidemiology, 43
South Beach™, 176
Spondyloarthropathies, 10–11
SS, *see* Sjögren's syndrome
Strength training, 74
Symptom reports of SS, 236
Systemic lupus erythematosus (SLE), 3, 35, 49, 159
    ANAs in, 5
    antibodies against nuclear antigens, 5

autoantibody formation in, 5–6
and environmental exposures, 44
epidemiology, 49–52
immune complex formation and, 6
MHC and, 11
pathogenesis of, 49
prevention of CVD, a key feature, 95
Systemic lupus erythematosus, beneficial nutritional modifications
  caloric restriction, 160
  dehydroepiandrosterone, 163–164
  dietary fat intake, 161
  flaxseed, 163
  low-protein diets, 160
  plant herb, 163
  selenium, 162–163
  vitamin A, 162
  vitamin E, 162
  zinc, 163
Systemic lupus erythematosus, harmful nutritional substances
  alfalfa, 164–165
  echinacea, 165
  iron, 164
  noni juice (Morinda citrifolia), 165
Systemic lupus erythematosus, nutritional supplementation in, 159, 165
  beneficial nutritional modifications
    caloric restriction, 160
    dehydroepiandrosterone, 163–164
    dietary fat intake, 161
    flaxseed, 163
    low-protein diets, 160
    plant herb, 163
    selenium, 162–163
    vitamin A, 162
    vitamin E, 162
    zinc, 163
  harmful nutritional substances
    alfalfa, 164–165
    echinacea, 165
    iron, 164
    noni juice (Morinda citrifolia), 165
Systemic-onset JIA, 256–257
Systemic sclerosis, *see* Scleroderma

T

Takayasu's arteritis, 8
T-cell help, increased, 4
Tertiary prevention, rheumatic disease, 40
Th (T helper)2 cells, 12
  and cytokines, 12
Thunder god vine (Tripterygium wilfordii), 103
  achievement of therapeutic effect, 103
  beneficial effect, 103
Tofu, 175
Transforming growth factor (TGF), 130
Transthyretin (Prealbumin), 21
Tripterygium wilfordii hook F (TWH)
  toxicity, 163
  used for SLE and RA, 163
Tumor necrosis factor (TNF)-α, 116
  relationship between production of, whole-body protein breakdown, 118
Turmeric (Curuma longa), 105

U

Uric acid (urate), 169
  beer ingestion and, 178
  higher levels of serum urate (SU) in humans, 169–170
  high-protein diets associated with increased urinary, 175
  metabolism and insulin resistance, 171
  See also Gout; Hyperuricemia
Urinary creatinine, 22

V

Vasculitides, 8, 215–222
  autoantibodies formation in, 8–9
    association, 8
  cause, 8
  central nervous system, 219–220
  Churg-Strauss syndrome, 217
  cryoglobulinemic, 217–218
  defined, 215
  drug-induced, 219
  giant cell arteritis, 220–221
  and immune complexes, 8
  MHC and, 11–12
  microscopic polyangiitis, 217
  nutritional values and, 222
  other vasculitides, 221
  polyarteritis nodosa, 215–216
  Wegener's granulomatosis, 218–219
VDR, 131–132
Vegetarian diets, nutrition and fibromyalgia, 186–187
  antioxidants, 189–190
  food intake and their matched controls, 188
  intestinal microflora, 190
  raw-food diets and dietary supplements, 187–189
Vinegar preparations, 90
Vitamin A
  and its benefits for SLE, 162

Vitamin C, 97–98, 127, 129
  beneficial effects in OA, 129–130
  functions in biosynthesis of cartilage, 128
  high dose associated with arthritis, 130
  higher intake, reduced progression of OA, 129
  long-term exposure, 98
  OA and nutritional supplements, 127–131
  participation in GAG synthesis, 128
  study on its effect on OA, 130
    limitations, 130–131
Vitamin D, 22, 97, 131
  deficiency affecting other elements of OA, 132
  effects on chondrocytes in osteoarthritic
    cartilage, 131
  OA and nutritional supplements, 131–134
  relationship between, and cartilage loss
    in OA, 133
  risk of osteoporosis, 205–206
  role in OA and RA, 97
  supplements and its use, 133–134
Vitamin E, 134, 162, 206
  blocking formation of AA, 134
  controversial usage, 162
  effects of, on chondrocytes, 134
  increasing cardiovascular disease (CVD), 162
  and its benefits for SLE, 162
  OA and nutritional supplements, 134–135
  sources of, 134
  trials on effects of, 135
Vitamin K, 99, 135–136
  bone and cartilage effects, 136
  deficiency, 137
  OA and nutritional supplements, 135–137
Vitamins, 97
  deficiencies diseases, 97

glucosamine and chondroitin, 99–101
  treatment of OA, 99–101
Vitamin C, 97–99
  long-term exposure, 98
Vitamin D, 97
  role in OA and RA, 97
Vitamin K, 99

W

Waist circumference measurement, 19
Walking, as physical activity, 77
Wegener's granulomatosis (WG), 5, 8, 218–219
  ANCAs pathogenic role, 9
  symptoms and treatment of, 218–219
WG, see Wegener's granulomatosis
Willow bark (salix sp), 102
  refined product of, see Aspirin (acetylsalicylic
    acid)

X

Xeropthalmia (KCS), 231
Xerostomia, 231
  effects of, on dentition, 232
    risk of dental caries, 232
  effects of, on diet and nutrition, 234

Z

Zinc
  and its benefits for SLE, 163
  role in T-cell development and thymic
    atrophy, 163
Zone™, 176

About the Editor

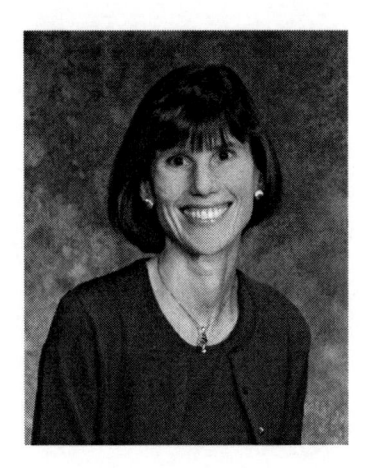

Dr. Laura A. Coleman is a Project Scientist in the Epidemiology Research Center at the Marshfield Clinic Research Foundation in Marshfield, WI. Prior to obtaining her doctorate in Human Nutrition Science from the Friedman School of Nutrition Science and Policy, Tufts University, Boston, MA, where she concentrated on nutrition and immunology, Dr. Coleman worked as a clinical dietitian at Massachusetts General Hospital. She has written multiple peer-reviewed articles and book chapters on nutrition and rheumatic disease over the past decade, focusing primarily on systemic lupus erythematosus and rheumatoid arthritis. She currently serves on the Advisory Board for the Lupus Foundation of America's award-winning publication, Lupus Now.

About the Series Editor

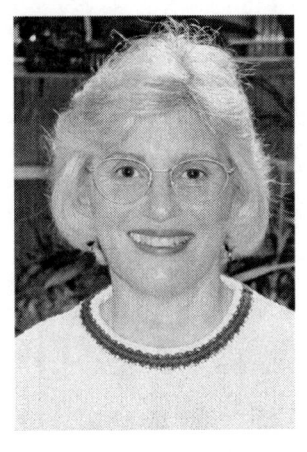

Dr. Adrianne Bendich is Clinical Director of Calcium Research at GlaxoSmithKline Consumer Healthcare, where she is responsible for leading the innovation and medical programs in support of several leading consumer brands including TUMS and Os-Cal. Dr. Bendich has primary responsibility for the coordination of GSK's support for the Women's Health Initiative (WHI) intervention study. Prior to joining GlaxoSmithKline, Dr. Bendich was at Roche Vitamins Inc., and was involved with the groundbreaking clinical studies proving that folic acid-containing multivitamins significantly reduce major classes of birth defects. Dr. Bendich has co-authored more than 100 major clinical research studies in the area of preventive nutrition.

Dr. Bendich is recognized as a leading authority on antioxidants, nutrition and bone health, immunity, and pregnancy outcomes, vitamin safety, and the cost-effectiveness of vitamin/mineral supplementation.

In addition to serving as Series Editor for Humana Press and initiating the development of the 20 currently published books in the *Nutrition and Health*™ series, Dr. Bendich is the editor of 11 books, including *Preventive Nutrition: The Comprehensive Guide for Health Professionals*. She also serves as Associate Editor for *Nutrition: The International Journal of Applied and Basic Nutritional Sciences*, and Dr. Bendich is on the Editorial Board of the *Journal of Women's Health and Gender-Based Medicine*, as well as a past member of the Board of Directors of the American College of Nutrition. Dr. Bendich also serves on the Program Advisory Committee for HelenKeller International.

Dr. Bendich was the recipient of the Roche Research Award, was a Tribute to Women and Industry Awardee, and a recipient of the Burroughs Wellcome Visiting Professorship in Basic Medical Sciences, 2000–2001. Dr. Bendich holds academic appointments as Adjunct Professor in the Department of Preventive Medicine and Community Health at UMDNJ, Institute of Nutrition, Columbia University P&S, and Adjunct Research Professor, Rutgers University, Newark Campus. She is listed in *Who's Who in American Women*.